150 Years of ObamaCare

150 Years of ObamaCare

Daniel E. Dawes

Foreword by David Satcher, MD, PhD,
16th US Surgeon General

Johns Hopkins University Press / Baltimore

© 2016 Johns Hopkins University Press
All rights reserved. Published 2016
Printed in the United States of America on acid-free paper
9 8 7 6 5 4 3 2 1

Johns Hopkins University Press
2715 North Charles Street
Baltimore, Maryland 21218-4363
www.press.jhu.edu

Library of Congress Cataloging-in-Publication Data

Dawes, Daniel E., 1980-, author.
 150 years of ObamaCare / Daniel E. Dawes ; foreword by David Satcher.
  p. ; cm.
 One hundred fifty years of ObamaCare
 Includes bibliographical references and index.
 ISBN 978-1-4214-1963-3 (hardcover : alk. paper) — ISBN 1-4214-1963-7
(hardcover : alk. paper) — ISBN 978-1-4214-1964-0 (electronic) — ISBN
1-4214-1964-5 (electronic)
 I. Title.   II. Title: One hundred fifty years of ObamaCare.
 [DNLM: 1. United States. Patient Protection and Affordable Care Act.
2. Health Care Reform—trends—United States.   3. Health Care Reform—
history—United States.   4. History, 21st Century—United States.   5. Insurance,
Health—history—United States.   6. Insurance, Health—trends—United States.
WA 540.AA1]
 RA395.A3
 362.1'04250973—dc23   2015028201

A catalog record for this book is available from the British Library.

*Special discounts are available for bulk purchases of this book. For more information,
please contact Special Sales at 410-516-6936 or specialsales@press.jhu.edu.*

Johns Hopkins University Press uses environmentally friendly book materials,
including recycled text paper that is composed of at least 30 percent post-
consumer waste, whenever possible.

To all health equity champions, past, present, and future

Contents

Foreword

So let us begin anew—remembering on both sides that civility
is not a sign of weakness, and sincerity is always subject to
proof. Let us never negotiate out of fear. But let us never fear to
negotiate. Let both sides explore what problems unite us instead
of belaboring those problems which divide us. . . . In your hands,
my fellow citizens, more than mine, will rest the final success or
failure of our course.—*President John F. Kennedy, inaugural address
given January 20, 1961*

Few people would probably disagree that the health reform debate has been exceptionally contentious and polarizing. The extreme partisan bickering has spilled over into mainstream conversations, causing
widespread confusion and angst among communities across the country.
Some argue that this debate, as profound and necessary as it is, cannot be
reconciled. They point to the intensity of the struggle to pass the law and
now the unyielding assault on the law as it is being implemented.

Today, we are at an inflection point, with many of the health reforms
either already implemented or almost implemented. However, with unwavering opposition to the Affordable Care Act (ACA) and attempts to
dismantle the very core of this law, is it even possible to overcome this
acrimonious debate and objectively examine what is working and what
could be changed to ensure that all Americans have access to affordable
patient-centered care, appropriate treatments, and preventive services? Indeed, the ACA is a comprehensive and complex law, which has taken generations to finally produce. Its rich history of advocacy, negotiations, and
ultimate evolution certainly merits our thoughtful attention in order to
understand what the law entails, how it goes about accomplishing its objectives, and the impact it has had to date.

Perhaps in such a time as this, with emotions at an all-time high in favor or against the health reform law, it would be prudent to heed President Kennedy's admonition to stop belaboring those problems that divide us and instead explore what problems unite us, because the success of this law's implementation is in our hands. We have the power to ensure not only that this law is implemented but that it is implemented in a manner that will have the most positive impact on communities across the nation.

I encountered a major challenge with our health system early in my life. At the age of two, I suffered a severe and life-threatening illness while growing up on a farm outside of Anniston, Alabama. A combination of race and poverty virtually shut my family and others out of the health care system. Fortunately, the one black physician in the area, Dr. Fred Jackson, agreed to come out to the farm on his day off to see me. He doubted that I would survive but instructed my parents on how to give me the best chance of survival. I did survive, but I never met Dr. Jackson after that encounter because he died of a stroke that same year. He was fifty-four years of age. But, out of that encounter, I developed a desire to be a physician and a passion to make health care better for everyone—a passion that has characterized my career to this day.

Through public service and leadership roles as the former director of the Centers for Disease Control and Prevention, US assistant secretary of Health and Human Services, and 16th US surgeon general, I saw the full scope of the impact that our fragmented health care system, with its lack of attention to population health, was having on our nation. During my tenure in public service, I gained firsthand experience in some of the intricacies involved with repairing a broken health care system. As surgeon general I continued the battle against smoking and worked tirelessly to address pressing public health issues, including obesity, oral health, mental and behavioral health, sexual health, and violence. We conducted large-scale studies to examine these particular issues and institute appropriate public policies and strategies to effect positive changes.

As a result of rigorous scientific investigations, we were able to produce landmark reports, including *Mental Health: A Report of the Surgeon General* (1999), *Oral Health in America: A Report of the Surgeon General* (2000), and *The Surgeon General's Call to Action to Promote Sexual Health* (2001), highlighting issues that were critical to improving health outcomes across the nation but long neglected because people were fearful of discussing them. These reports as well as other studies helped to inform proposed and existing health policies such as the Mental Health Parity and Addiction Equity Act, the Ryan White CARE Act, and the Child Healthcare Crisis Relief Act. However, I am most proud that these studies played a role in informing and shaping the historic health reform law that was enacted on March 23, 2010. Today we stand firmly at the threshold of a historically momentous opportunity to delineate a national agenda to promote health and health care for all Americans. The enactment of the Affordable Care Act represents both a culmination of enduring legislative and health policy efforts and a reinvigorated infrastructure that expands access to one of the most essential and basic human rights—health. It is the first major law that comprehensively addresses the complexities inherent in our health care system, including its multidimensional workforce, delivery of care, health equity, prevention, and public health issues that are important for diverse populations. Because of the ACA, I am optimistic that we will make significant strides in improving the health of individuals, families, and communities in our nation.

An Institute of Medicine book, *US Health in International Perspective: Shorter Lives, Poorer Health* (2013), documented the alarming implications of the poor health status of our population. This landmark report helps to explicate from a global perspective comparisons among seventeen peer countries of life expectancy, selected medical conditions, and health outcomes, particularly infant mortality and low birth weight, injuries and homicides, disability, adolescent pregnancy and sexually transmitted infections, HIV and AIDS, drug-related deaths, obesity and diabetes, heart disease, and chronic lung disease. One notable finding was that individuals who are most negatively impacted, suffer the greatest, and are at highest risk for deleterious outcomes are people of lower socioeconomic status who live in underserved, vulnerable, and impoverished communities. These harsh realities certainly warrant further examination and reinforce the need to implement the reforms embodied in the Affordable Care Act so that America can stand unchallenged as a leader in the quest for global health equity.

Equity in health ideally extends to all people a fair opportunity to attain their full health potential; more pragmatically, no one should be disadvantaged from achieving this potential (WHO, 1985). In many nations, social justice, environmental, and economic issues impact an individual's livelihood, exposure to illness, and risk of early mortality, according to a 2008 report of the World Health Organization's Commission on Social Determinants of Health, which was established in 2005. When extreme differences in health are significantly associated with social disadvantages, the differences can be labeled as health inequities; and in most cases these differences are (1) systematic and avoidable; (2) facilitated and exacerbated by circumstances in which people live, work, and contend with illness; and (3) intensified by political, economic, or social influences (WHO, 2008). Even in countries such as the United States, which have economic power and communities with adequate resources, persons belonging to lower socioeconomic levels experience the worst health outcomes (WHO, 2008).

It is imperative that policy makers, public health professionals, researchers, and clinicians embrace lead roles to bridge this gap between the rich and the poor by promoting health equity and setting guidelines for global health initiatives. To address health inequities, social justice must be expanded to reach people on a larger and more inclusive scale. We need leaders who will actively promote the three Commission on Social Determinants of Health principles of action: (1) enhance daily living conditions in which people are born, grow, live, work, and age; (2) address inequitable distribution of power, money, and resources; and (3) accurately measure the issues of, assess action plans addressing, increase the knowledge base around, create a workforce trained in, and increase awareness about social determinants of health. Moreover, one of the overarching goals for our own country's public health agenda, Healthy People 2020, is to "achieve health equity, eliminate disparities, and improve the health of all groups" (DHHS, 2010). This can be accomplished with ethical leaders and policy makers with a bipartisan orientation at the helm.

Health equity is the "attainment of the highest level of health for all people" (DHHS, 2011), and clinical practice, research, prevention initiatives, and advocacy have unique yet complementary roles to play in reaching this goal. Working collaboratively, health professionals, scholars, health advocates, researchers, business leaders, faith leaders, legal professionals, and policy makers both domestically and internationally can help our efforts to achieve health equity. Ethical leadership is one key to our success, and we must not leave their emergence to chance alone. Leaders must exercise civility and continually learn more about themselves and those they lead, as well as the cause for which they work. Focused initiatives and cross-cultural collaborations will continue to transform the science of ethical decision making and discovery in health policy research, health promotion, and practice. This is especially crucial if we are to realize the goals engendered in the health reform law.

This book, *150 Years of ObamaCare*, is long overdue and provides an engaging narrative of the struggle to pass health reform and elevate health equity across the United States. A vital resource for greater insight into an often misunderstood and distrusted policy making process, *150 Years of ObamaCare* provides an honest assessment of the health care law and an unparalleled explanation of its provisions, especially those impacting vulnerable populations. It depicts the persistence, passion, and patience required to inform health policy in the United States with the goal of eliminating health disparities and promoting global health equity.

David Satcher, MD, PhD
16th US Surgeon General

BIBLIOGRAPHY

Institute of Medicine (2013). *US Health in International Perspective: Shorter Lives, Poorer Health*. Washington, DC: National Academies Press.

US Department of Health and Human Services (2010). *Healthy People 2020*. Washington, DC: Author. healthypeople.gov.

US Department of Health and Human Services (2011). *HHS Action Plan to Reduce Racial and Ethnic Health Disparities: A Nation Free of Disparities in Health and Health Care*. Washington, DC: Author.

World Health Organization (1985). *Targets for Health for All*. Copenhagen: World Health Organization Regional Office for Europe.

World Health Organization, Commission on Social Determinants of Health (2008). *Closing the Gap in a Generation: Health Equity through Action on the Social Determinants of Health*. Final report of the Commission on Social Determinants of Health. Geneva: Author.

Preface

The Honorable Cecil Charlton once said that, when an opportunity presents itself, you have got to grab hold of it, for you never know if and when it will come back around. When health reform discussions were initiated in the spring of 2008 by the Senate Finance Committee, just months before the presidential election, health reform advocates knew it was a once-in-a-lifetime opportunity to pass legislation comprehensively addressing health reforms that had eluded prior generations. In 2007, even before that hearing took place, congressional staff and external advocates who were working on the Paul Wellstone and Pete Domenici Mental Health Parity and Addiction Equity Act, a health insurance reform statute, were confident that, in the next Congress, they would have the unique opportunity to tackle comprehensive health reform once again. Advocates quickly and diligently organized, strategized, and advocated for this legislation once the 111th Congress convened in January 2009 and Barack Obama was sworn in as the forty-fourth president of the United States of America.

For many advocates, the drive to realize health reform ultimately resulted from personal experiences involving access to health care in the United States. In the summer of 2002, I found myself assigned to work in the emergency room of a hospital in Ft. Lauderdale, Florida, where I got an up-close look at the massive health problems faced by underserved communities in South Florida. My first experience with the health care system involved a patient who was a Haitian immigrant. She was obviously in a great deal of pain, but each time she tried to tell the staff in the emergency room about her problem, they responded with nothing more than blank stares. Unfortunately, this patient could speak only Haitian Creole. As I watched her trying to make herself understood, I could not help but think, Oh my gosh! What if her condition is life threatening? Every minute, every second would be critical. That afternoon was a revelation for me of just how vulnerable many patients really are and how complicated health care delivery could be in the United States.

My interest in health care reform was further piqued when I discovered the hardships many people in my own community were facing. Nowhere is that hardship more evident, I soon learned, than in health care—where lack of money or insurance and disparities in care can deprive desperately ill patients of the quality care, treatment, and medicines they need to survive and thrive. Indeed, the health disparities confronting vulnerable populations are many and varied as well and are driven in large part by the social, political, and physical determinants of health. People in these populations may experience symptoms that go undiagnosed, underdiagnosed, or misdiagnosed for cultural, linguistic, or other reasons. Oftentimes, these health disparities result from laws and policies adopted without meaningful assessment of their impact on vulnerable populations or on health equity overall.

With growing ethnic and cultural diversity in our country and with the failure to reduce or eliminate risk factors that can influence health outcomes, it was apparent to me that we had to develop, promulgate, and implement health laws, policies, and programs that advance health equity among vulnerable, underserved, and marginalized populations. The negotiations over health reform, or "ObamaCare," provided advocates the perfect vehicle to elevate health equity, increase health care access, improve the delivery of care, and prioritize prevention and early interventions to reduce the impact of chronic diseases on urban, rural, and frontier communities across the United States. When the news broke around 10:30 p.m. on March 21, 2010, that the US House of Representatives had just passed the Patient Protection and Affordable Care Act by the incredibly slim margin of 219-212, health equity champions were ecstatic. All day long the House had been arguing over HR 3590, which was its version of President Obama's health care reform package. The vote was agonizingly close, right up to the last minute, but the results were now clear. Comprehensive health care reform was law, and I started jumping for joy. For the past two years, I had worked directly with hundreds of coalitions, associations, and organizations to develop this legislation and ensure that it prioritized health equity.

Our advocacy efforts brought together a diverse group of stakeholders to collaboratively accomplish one of the most, if not *the* most, challenging and ambitious legislative feats in the history of the United States. During health reform negotiations I was at the helm of policy efforts leading the largest group on health reform and health equity—the National Working Group on Health Disparities and Health Reform—a diverse collective that included more than three hundred major organizations. This incredible group of stakeholders fought to secure health equity for vulnerable populations in this legislation, including organizations and coalitions representing women; children and youth; racial and ethnic minorities; lesbian, gay, bisexual, and transgender (LGBT) individuals; older adults; people with disabilities; veterans; faith-based organizations; health care providers; insurers; public health professionals; tribal, frontier, and rural communities; and people of lower socioeconomic status. This group worked cooperatively to develop and implement a master plan for health reform and health equity—working in concert with champions in the White House and Congress. This group of talented leaders and health policy experts was sought after for advice during the process to ensure that legislative proposals addressed key issues impacting our communities.

Health policy has been and is still, arguably, one of the most contentious areas in public policy. Everyone has had at least some experience with the health care system, and advocates on either side of the debate are passionate and vocal about their cause. For more than a century and a half there have been bitter struggles over advancing health care access and improving delivery of care in this country. So how did advocates of health reform and health equity in 2010 achieve the most significant milestone in United States health law and policy?

I have written this untold story to draw back the curtains and offer an insider's look into the crafting of the landmark Affordable Care Act. I present an authoritative account of reform history that debunks prevailing narratives. I also provide a comprehensive and unprecedented review of the health equity movement and the little-known leadership efforts to reform mental health, minority health, and universal health policies.

In an increasingly polarized political environment, ObamaCare has been caught in the cross fire of the partisan struggle, making it difficult to separate fact from fiction. "Government takeover." "Death panels." It can be difficult to figure out the truth in an environment full of misinformation where health care reform detractors have reduced the health care law to talking points and negative propaganda in order to score political gains. This book chronicles ObamaCare's development, promotion, and implementation; provides an engaging and objective examination of the health care statute and its implications; offers a clear analysis of the legal, political, and historical issues impacting this law and a thoughtful and accurate explanation of the complex legal language; and sheds light on a process often criticized as obscure and cloaked in secrecy. It recounts not only the process by which this law was developed but its implementation, breaking down key issues currently impacting the Affordable Care Act.

The book is the culmination of tireless health equity leadership and advocacy and is intended to take readers on the journey of health care transformation in the United States. It highlights and explores the strengths and weaknesses of the enduring campaign and continuous struggles for health care in America. It examines the breadth of existing health equity focused policies and laws and the level of advocacy involved in getting them passed. It provides insight into how we, as advocates, contributed in passing, defending, and implementing the ACA and illustrates the strategies that were developed and executed by proponents of health reform, including policy makers and advocates, to stimulate and sustain the necessary political will. In *150 Years of ObamaCare*, you will find unparalleled clarity about the health care law for anyone interested in learning what it contains or needing clarification about certain elements—essentially providing an even-handed and honest analysis and appraisal of the Affordable Care Act. This book also discusses the dramatic events when passage of the ACA nearly failed as well as examines the next steps in the health equity movement.

I wrote *150 Years of ObamaCare* so that future generations of health equity advocates, students, and scholars can learn from our efforts, build upon our successes—understanding what strategies we employed and why, what challenges we faced internally and externally, and how we overcame them. As Vice President Joe Biden acknowledged during the signing ceremony for the health reform law, "History is not merely what is printed in textbooks. It doesn't begin or end with the stroke of a pen. History is made. History is made when men and women decide that there is a greater risk in accepting a situation that we cannot bear than in steeling our spine and embracing the promise of change. That's when history is made."[1] This book was written to highlight how history was made, to put readers in the front seat and help them get a clearer view of the incredible turning points in the health equity movement so that we can continue to effect the changes necessary to improve the health of all communities.

NOTE

1. Barack Obama and Joe Biden, "Remarks by the President and Vice President at Signing of the Health Insurance Reform Bill," press release, March 23, 2010, https://www.whitehouse.gov/the-press-office/remarks-president -and-vice-president-signing-health-insurance-reform-bill.

150 Years of ObamaCare

1

Making the Case for Health Reform

We need to focus on the uninsured and those who suffer from health care disparities that we so inadequately addressed in the past.—*Senator William H. Frist, US Senate majority leader, on his priorities for the 108th Congress*

It was Thursday, June 28, 2012, and I was rushing to the airport to catch a flight for a meeting in Washington, DC. That morning, the US Supreme Court was expected to release its decision on the landmark health reform law, and I had asked several people to contact me immediately if they heard any news. As I cleared security at the Atlanta Hartsfield International Airport I started receiving phone calls and messages, but I was running to get to my gate. My heart was racing, as I had a gut feeling these calls were to tell me the fate of the Affordable Care Act, which was hanging in the balance. I ignored them, not yet ready to hear the news. When I finally got to my gate, the airline was calling zone 1. My father had called me four times so I decided to call him back first. I will never forget his words when he answered, "They overturned the ObamaCare law! They say it's unconstitutional!"

I was stunned, in a state of disbelief and grief. Though it was unlike me to yell in an airport, I screamed, "What?! Why?!" and thought to myself this could not be happening. After ending our conversation I checked my text messages and saw more confirmation of what my father said, the Supreme Court overturned President Obama's signature health law. Text after text repeated this news and ended with condolences, as though I had just lost a loved one. The gate agents had long ago called my zone, but I would not get on the plane. I was trying to find the nearest television to see what was being reported, but no television was nearby. Finally, I had to accept that if I did not get on the plane, I would be left behind, so I hurried onto the plane, stowed my luggage, buckled my seatbelt, and was about to turn my phone off when I got one more text: "You must be so relieved! Congratulations! Thank God."

I was perplexed. Why would I be happy with the Supreme Court holding the Affordable Care Act unconstitutional? I was even more puzzled since the message came from a fellow health reform champion. Unfortunately, I didn't have time to follow up and ask her what she meant, as the flight attendant had just ordered us to turn off our cell phones. Before this trip, I had never purchased wireless access, but as soon as I could turn my iPad on, I purchased in-flight Wi-Fi so I could find out what happened. I soon realized that there was widespread confusion about the Supreme Court's decision. Several major news networks erroneously reported that the law had been overturned. They had read the first part of the ruling, which said that the law's individual mandate could not be upheld under the Commerce Clause of the Constitution. However, they missed the crucial part of the ruling, hidden deep in the opinion, that said it could be upheld as a tax under the Taxing Clause. One on-air correspondent, in acknowledging the mistake, attributed it to the Court's "very confusing, large opinion."[1]

As I sat back to read Chief Justice Roberts's opinion myself, I could not help but agree. Even as a lawyer, I had to closely and carefully read all the way through the Court's decision to determine its impact and implications because sometimes what counts is not immediately apparent. As I read the opinion and realized that the key provisions of the Affordable Care Act had been upheld, I felt euphoric and unspeakably relieved that years of hard work had not gone to waste. To appreciate the roller coaster of emotions, you would need to have been there from the beginning—be part of the vexing journey to pass this comprehensive health care statute intended to tackle the high uninsured rates, the fragmentation in delivering care, and so many other problems inherent in our health care system. As health policy developers, we are always told never to get too attached to our bills, but this was different. Too many people from all walks of life were depending on this law—their lives, their health, and their well-being literally depended on its passage and implementation.

Consider, for example, the rabbi in Florida who made a blog post seeking a younger woman to marry him so he could get cheaper health insurance coverage. Or the former police officer in Georgia who was facing "'severe health' problems and homelessness" and robbed a bank with the intention of going to federal prison so he could finally get care and treatment. This officer who had served in his police department for fifteen years and had been jobless for more than a year "couldn't think of any other way to get help." In a similar incident, a North Carolina man robbed a bank for one dollar with the intention of going to prison in order to gain access to health services. The man had a growth on his chest and two ruptured disks and could not afford health care. Three years prior, he had been laid off from a major company after working there for seventeen years. Since that time, he was able to secure only part-time jobs that did not provide insurance coverage.[2] These stories, of people succumbing to desperate, il-legal, even life-threatening measures highlight the fundamental weaknesses of our health care system and how critically reform was needed.

Prior to the passage of the landmark health reform law, more than fifty million Americans lacked health insurance, the majority of these individ-uals among the ranks of the working poor. More than fifty-seven million people had been determined to have a preexisting condition, and many of these individuals were denied health insurance coverage on that basis. Be-fore the ACA was enacted, insurers would rescind coverage to individuals who needed care the most or find any mistake in their applications to deny them coverage. And approximately forty-five thousand people in the United States were dying each year because they lacked health insurance, equat-ing to about five individuals every hour.[3]

For consumers who had health insurance coverage and did not think reforms would positively impact them, the opposite was true—nearly 40 percent of the health care costs of the uninsured were being passed on to consumers who did have health insurance coverage, in the form of higher premiums. Moreover, the high costs of health care were directly impacting businesses and consumers, as both the family and employer shares of employer-based coverage nearly doubled from 2001 to 2010. The United States was spending far more on medical care than any other in-dustrialized nation but ranked twenty-seventh among thirty-four Orga-nisation for Economic Co-operation and Development countries in terms of life expectancy.[4]

Seven out of ten deaths in the United States were related to prevent-able diseases such as obesity, diabetes, high blood pressure, heart disease, and cancer, and 75 percent of our health care dollars were being spent treating them. However, only three cents of each dollar spent on health care (total public and private) were going toward prevention. Altogether, the five leading causes of death in the United States—heart disease, cancer, uninten-tional injuries, chronic lower respiratory diseases, and stroke—accounted for 63 percent of all deaths, but up to 40 percent of these annual deaths

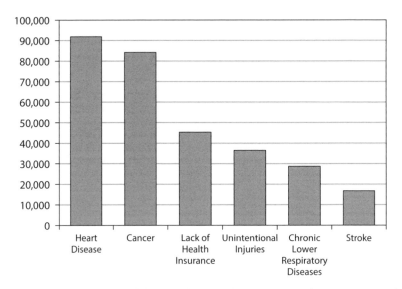

Figure 1.1. Leading causes of death in the United States. Centers for Disease Control and Prevention, "Up to 40 Percent of Annual Deaths from Each of Five Leading US Causes Are Preventable"; Wilper et al., "Health Insurance and Mortality in US Adults."

were preventable according to the Centers for Disease Control and Prevention. The total number of preventable deaths due to lack of health insurance displaces unintentional injuries as the third leading cause of preventable death.[5] This does not even include the number of preventable deaths due to medication errors, hospital acquired conditions, or other issues.

There were also considerable disparities in health status and health care among vulnerable populations. Members of underserved populations, such as racial and ethnic minorities, experience higher mortality rates and earlier onset of diseases. They also receive lower-quality health care and worse health outcomes. African American women have the highest death rates from heart disease, breast and lung cancer, stroke, and pregnancy among women of all racial and ethnic backgrounds. Hispanics have poorer quality of care than non-Hispanic whites for about 40 percent of quality measures, including not receiving screening for cancer or cardiovascular risk factors. American Indians and Alaska Natives have a suicide rate that is 50 percent higher than the national average, and Asian Americans have a high prevalence of chronic obstructive pulmonary disease, hepatitis B, tuberculosis, and liver disease.[6]

In general, people with disabilities are more likely to have difficulty or experience delays in accessing vital health services, including oral health care. Individuals with serious mental illness die on average twenty-five years earlier than the general population, at fifty-three years of age. Lesbian, gay, bisexual, and transgender individuals also experience disproportionate burden from discrimination and disease. They are approximately two and a half times more likely than heterosexuals to have a mental health disorder in their lifetime, and studies have shown that discrimination against LGBT persons has been associated with high rates of depression, substance use, and suicide.[7]

Studies have also shown that where you work, live, learn, pray, and play has a significant impact on your overall health status. Rural populations across the country have long struggled with obtaining primary care and hospital services. Depending on their geographic location, they may even endure disproportionate rates of chronic diseases or higher burden from behavioral health risks. For instance, rural communities in the South have long experienced higher rates of poverty, smoking, physical inactivity, and death due to heart disease; rural communities in the West have higher rates of alcohol abuse and suicide; and rural communities in the Northeast have higher rates of total tooth loss.[8]

The consequences of health care disparities are evident in experiences like that of a homeless woman in Missouri who sought care in a hospital emergency room. After being examined by a doctor, she was told she was healthy enough to go to jail when she refused to leave. She complained of pain in her legs, but police thought she was on drugs and arrested her for trespassing. She was carried into jail by her arms and ankles, where her body slackened and she died. An autopsy later revealed that she died from blood clots that had formed in her legs and traveled to her lungs. One HIV-positive man recounted an episode when a hospital denied him treatments and visitors and a doctor stated, "This is what he gets for going against God's will." A three-year-old girl was denied a lifesaving kidney transplant because she had a developmental disability, and a twelve-year-old boy died when his dental issue was left untreated due to lack of coverage and he succumbed to a very severe brain infection. Disproportionalities experienced by vulnerable groups lead to approximately eighty-three thousand deaths and more than $300 billion in costs to the country per year.[9]

These experiences and statistics provide only a glimpse of why we needed health reform and why it was so crucial that the Affordable Care

Act be upheld. For those of us with health insurance and access to care, it would be easy to lose sight of the individuals who struggle every day without coverage. It would be easy and unconscionable to ignore the dangerous and desperate attempts some individuals engage in to gain access to critical health services, treatments, or preventive care. It would even be easy to overlook the discriminatory and despicable treatment certain groups have experienced and continue to endure in health systems across the nation. But, as health equity advocates, we strive to attain the highest level of health for all people—to ensure that individuals and groups are not overlooked, that they have equitable access to quality, patient-centered care, as well as preventive services.[10] Stated differently, there is a public health benefit in eliminating legal and policy barriers to health equity. We know how important it is to advocate for vulnerable groups, to fight for resources for them, to ensure their voices are heard. We recognize the burden not only in lives lost but in the severe national economic impact of neglecting the health needs of underresourced communities.

Dr. Martin Luther King Jr. wrote in his "Letter from a Birmingham Jail" that "in any nonviolent campaign there are four basic steps: collection of the facts to determine whether injustices exist; negotiation; self-purification; and direct action."[11] This described his civil rights campaign, and it still rang true forty-five years later during the advocacy effort around the Affordable Care Act. Early on in the process, health equity advocates set out to apply Dr. King's teachings and decided to create a working group of committed champions for health reform and health equity. We were determined to work diligently and tirelessly to ensure the issue was prioritized in health reform negotiations. For too long, health equity had been relegated to a secondary position in health policy, but we believed it was the right time to propel it to the forefront. Armed with convincing data from studies on the impact of health disparities, we set out to demonstrate that this was an issue worth addressing finally in a comprehensive manner.

To achieve any significant reform the stars have to align perfectly. As we will later see, a bill can get through Congress and be vetoed by the president, or a bill can even be enacted and then fail to be implemented by the next administration. Sometimes, a bill can be signed into law by a president and upheld by successive administrations, but then the Supreme Court or an appellate court overturns the law. Policy making and advocacy can take countless hours, days, weeks, and even years of sacrifice and hard work. Every sentence, every word, every punctuation mark has a purpose and may convey a particular meaning. Of course, deciphering legislative language can be difficult and frustrating, which is why President Bill Clinton once acknowledged in a speech to college students, "I think that it's very important to understand we live in a time when, for a whole variety of reasons, policy making tends to be dimly understood, often distrusted and disconnected from the consequences of the policies being implemented."[12]

Perhaps no recent law has elicited more confusion, distrust, and disconnect than the health reform law. In fact, President Clinton went on to state that he intensely felt this was the case "in the development, the passage, and the implementation of the Affordable Care Act."[13] This was certainly my experience, and I hope this book will help demystify some of the policy making process in passing the ACA. This is the story of more than a century and a half of the resolve, patience, and drive it took to advance a health equity agenda in the United States.

NOTES

1. Fung and Mirkinson, "Supreme Court Health Care Ruling."

2. Galewitz, "For Love or Insurance?"; "Ex-Cop Admits to Robbing Bank to Get Health Benefits in Federal Prison"; Park, "Man Says He Robbed Bank to Get Health Care."

3. Wilper et al., "Health Insurance and Mortality in US Adults."

4. Organisation for Economic Co-operation and Development, *Health at a Glance 2011.*

5. Centers for Disease Control and Prevention, "Up to 40 Percent of Annual Deaths from Each of Five Leading US Causes Are Preventable"; Wilper et al., "Health Insurance and Mortality in US Adults."

6. US Department of Health and Human Services, Office of Minority Health, Minority Population Profiles, 2015.

7. US Department of Health and Human Services, *Healthy People 2020.*

8. Hartley, "Rural Health Disparities, Population Health, and Rural Culture."

9. Park, "Hospital"; Fry, "Doctors with Gay Bias Denied Meds, Man Says"; "Serious Issues in Disabled Girl Transplant Case"; Owings, "Toothache Leads to Boy's Death"; Satcher et al., "What If We Were Equal?"; LaVeist, Gaskin, and Richard, *Economic Burden of Health Inequalities in the United States.*

10. US Department of Health and Human Services, *Healthy People 2020.*

11. King, "Letter from a Birmingham Jail."

12. Walshe and Kreutz, "Bill Clinton Accuses Political Press of 'Blindness.'"

13. Ibid.

BIBLIOGRAPHY

Centers for Disease Control and Prevention, "Up to 40 Percent of Annual Deaths from Each of Five Leading US Causes Are Preventable." Press release, May 1, 2014. http://www.cdc.gov/media/releases/2014/p0501-preventable-deaths .html.

"Ex-Cop Admits to Robbing Bank to Get Health Benefits in Federal Prison." *CBS Atlanta News*, February 24, 2012.

Fry, Chris. "Doctors with Gay Bias Denied Meds, Man Says." Courthouse News Service, June 1, 2012, http://www.courthousenews.com/2012/06/01/47019 .htm.

Fung, K., and J. Mirkinson. "Supreme Court Health Care Ruling: CNN, Fox News Wrong on Individual Mandate" (video). *Huffington Post*, June 28, 2012. http://www.huffingtonpost.com/2012/06/28/cnn-supreme-court-health-care -individual-mandate_n_1633950.html.

Galewitz, Phil. "For Love or Insurance? Rabbi Seeks Young Wife to Lower Health Costs." NPR, August 17, 2011. http://www.npr.org/sections/health -shots/2011/08/17/139719331/for-love-or-insurance-rabbi-seeks-young-wife -to-lower-health-costs.

Hartley, David. "Rural Health Disparities, Population Health, and Rural Culture." *American Journal of Public Health* 94, no. 10 (October 2004): 1675–1678.

King, Martin Luther, Jr. "Letter from a Birmingham Jail." April 16, 1963.

LaVeist, T., D. Gaskin, and P. Richard. *The Economic Burden of Health Inequalities in the United States.* Joint Center for Political and Economic Studies Report, September 2009.

National Federation of Independent Business v. Sebelius, 132 U.S. 2566 (2012).

Organisation for Economic Co-operation and Development. *Health at a Glance 2011: OECD Indicators.* Geneva: OECD Publishing, 2011. http://dx.doi.org/10 .1787/health_glance-2011-en.

Owings, Laura. "Toothache Leads to Boy's Death." *ABC News*, March 5, 2007.

Park, Madison. "Hospital: Mom Booted from ER Who Died in Jail Was Treated Appropriately." *NBC News*, March 29, 2012. http://usnews.nbcnews.com/ _news/2012/03/29/10926817-hospital-mom-booted-from-er-who-died-in-jail -was-treated-appropriately?lite.

———. "Man Says He Robbed Bank to Get Health Care." *The Chart* (blog). CNN. June 21, 2011. http://thechart.blogs.cnn.com/2011/06/21/man-says-he -robbed-bank-to-get-health-care/comment-page-6/.

Satcher, D., et al. "What If We Were Equal? A Comparison of the Black-White Mortality Gap in 1960 and 2000." *Health Affairs* 24, no. 2 (2005): 459–464.

"Serious Issues in Disabled Girl Transplant Case." *NBC News*, January 17, 2012. http://vitals.nbcnews.com/_news/2012/01/17/10175611-serious-issues-in -disabled-girl-transplant-case.

US Department of Health and Human Services. *Healthy People 2020*. Washington, DC: US Department of Health and Human Services, 2010. healthypeople.gov.

US Department of Health and Human Services, Office of Minority Health. Minority Population Profiles, 2015. http://minorityhealth.hhs.gov/omh/browse.aspx?lvl=2&lvlid=26.

Walshe, S., and L. Kreutz. "Bill Clinton Accuses Political Press of 'Blindness.'" *ABC News*, April 30, 2014. http://abcnews.go.com/blogs/politics/2014/04/bill-clinton-accuses-political-press-of-blindness/.

Wilper, Andrew P., et al. "Health Insurance and Mortality in US Adults." *American Journal of Public Health* 99, no. 12 (2009): 2289-2295.

2

Past Meets Present
The Historical Roots of ObamaCare

If you would understand anything, observe its beginning and development.—Aristotle

A father had children who were always arguing among themselves. When his appeals failed to assuage their disputes, he decided to give them a practical lesson on the consequence of disunity. He told them each to bring him a bundle of sticks. He placed a bundle into each child's hands and told them to break it in pieces. Each child tried with all of his or her might, but was not able to break the bundle. He then opened the bundle, took the sticks apart, one by one, and put one stick in each child's hands. This time they broke them easily. Once the sticks were broken, he addressed them in these words: "If you are of one mind, and unite to assist each other, you will be as this bundle, uninjured by all the attempts of your enemies; but if you are divided among yourselves, you will be broken as easily as these sticks."[1] This is the story of the competing advocacy groups that united in 2010 to achieve comprehensive health reform after trying to achieve their own piecemeal reforms for more than 150 years without much success.

Although discussions have focused primarily on universal health coverage, the Affordable Care Act is a comprehensive and reticulated statute that includes numerous other health policies impacting groups that have long fought for equity in health care. Before its passage, advocates for mental health, minority health, and other causes labored tirelessly to develop, introduce, pass, and implement legislation intended to benefit their own respective groups. They often advocated independently for their own priorities, employing autonomous campaigns and strategies, and were met with limited progress. When one group successfully lobbied for its priorities, another group found itself on the losing end of the fight.

But even those groups that achieved their advocacy efforts often found their victories short lived. Once the political winds shifted, or as time passed and priorities changed within an administration or Congress, legislation would be halted or statutes repealed. Sometimes a bill passed in one chamber of Congress but failed to pass in the other, or it passed both chambers of Congress but was then vetoed by the president. And even legislation that had been signed into law by one president could be repealed by Congress, overturned by a court, or defunded by a subsequent administration. Success was often tempered when advocates lost the political will to continue pushing the agenda or became disengaged from the process. Or, as has been the case with major advocacy campaigns throughout the decades, progress waned because advocates with competing interests failed to come together and harness the power of collaboration. As President John F. Kennedy reminded the nation when he was first elected: "United there is little we cannot do in a host of cooperative ventures. Divided there is little we can do, for we dare not meet a powerful challenge at odds and split asunder."[2]

Early on, mental health and minority health advocates realized tremendous progress in the mid-1800s, only to have their gains wiped out by a president or by the Supreme Court. For both groups, it would take almost a century before noteworthy gains in federal policy were achieved in piecemeal fashion. By contrast, advocates for universal health saw consistent attention to their priority from the turn of the twentieth century until the present by various administrations and congresses. Today, the health reform bill that President Obama signed into law—the Affordable Care Act—could be seen as a crowning achievement for each group working collaboratively to accomplish its priorities.

To understand the entire picture, we need to revisit the past for a moment and take a closer look at how health reform efforts began, developed, and were executed. Indeed, the various attempts throughout history to pass health reform legislation demonstrate why health reform advocates employed certain strategies and tactics to pass the Affordable Care Act in 2010. This chapter reveals the impact that various White House administrations, Congresses, and courts have had on policies intended to bolster health equity. This chapter also discusses previous advocacy efforts to increase access to health services and advance a health equity agenda. It highlights some of the great achievements and bitter disappointments in developing and implementing health laws and policies over the years, and shows how health reform finally materialized.

Comprehensive Health Policy Timeline

Major laws related to health care reform appear in bold.

1798 – President John Adams signed into law the Act for Relief of Sick and Disabled Seamen.

1854 – Congress passed the Bill for the Benefit of the Indigent Insane but vetoed by President Pierce.

1865 – The Freedmen's Bureau Act was signed into law.

1869 – Congress failed to reauthorize Freedmen's Bureau.

1872 – Freedmen's Bureau officially closed.

1875 – Civil Rights Act of 1875 was signed into law.

1883 – Civil Rights Act of 1875 ruled unconstitutional by the US Supreme Court.

1896 – *Plessy v. Ferguson* decided by the US Supreme Court promoting separate-but-equal doctrine.

EARLY 20th CENTURY

1912 – President Theodore Roosevelt endorsed social insurance as part of his platform, including health insurance, but lost election.

1912 – President William Howard Taft established the Children's Bureau, which began a nationwide investigation of maternal and infant mortality rates.

1915 – National Negro Health Week established.

1921 – President Warren G. Harding signed the Sheppard-Towner Maternity and Infancy Protection Act, which provided funding to states to establish and run prenatal and child health centers based on the work done by the Children's Bureau. It expired eight years later in 1929 and was not reauthorized because of the stock market crash.

1927 – President Calvin Coolidge established the Committee on the Cost of Medical Care to investigate the health care system, but recommendations from this committee were put on hold because of the stock market crash in 1929.

1932 – The US Public Health Service opened the Office of Negro Health Work.

1935 – President Franklin D. Roosevelt signed the Social Security Act but abandoned the inclusion of national health insurance coverage because of strong opposition.

1936 – FDR established by executive order the Interdepartmental Committee to Coordinate Health and Welfare Activities to assess the health care needs of the people.

MID-20th CENTURY

1940 – FDR enacted the Lanham Act, which provided federal funding to communities impacted by the defense industry so that they could improve their infrastructure, including health care facilities.

1942 – President FDR signed Executive Order 9079, Making Certain Public Health Service Hospitals Available for the Care and Treatment of Insane Persons.

1945 – President Harry S. Truman argued that the federal government should play a role in health care during a special address to Congress. After his speech the Murray-Wagner-Dingell bill authors redrafted their legislation to include President Truman's health care proposal.

1946 – President Truman signed the Hospital Survey and Construction Act, also referred to as the Hill-Burton Act.

1946 – President Truman signed the National Mental Health Act into law.

1949 – National Institute of Mental Health established.

1955 – President Eisenhower signed the Mental Health Study Act, leading to the establishment of the Joint Commission on Mental Illness and Mental Health.

1956 – President Eisenhower argued for federal reinsurance under which the federal government would subsidize partial payment of premiums for low-income individuals.

1956 – *Eaton v. Board of Managers of the James Walker Memorial Hospital* initiated by NAACP to challenge the separate-but-equal doctrine supported by the Hill-Burton Act.

1960s

1960 – President-elect John F. Kennedy appointed the presidential Task Force on Health and Social Security for the American People, which recommended

Comprehensive Health Policy Timeline

private health insurance for older adults.

1961 – President Dwight D. Eisenhower's Joint Commission on Mental Illness and Mental Health released comprehensive report.

1962 – *Simkins v. Moses H. Cone Memorial Hospital* initiated by the NAACP to challenge the separate-but-equal doctrine in health care privileges.

1963 – President Kennedy signed the Mental Retardation Facilities and Community Mental Health Centers Construction Act.

1964 – Civil Rights Act of 1964 signed into law.

1965 – President Lyndon B. Johnson signed the Medicare and Medicaid legislation into law.

1970s

1971 – Sen. Edward M. "Ted" Kennedy introduced a health insurance reform statute, which was countered by a proposal from President Richard Nixon a few months after titled National Health Insurance Partnership Act.

1971 – Congressional Black Caucus established.

1973 – President Nixon signed into law the Health Maintenance Organization Act.

1974 – President Gerald Ford prioritized universal health insurance, and set a goal of passing the Kennedy-Mills plan that year.

1976 – Congressional Hispanic Caucus established.

1977 – President Jimmy Carter issued an executive order establishing the President's Commission on Mental Health.

1978 – President's Commission on Mental Health produced seminal report.

1978 – Congressional Black Caucus Health Braintrust established.

1979 – President Carter developed national health insurance plan and delivered it to Congress.

1979 – First hearing on minority health held in the US Senate by Senator Kennedy.

1979 – Patricia Roberts Harris appointed first African American secretary of Health, Education, and Welfare.

1980s

1980 – President Carter signed the Mental Health Systems Act.

1981 – President Ronald Reagan signed the Omnibus Budget Reconciliation Act, which rendered most of the Mental Health Systems Act moot.

1983 – External groups presented reports on minority health and health disparities to Secretary Margaret Heckler.

1983 – Secretary Heckler recognized significant gaps in minority health.

1984 – Secretary Heckler established the Task Force on Black and Minority Health.

1985 – The Emergency Medical Treatment and Active Labor Act was signed into law.

1985 – Landmark *Report of the Secretary's Task Force on Black and Minority Health* released.

1986 – Office of Minority Health created at HHS.

1989 – Minority Health Bill introduced by Rep. Louis Stokes and Sen. Kennedy.

1989 – President George H. W. Bush developed a comprehensive health insurance proposal, but it was set aside because of pressing international issues.

1990s

1990 – President Bush signed into law the Americans with Disabilities Act.

1990 – *Healthy People 2000* released, prioritizing "reduction of health disparities."

1990 – Congress passed the Disadvantaged Minority Health Improvement Act of 1990.

1990 – The Office of Research on Minority Health established.

1991 – Congress appropriated $1 million to support health disparities research.

1992 – The Minority Health Initiative was launched and allocated $45 million for programs geared to addressing health disparities.

1993 – President Bill Clinton convened the White House Task Force on Health Reform and appointed First Lady Hillary Clinton as chair.

1993 – Democratic Sen. George Mitchell introduced a 1,370-page bipartisan bill with 29 cosponsors

Comprehensive Health Policy Timeline

entitled the Health Security Act, which was the embodiment of the Clinton plan. That same day, Republican Sen. John Chafee introduced the bipartisan Health Equity and Access Reform Today Act with 20 cosponsors.

1994 – The Clinton plan was defeated.

1994 – Congressional Asian Pacific American Caucus established.

1996 – President Clinton signed into law the Mental Health Parity Act.

1998 – Minority HIV/AIDS Initiative began with $156 million in funding from Congress.

1999 – The REACH program is created at the Centers for Disease Control and Prevention.

1999 – The Clinton administration released *Mental Health: A Report of the Surgeon General*.

2000s

2000 – *Healthy People 2010* released, prioritizing "elimination of health disparities."

2000 – Congress passed the Minority Health and Health Disparities Research and Education Act

2001 – Institute of Medicine report *Crossing the Quality Chasm: A New Health System for the 21st Century* released.

2001 – The Clinton administration released report titled *Mental Health: Culture, Race and Ethnicity*.

2002 – President George W. Bush established the New Freedom Commission on Mental Health.

2002 – IOM report *Unequal Treatment: Confronting Racial and Ethnic Disparities in Health Care* released.

2003 – The New Freedom Commission on Mental Health report *Achieving the Promise: Transforming Mental Health Care in America* released.

2003 – Agency for Healthcare Research & Quality released the first *National Healthcare Disparities Report*.

2003 – The NIH *Strategic Research Plan and Budget to Reduce and Ultimately Eliminate Health Disparities* was issued.

2007 – President Bush proposed a plan to address health insurance coverage.

2008 – President Bush signed the Paul Wellstone and Pete Domenici Mental Health Parity and Addiction Equity Act.

2008 – President Bush signed into law the Americans with Disabilities Act Amendments Act.

2009 – President Barack Obama signed the American Recovery and Reinvestment Act.

2009 – National Working Group on Health Disparities and Health Reform created.

2009 – President Obama and the Tri-Caucus declared support for addressing health disparities in a comprehensive health reform package.

2009 – The Joint Center report *The Economic Burden of Health Disparities in the United States* released.

2010s

2010 – President Obama signed the Patient Protection and Affordable Care Act into law, the first comprehensive health reform enacted.

2010 – *Healthy People 2020* released prioritizing achievement of health equity, elimination of disparities, and improvement in the health of all groups.

2015 – President Obama signed into law the Medicare Access and CHIP Reauthorization Act, which extended many of the health reform programs from the ACA and expanded delivery and payment reforms.

Mental Health

The mental health problems facing our country are the problems of all citizens. The people with these problems are ourselves, our families, our neighbors and our friends.—*Rosalynn Carter, 1979 Senate testimony on the need to support mental health programs*

Mental Health: The Early Struggle to Increase Federal Responsiveness

The history of the government's involvement in mental health issues in the United States neatly illustrates the struggles advocates have endured throughout the last century and a half. It is a powerful reminder that even when it seems that health equity advocates have taken two steps forward, the political tides may change and push us backward four steps.

In the early 1800s, Dorothea Dix, a schoolteacher from Cambridge, Massachusetts, was inspired to take up the cause of those who had mental health challenges. She spent years traveling to several states and urging legislatures to provide adequate institutions to treat and care for these individuals. In the course of this work, Dix had learned that many states were unable or unwilling to bear the cost of these institutions; she decided then to turn to the federal government to provide aid. In 1848 Dix urged Congress to authorize a grant of five million acres of public lands, which would be sold and the proceeds used "as a perpetual fund for the care of the indigent insane." She believed that Congress might provide the grants, as they had done so for the building of roads, educational purposes, and for other domestic improvements. However, no action was taken on the proposal.[3]

In 1850, Dix again brought forward her proposal, this time requesting ten million acres of land. Debate on the bill revolved around conflicting views about how federal public lands should be used, with little to no attention paid to the needs of the mentally ill. Only Senator William Dawson of Georgia argued for the bill on the basis of its humanitarian intent, saying, "We cannot do a more charitable act than that which is proposed by this bill." The bill passed in the Senate but was deferred in the House. Dix advocated for the bill again in 1852, but no action was taken in either chamber of Congress. Finally, in 1854 Dix successfully lobbied for the Bill for the Benefit of the Indigent Insane, after having achieved many successes in various states by acquiring state funding to increase mental health care services. She had done so after developing reports on substandard mental health care for each state she visited, which led to the creation and passage of bills to establish psychiatric facilities. The congressional Bill for the Benefit of the Indigent Insane finally passed the Senate and the House and was sent to President Franklin Pierce to be signed into law.[4]

Instead of signing the bill, however, President Pierce vetoed the legislation. He believed that it would be unconstitutional to regard health as anything but a private matter in which government should not become involved.

> I readily and, I trust, feelingly acknowledge the duty incumbent on us all as men and citizens, and as among the highest and holiest of our duties, to provide for those who, in the mysterious order of Providence, are subject to want and to disease of body or mind; but I can not find any authority in the Constitution for making the Federal Government the great almoner of public charity throughout the United States. To do so would, in my judgment, be contrary to the letter and spirit of the Constitution and subversive of the whole theory upon which the Union of these States is founded.[5]

Pierce's veto set the policy of extremely limited federal participation or nonparticipation in the realm of mental health and social welfare for the next almost one hundred years. This essentially resulted in a tug-of-war between state and local governments, where states assumed responsibility for mental health care by building and operating asylums and local governments would pay for episodes of care. Then, in 1942, President Franklin Delano Roosevelt signed Executive Order 9079, Making Certain Public Health Service Hospitals Available for the Care and Treatment of Insane Persons. The order authorized the transfer of mentally ill patients to Public Health Service Hospitals in Lexington, Kentucky, and Fort Worth, Texas.

Four years later, President Harry Truman enacted the National Mental Health Act of 1946, which for the first time in US history provided a significant amount of funding for research into the causes, prevention, and treatment of mental illness. The National Mental Health Act led to the creation in 1949 of the National Institute of Mental Health and helped to bolster the community mental health movement, which pushed for deinstitutionalization and integration in order to treat patients in their communities rather than in psychiatric hospitals. A decade later in 1955, President Eisenhower signed the Mental Health Study Act, leading to the establishment of the Joint Commission on Mental Illness and Mental Health, which was tasked with assessing the available resources for tackling mental illness and providing recommendations to address this issue.[6]

The next major mental health legislation came in 1963, when President John F. Kennedy signed the Community Mental Health Act (also known as the Mental Retardation Facilities and Community Mental Health Centers Construction Act of 1963). The law provided the first federal funding for developing a network of community mental health centers as an alternative to institutionalization, drastically changing the delivery of mental health services. The basis of this act was a report issued in 1961 by Eisenhower's Joint Commission on Mental Illness and Mental Health, showing that people with mental health challenges could be treated more effectively in community settings than in traditional psychiatric institutions and hospitals. The Social Security Amendments of 1965 further sustained community mental health centers by allocating staff funding, and they established the framework for a new commission, the Joint Commission on the Mental Health of Children, charged with examining children's mental health issues and recommending a national action plan to address them. The progress achieved by the Truman, Eisenhower, and Kennedy administrations in bolstering community mental health was diminished, however, with the election of President Richard M. Nixon, who tried to defund the community mental health centers. The centers had been authorized $260 million in funding from 1965 to 1969; under Nixon, they received only $50 million from 1970 to 1973.[7]

Achieving Comprehensive Mental Health Reform for a Few Months

The election of President Jimmy Carter in 1977 was a major step forward for federal involvement in the mental health system. When he was the governor of Georgia, Carter had established the Commission to Improve Services to the Mentally and Emotionally Retarded and appointed his wife, Rosalynn, to the commission. One tremendous success during his governorship was an approximately 30 percent decrease in the number of hospitalized patients in Georgia. Mrs. Carter decided that if her husband were elected president, she would continue to focus on mental health reform, hoping that the beneficial results of deinstitutionalization and the creation of community mental health centers in Georgia could be repeated on a national level. Soon after his election, Carter issued an executive order establishing the President's Commission on Mental Health, the first-ever commission dealing comprehensively with the mental health system. It was tasked with determining whether the mentally ill were underserved, what the proper role of the federal government was, what kind

Mental Health Policy Timeline

Major laws related to health care reform appear in bold.

PRE-20th CENTURY

1854 - Congress passed the Bill for the Benefit of the Indigent Insane, but it was vetoed by President Franklin Pierce.

1940s

1942 - President Franklin D. Roosevelt signed Executive Order 9079, Making Certain Public Health Service Hospitals Available for the Care and Treatment of Insane Persons.

1946 - President Harry S. Truman signed the National Mental Health Act into law.

1949 - National Institute of Mental Health established.

1950s

1955 - President Dwight D. Eisenhower signed the Mental Health Study Act, leading to the establishment of the Joint Commission on Mental Illness and Mental Health.

1960s

1961 - President Eisenhower's Joint Commission on Mental Illness and Mental Health released comprehensive report.

1963 - President John F. Kennedy signed the Mental Retardation Facilities and Community Mental Health Centers Construction Act.

1970s

1977 - President Jimmy Carter issued executive order establishing President's Commission on Mental Health.

1978 - President's Commission on Mental Health produced seminal report.

1980s

1980 - President Carter signed Mental Health Systems Act.

1981 - President Ronald Reagan signed Omnibus Budget Reconciliation Act, which rendered most of Mental Health Systems Act moot.

1990s

1990 - President George H. W. Bush signed into law Americans with Disabilities Act.

1996 - President Bill Clinton signed into law Mental Health Parity Act.

1999 - The Clinton administration released report titled *Mental Health: A Report of the Surgeon General*.

2000s

2001 - The Clinton administration released report titled *Mental Health: Culture, Race and Ethnicity*.

2002 - President George W. Bush announced establishment of New Freedom Commission on Mental Health.

2003 - New Freedom Commission on Mental Health released report titled *Achieving the Promise: Transforming Mental Health Care in America*.

2008 - President Bush signed Paul Wellstone and Pete Domenici Mental Health Parity and Addiction Equity Act.

2008 - President Bush signed into law Americans with Disabilities Act Amendments Act.

2009 - **President Barack Obama signed American Recovery and Reinvestment Act, laying the foundation for health reform.**

2010s

2010 - **President Obama signed Patient Protection and Affordable Care Act into law, the first time comprehensive health reform enacted.**

2015 - **President Obama signed into law Medicare Access and CHIP Reauthorization Act, which extended many health reform programs from the ACA and expanded delivery and payment reforms.**

of research was needed, and whether a unified approach to mental health could be developed, among other issues.[8]

The President's Commission on Mental Health produced a seminal report in 1978 that committed to the goal of making high-quality mental health care available and affordable to those who need it in the least restrictive setting with strengthened personal and community supports. It recommended a federal program that would create new community mental health services, particularly in underserved areas, and would encourage mental health specialists to work in those areas and ensure their training and knowledge were suitable for the needs of those populations. The report urged closing large psychiatric hospitals in favor of more comprehensive and integrated care that included community-based services and small state hospitals. After receiving the report, Carter directed the head of the Department of Health, Education, and Welfare, Secretary Patricia Roberts Harris, to draft model legislation that would implement its recommendations.[9]

Exactly 125 years after Franklin Pierce vetoed a mental health reform legislation that early advocates had spent their lives trying to get passed, President Carter in May of 1979 sent a message to Congress along with a draft mental health systems act that would establish "a new partnership between the federal government and the states in the planning and provision of mental health services." Passage of the final bill would take almost a year and a half. The Mental Health Systems Act of 1980 aimed to restructure the community mental health center program and improve services for people with mental illness. It required states to establish community mental health centers, providing inpatient, outpatient, and emergency services as well as consultation and education. Carter signed the act into law on October 7, 1980, saying at the time, "This is the most important piece of Federal mental health legislation since President John Kennedy signed the Mental Retardation Facilities and Community Mental Health Centers Construction Act 17 years ago."[10]

The Mental Health Systems Act became law one month before the 1980 presidential election, which Carter lost to Republican Ronald Reagan. Immediately after he was inaugurated, President Reagan set about dismantling many of the achievements of the Carter administration. Within months of its enactment, President Reagan signed into law the Omnibus Budget Reconciliation Act in the summer of 1981, which repealed or rendered most provisions of the Mental Health Systems Act moot. The act authorized instead federal block grants to the states for mental health services.

The grants provided the states only 75–80 percent of what they would have received under the Mental Health Systems Act. Reagan effectively ended federal funding of community treatment for the mentally ill, shifting the burden to individual state governments.

Strengthening Individual Protections for People with Mental Health Issues: The Americans with Disabilities Act

In 1990, President George H. W. Bush signed into law the Americans with Disabilities Act (ADA), which guaranteed individuals with disabilities, including people with mental health issues, equal access to employment; government services including transportation, public accommodations, telecommunications; and other services such as insurance. Then, eighteen years later in 2008, his son, President George W. Bush signed into law the Americans with Disabilities Act Amendments Act, which gave broader protections to workers with disabilities by clarifying and expanding the definition of disability in the original ADA of 1990. The second Bush administration, working in conjunction with mental health champions in Congress, realized that over time the US Supreme Court had eroded many of the protections in the 1990 law and had narrowed the definition of disability under the law.[11] The law as Congress originally intended it had been terribly weakened when court after court decided that individuals with various impairments, including cognitive impairments, were not disabled for the purposes of the ADA. Senator Edward Kennedy (D-MA) was determined to fix these judicial errors and delegated the effort to Senator Tom Harkin (D-IA) of Iowa.

Under Harkin's leadership, Congress set out to strengthen the ADA after the National Council on Disability released a report in 2004, *Righting the Americans with Disabilities Act*. On the House side, in 2006, Congressmen Jim Sensenbrenner (R-WI) and Steny Hoyer (D-MD) worked together to draft legislation rectifying this issue, and introduced their bill on September 29. The Senate followed with a new version in the following Congress, introduced by Harkin and Senator Arlen Specter (R-PA). Early on, disability advocates decided to call a meeting of the leading disability groups in Washington, DC, to decide whether they were going to work together and strengthen the ADA, and to determine the specific changes they were seeking.

The ground rule was laid that, once reopened, advocates would not use the ADA as a vehicle to push other agendas or priorities; their job was simply to address where the courts had gone wrong. After spending several years working to strengthen the ADA, in 2008, the disability advocacy groups found out that there was heavy opposition to the new bill from the US Chamber of Commerce, the Society for Human Resource Management, and other business groups. These groups had lobbied against the ADA back in 1989 because they believed it would detrimentally impact small businesses, and they were again concerned about the scope of the proposed fix. After six months of intense negotiations, there was finally a breakthrough and the disability advocacy groups and the business community came to an agreement on what the final legislation should look like. This was a significant milestone to see two fiercely opposing groups coming together to tell Congress to pass this bill and the Bush administration to sign it into law.

Strengthening Health Insurance Access for People with Mental Health Issues: The Mental Health Parity Act

The next major mental health legislation was enacted when the nation was again under a Democratic president. Bill Clinton in 1996 signed into law the Mental Health Parity Act (MHPA), which required that annual or lifetime dollar limits on mental health benefits be no lower than limits for medical and surgical benefits offered by a group health plan. Immediately after the MHPA was enacted, some insurers and employers began finding ways to sidestep the law or comply only to the extent required by the law. Their strategies included higher copays, higher deductibles, out-of-pocket maximums, caps on the number of visits with a care provider or number of days in a hospital visit.

Approximately three years after President Clinton signed the MHPA into law, his administration released a major report on mental health in 1999 titled *Mental Health: A Report of the Surgeon General*, which highlighted the complex issues impacting mental health in the United States. Three years after the report was released, President George W. Bush announced the establishment of the New Freedom Commission on Mental Health on April 29, 2002. This commission was charged with studying the mental health service delivery system to determine how effective it was in meeting the needs of people with serious mental illnesses and serious emotional disturbances as well as make recommendations for transforming the mental health system to meet the needs of vulnerable individuals. The George W. Bush administration was concerned about the gaps in care and wanted people with serious mental health issues to live, work, learn, and participate fully in their communities. On July 22, 2003, this commission developed a comprehensive report, *Achieving the Promise: Transforming Mental Health Care in America*, which would prove influential and highly valuable during the 2007 negotiations to strengthen the Mental Health Parity Act spearheaded by a bipartisan group of congressional mental health champions.

In 2007, Senator Kennedy and two Republican colleagues, Senators Pete Domenici of New Mexico and Senator Mike Enzi of Wyoming, initiated efforts to address the inherent weakness of the 1996 mental health parity law. Domenici, who had a daughter with schizophrenia, was expected to retire at the end of 2008 and believed strongly that the MHPA should be strengthened to provide protections to individuals experiencing discrimination in mental health benefits. Kennedy, who chaired the Senate Health, Education, Labor and Pensions (HELP) Committee, and Enzi, its ranking member, supported Domenici's desire to see the MHPA strengthened and wanted this achievement to become part of his legacy.

Similar to the process for passing the ADA under Senator Harkin's leadership, congressional staff decided to convene meetings with all major stakeholders. These stakeholders included insurance companies, employer groups, and mental and behavioral health associations, including the American Psychological Association, American Psychiatric Association, National Alliance on Mental Illness, American Benefits Council, National Retail Federation, Mental Health America, and the Association for Behavioral Health and Wellness. Lobbyists for the American Psychological Association and Aetna insurance company were chosen by congressional staff to be the points of contact for each side. On February 12, 2007, Senator Domenici introduced the Mental Health Parity Act of 2007. On the House side, Patrick Kennedy (D-RI) and Jim Ramstad (R-MI) worked in concert with Senator Kennedy to champion the legislation and develop and execute the legislative strategies to get it passed. The House's version of the bill was intentionally broader in scope than the Senate bill and caused the insurers and employers to deem it far too overreaching early in the negotiations. As a result, all stakeholders continued to work closely with the Senate HELP Committee to negotiate the bill and produce a mutually acceptable version that would pass both the House and Senate and be approved by the Bush administration.

The bill did not require health insurers or employers to provide mental health and substance use benefits, but if they did offer such benefits, they had to be on par with medical and surgical benefits. A year later, after almost two years of intense negotiations among all parties, President George W. Bush signed the Paul Wellstone and Pete Domenici Mental Health Parity and Addiction Equity Act of 2008 into law. Although it did not mandate health benefits in general, proponents believed that mandatory health benefits would be possible in the next administration. Congressional staff who worked on the act were proud of having achieved some health insurance reform, but they still had an eye to more comprehensive health reform. The lessons learned from this process would prove crucial a few years later during the fight for health reform.

Minority Health

Of all the forms of inequality, injustice in health care is the most shocking and inhumane.—*Dr. Martin Luther King Jr., in a speech to the Medical Committee for Human Rights, 1966.*

Almost 150 years after the Civil War ended, Senator Edward M. Kennedy declared, "How we respond to the minority health crisis is a basic measure of the depth of the nation's actual commitment to the ideals of liberty and justice for all."[12] From that perspective, our nation's actual commitment to liberty and justice for all is problematic at best, given the frustratingly inadequate response to minority health issues over the decades following the Civil War. While discrimination in health services has become less overt over time, the disproportionalities and inequities experienced by vulnerable populations continue to widen at alarming rates. This result is, arguably, due in part to the impact of health laws and policies on vulnerable and underserved groups, which have hampered or advanced health equity for generations.

Freedmen's Bureau: The Federal Government's First Response to the Minority Health Crisis

One of the most significant early policies concerning the health of minorities was the Freedmen's Bureau legislation. After the Civil War ended, when slaves had been emancipated and were moving into cities in large numbers, a health crisis was created that required the federal government's involvement. In 1865, Congress grudgingly created the Freedmen's Bureau, formally known as the Bureau of Refugees, Freedmen and Abandoned Lands. Interestingly and somewhat ironically, to pass a bill that would benefit individuals who had formerly been enslaved, congressional sympathizers had to include language supportive of former Confederate soldiers who were displaced as a result of the war. There simply was no appetite to pass legislation that would solely benefit freedpeople or former slaves who were not yet considered full citizens of the United States.

The Freedmen's Bureau was a federal agency that aided former slaves during the post-Civil War Reconstruction era. Its purpose was to provide food and medical care to freedpeople and poor whites in war-torn areas, regulate the labor of the freedpeople, administer justice, manage land confiscated during the war, and establish schools for the freedpeople. In 1866, newly elected president Andrew Johnson vetoed a bill intended to increase the power of the Freedmen's Bureau. The bill was subsequently reintroduced and passed by Congress later in 1866, and the Bureau was reauthorized by Congress every year until 1869, one year after the Fourteenth Amendment to the US Constitution was ratified declaring all former slaves US citizens.[13]

The 1865 legislation created and funded the Medical Division to address the needs of the newly freed slaves. The bureau established hospitals and dispensaries throughout the South, for the most part using existing buildings such as abandoned mansions. The bureau's doctors also provided home visits, through which patients with less acute illnesses could receive care. During the less than seven years of the Freedmen's Bureau's existence, the Medical Division established more than ninety hospitals and other health facilities throughout the South, providing care to well over five hundred thousand patients.[14] The facilities, however, suffered insufficient funding, supplies, and staff. The bureau often struggled with recruiting physicians, nurses, and other health professionals, and the health professionals it was able to recruit were frequently inexperienced or unqualified. Conditions in some of the hospitals were so unsanitary that they resulted in illnesses and deaths, lacking funds to address this issue much less buy proper food for patients.

While the Freedmen's Bureau did fall short of providing quality health care to millions of former slaves, because of the racial politics of that time, in June 1872, Congress voted to completely shut the bureau down by the end of that month. This decision would serve as one of the rarest, if not the rarest, congressional action that successfully dismantled a health care program that had already been implemented for several years. The impact of that decision would be felt by generations of African American families for almost a century and a half. Millions of African Americans would find themselves unable to access care when they needed it the most. In the era of Jim Crow laws, many hospitals and other health care facilities refused to provide care or lifesaving treatments to African Americans. Not surprisingly, hospitals that were established by African American physicians during the Jim Crow era were also underresourced. And in many respects, safety-net hospitals and clinics that serve the most vulnerable communities even today continue to struggle with insufficient resources.

With the advent and imposition of Jim Crow laws and policies during the late 1800s and early 1900s, racist studies were conducted and the results were promulgated, arguing that African Americans had poorer health because they were an inferior race. Prominent African American leaders and scientists refuted those assertions and conducted their own research to show why there were terrible disparities in health status between blacks and whites, including the notable W. E. B. Du Bois, who edited a scientific volume titled *The Health and Physique of the Negro American*. In conjunction with black business organizations and groups such as the National Urban League, the National Association for the Advancement of Colored People (NAACP), the National Medical Association, and the National Dental Association, African American leaders held conferences and created reports on the topic.[15]

In 1915, under the leadership of Booker T. Washington, the founder of Tuskegee Institute, a National Health Improvement Week was launched, which later became known as National Negro Health Week during the first week of April. This public health campaign was launched to increase awareness and education about healthy lifestyles among African Americans since at that time the health status of blacks was decades behind that of whites. In fact, 45 percent of all deaths among African Americans were deemed preventable, 450,000 African Americans were estimated to be seriously ill or had a disability all the time, and it was costing our nation tens of millions of dollars. From the National Negro Health Week evolved a National Negro Health Movement that lasted thirty-five years and incorporated community development and engagement, health education, professional training, and health policy initiatives. Years later this nationally recognized week was elevated to a whole month and was designated National Minority Health Month, which is now recognized each year during April.

Blatant Discrimination in Health Care

In autumn of 1931, Juliette Derricotte, the dean of women at Fisk University, a historically black university located in Tennessee, was involved in a serious car accident while traveling through Dalton, Georgia, a city nestled in the foothills of the Blue Ridge Mountains in northwest Georgia. A white physician did his best to stabilize her and provided care for her in his office, but when he tried desperately to admit Ms. Derricotte to the hospital for more aggressive care, the hospital refused because she was black. She was later transferred to the black ward of a hospital in Chattanooga, Tennessee, but the care that could have saved her life came too late and she died.

The NAACP was outraged and used this story to highlight the impact of racial discrimination in health care, hoping to draw support for desegregating hospitals in America. It publicized the story in newspapers across the country—targeting both blacks and whites.[16] One year after Ms. Derricotte's death in 1932, the US Public Health Service established the Office of Negro Health Work under the leadership of Dr. Roscoe G. Brown, an African American dentist. This new office represented the second time since the creation of the Freedmen's Bureau that the federal government established an entity that was aimed at addressing African American health. Unlike the Freedmen's Bureau, which lasted less than seven years, the Office of Negro Health Work lasted almost two decades until it was disbanded in 1951 along with the National Negro Health Movement, which came under the Office of Negro Health Work.

Drawing back a veil on the disturbing past and indefensible apathy demonstrated by lawmakers through the ensuing years, Congress finally mustered the support to pass another bill eighty years after the Civil War intended to increase access to care for racial and ethnic minorities. One of the first major attempts by the federal government to prohibit discrimination in health care based on race, color, national origin, or creed was achieved by President Harry Truman when he signed into law the Hospital Survey and Construction Act on August 13, 1946. The Hill-Burton Act, as it is commonly referred to, provided federal aid to the states to establish or modernize hospitals and other health facilities that had deteriorated during the Great Depression and World War II.

The law was designed to reduce inequities in access to hospital care and ensured that the poorer states would receive more federal aid. The statute included a Community Service Assurance provision, requiring facilities to provide services to residents of their area without discrimination on the basis of race, national origin, or creed, but this did not mean hospitals were required to integrate. They could still segregate patients by race, but they could not deny treatment or services based on race or provide lower quality care because of race. Prior to this law many minorities, including Juliette Derricotte, were denied care and treatment at segregated hospitals across the United States. After the enactment of this law, health care conditions markedly improved. However, there were still numerous stories of minorities not only being prevented from gaining access to care, but dying because of segregated care.

As the civil rights movement gained steam in the 1950s, advocates were convinced that the federal doctrine of "separate but equal," as espoused in the 1896 case *Plessy v. Ferguson*, was unconstitutional, that it was resulting in the provision of inferior care, and was a major reason for the lower health status of minorities. Most of the legal challenges to this federal doctrine initially focused on education, and then widened to include public transportation, housing, health care, and employment. Ten years after the enactment of the Hill-Burton Act, the NAACP in 1956 challenged its separate-but-equal provision in *Eaton v. Board of Managers of the James Walker Memorial Hospital* but lost their case at the district and appellate level.[17] Undeterred, the NAACP filed another case six years later, *Simkins v. Moses H. Cone Memorial Hospital,* challenging the separate-but-equal doctrine when an African American dentist was denied privileges at a hospital that admitted African American patients and received Hill-Burton Act funding. Again, the NAACP lost its case at the district level, but this time it won at the appellate level, which meant that hospitals could no longer segregate patients or deny minorities admission to hospitals that had received Hill-Burton Act funding. In both instances, the US Supreme Court declined to review the cases or grant certiorari.

Strengthening the Prohibition against Discrimination in Health Care: The Civil Rights Act of 1964

Under the *Simkins* holding, hospitals that did not receive Hill-Burton Act funding could still legally discriminate or voluntarily desegregate. This changed when Congress passed and President Lyndon B. Johnson enacted the Civil Rights Act of 1964, which prohibited excluding, denying benefits, or discriminating against individuals based on race, color or national origin under any program or activity receiving federal funding. The Civil Rights Act of 1964 provided a general prohibition against discrimination based on race, color, or national origin unlike the Hill-Burton Act, which conditioned compliance of its antidiscrimination provision on whether one accepted funds authorized under that statute.

Decades earlier, Congress had attempted to prohibit discrimination in public accommodations by passing the Civil Rights Act of 1875, which was signed into law by President Ulysses S. Grant.[18] However, the Supreme Court overwhelmingly ruled that the law was unconstitutional a few years later holding, "On the whole, we are of opinion that no countenance of authority for the passage of the law in question can be found in either the Thirteenth or Fourteenth Amendment of the Constitution; and no other ground of authority for its passage being suggested, it must necessarily be declared void, at least so far as its operation in the several States is concerned." The Court held this opinion on the grounds that the Civil Rights Act of 1875 did not counteract or provide redress specifically against state laws but interfered in private interactions among citizens.[19]

Upon closer examination, there are clear parallels between the Civil Rights Act of 1964 and the 1875 civil rights statute that was overturned in 1883. Civil rights advocates in the 1960s actually incorporated provisions from the 1875 statute into the 1964 statute. Although advocates were more than likely shocked, bitterly disappointed, and disheartened by the Supreme Court's decision in 1883, they nevertheless persevered and pushed for policies that would require equal treatment in public accommodations even though their efforts took almost a hundred years to materialize.

The Civil Rights Act of 1964 made great strides in increasing minorities' access to health services; however, many hospitals resisted integration and used various tactics to avoid complying with the law. It was not until the advent of Medicare and Medicaid, which conditioned receipt of payments on whether a hospital desegregated, that hospitals realized the federal government was serious about integrating health care facilities. As a result, "within a few months, hospitals across the United States integrated their medical staffs, waiting rooms, and patient floors."[20] Most hospitals could not afford to lose Medicare payments since many major private health insurance plans refused to pay for services to adults sixty-five years and older. As the nation moves beyond the fiftieth anniversary of the Civil Rights Act of 1964 and the Medicare and Medicaid law, there is much to celebrate. The laws were a significant achievement, aimed at stamping out overt forms of discrimination; however, more subtle forms of discrimination and striking disparities persisted, and policies were needed to address those as well.

Paving the Way for Direct Federal Action
to Improve Minority Health

The 1960s and 1970s saw a remarkable change in attitude and policy from the federal government relative to the minority health crisis. The Congressional Black Caucus (CBC) was founded in 1971 by thirteen members of Congress.[21] Although there was one African American serving in the Senate, Edward Brooke, a Republican, he declined to join the CBC, stating that he could not serve just the African American cause, he had to serve all people in Massachusetts. The purpose of this new congressional caucus was to advance a civil rights agenda primarily through legislation in the House and promote economic, educational, and social issues that were important to African Americans. The CBC saw itself as the conscience of the Congress and the voice for minority and vulnerable communities. Its members understood that collectively they could accomplish so much more to "empower America's neglected citizens and to address their legislative concerns." Early on, the CBC adopted as their motto Congressman William Clay's (D-MO) perspective, "Black people have no permanent friends, no permanent enemies . . . just permanent interests."[22]

Two events led to the CBC's success early on. The first involved a major clash with President Nixon, who had repeatedly refused to meet with black members of Congress. This resulted in a widely publicized boycott of one of the president's State of the Union addresses and later led to an invitation to visit the White House to discuss various policy issues impacting the African American community.[23] The second instance dealt with intraparty politics and the lack of racial and ethnic diversity in leadership positions within the Democratic Party, which controlled the House and the Senate at the time. Although most of the CBC members were relatively new to Congress, they took issue with the seniority preference for committee leadership positions. It was not until they demanded that the Speaker increase the racial diversity of House committee appointments that their power and influence started to increase.

Even though the Supreme Court had banned segregation in public places such as hospitals and Congress had passed bills prohibiting discrimination against minorities and others in health care facilities, the Congressional Black Caucus soon realized that these laws alone would not completely address the minority health crisis. Policies were needed to bolster the diversity and cultural competence of the health professions and to increase access to health services for underserved communities. Consequently,

Congress authorized two critical programs: the Health Careers Opportunity Program and the Area Health Education Centers to encourage individuals from educationally or economically disadvantaged backgrounds to enter the health care professions.

Over time the CBC established various task forces and brain trusts to examine public policy issues impacting the African American community. Congressman Parren Mitchell (D-MD), who was one of the thirteen founding members of the CBC, was instrumental in developing a strategic agenda and increasing the CBC's clout. He served as chair of the caucus during the Ninety-Fifth Congress from 1977 to 1979. When he was chair, the CBC had established several brain trusts focused on housing, economic development, and other issues impacting African Americans.[24] Mitchell recognized, however, that the CBC also needed to establish a health brain trust to help the caucus navigate the complex health care and public health issues affecting African Americans. So he asked Congressman Louis Stokes (D-OH) to create and lead one in 1978.

Stokes, who had earlier served two consecutive terms as chair of the CBC when it was founded, played a significant role in shaping this caucus and its success. In 1971, Stokes successfully secured a seat on the powerful House Appropriations Committee and became the first African American during that time to gain a seat there. Because of his long tenure on the Appropriations Committee, he became known as one of its "cardinals." He later became chair of one of its Subcommittees for Veterans, HUD, and Independent Agencies—which at that time controlled more than $90 billion annually in federal funding. Using his influence on the Appropriations Committee, Stokes championed increasing health care access to all Americans, increasing the health status for minorities, and appropriately addressing chronic diseases that disproportionately impacted communities of color.

Mitchell and other leaders in the CBC believed that each member's expertise and strengths should be leveraged for the benefit of the caucus. As a result, Mitchell believed that Stokes would be able to pull together all the major leaders and experts in minority health, particularly African American health, and create a national network that would serve a tripartite purpose: provide sound advice and relevant information to the CBC so it could use this to develop appropriate legislation addressing issues affecting minorities, help determine the potential impact of bills on African Americans, and help the caucus advance its legislative priorities by mobilizing an extensive grassroots network around the country.

All of Stokes's experiences and advocacy to date convinced Mitchell that he was the most qualified to lead this effort and with the inclusion of Representatives Ronald Dellums (D-CA), who was a huge supporter of universal health; Harold Ford Sr. (D-TN) and Charles Rangel (D-NY), who were on the powerful Ways and Means Committee; and Mickey Leland (D-TX), a pharmacist who championed health care rights for communities of lower socioeconomic status and served on the Energy and Commerce Committee; the new Health Braintrust helped the CBC make tremendous gains in health policy.[25]

Once established, the CBC Health Braintrust held four major meetings a year and included more than six hundred experts in minority health from across the country at each meeting, including medical doctors, dentists, lawyers, nurses, social workers, psychologists, public health professionals, scientists, therapists, counselors, and other health policy experts. Stokes made it a priority to invite individuals from the federal agencies that were running various programs of interest to African Americans and other minority groups to come and present. He also recognized that he could not elevate minority health alone, and he invited Senator Edward Kennedy to join him in this effort. Kennedy graciously accepted his invitation to present at one of the CBC Health Braintrust meetings, and in 1979 Senator Kennedy decided to hold a hearing on minority health and health disparities in the Senate focused on the need to increase the diversity of the health care workforce.[26] This was the first time that the Senate had held a hearing on the issue in collaboration with the CBC Health Braintrust, helping to propel this issue further as a concern.

Congressman Dellums, who had been tasked with chairing a task force to examine issues across the country that were impacting black communities also recognized that the scope of the CBC's efforts was becoming overwhelming for the fledgling caucus, since it had neither the personnel nor the resources to tackle all of the issues it took on. He strongly believed that the CBC, to have the most impact and further its mission, needed to exert its influence and enable members to secure seats on key committees in Congress.

When legislation was introduced in the Appropriations Committee, Stokes and his staff would pull experts through the CBC Health Braintrust from all over the country to put pressure on congressional members either to support it or obstruct it.[27] Participants in the CBC Health Braintrust lived in Atlanta, Baltimore, Chicago, Cleveland, DC, Detroit, Los Angeles, St. Louis, and other cities. They were scattered across the United States and volunteered their time—often working through the weekends and formulating amendments and other responses to proposed legislation, hearings, and votes. Stokes also was a shrewd negotiator and developed a reputation as a fierce questioner. Every National Institutes of Health (NIH) director and other Health and Human Services (HHS) officials had to come before him to testify when he was on the Appropriations Committee. He queried each of them every time, "What are you doing in terms of minority health?" If they responded that they were doing something, he would ask, "Why aren't you doing more?" Each NIH director and HHS official dreaded having to answer these questions, but Stokes intentionally asked these questions to remind them that this was an important issue that they needed to pay close attention to.

In addition to the gains that were made in Congress by racial and ethnic minorities, the White House was also intentionally increasing the diversity of its cabinet and other senior officials. In the late 1970s, President Jimmy Carter, who had close ties with the Congressional Black Caucus appointed the first African American secretary of health and human services, Patricia Roberts Harris, who was a legal scholar, leader, and advocate for underserved and disenfranchised communities. Between 1977 and 1979 she had served as secretary of housing and urban development before being appointed to her highest cabinet post as secretary of health, education, and welfare (the department was renamed Health and Human Services during her tenure).

She was the first African American woman to serve in the US cabinet and was instrumental in protecting social programs during her tenure. Harris staunchly supported prevention and public health initiatives, including childhood immunizations, tobacco prevention, breast feeding, breast cancer screenings, and other critical women's health issues. She was also a champion for minority health and used her tenacity and fierce negotiating skills to persuade members of Congress to increase funding for her department's priorities during a period of austerity and budget cutting. Overall, Harris, enjoyed relatively good relations with the CBC, and Congressman Stokes ensured that her departments received adequate funding for her minority health projects. Together with the new CBC Health Braintrust, Secretary Harris was instrumental in substantially elevating minority health at the federal level.

Five years after the CBC was established, the Congressional Hispanic Caucus (CHC) was founded in December 1976 by five Latino congressmen.[28] As the first chair of the CHC, Congressman Edward R. Roybal

(D-CA) led the new caucus, whose purpose was to address domestic and international issues and policies impacting Latinos and collectively develop a legislative agenda to tackle these issues and policy gaps. Unlike the CBC, the CHC initially operated as a legislative service organization of the US House of Representatives. This allowed it to receive a House account from which it could draw funds to pay staff and purchase supplies as well as have an office space in a congressional building. It was reorganized, however, as a congressional member organization soon after Republicans won the elections in 1994. They believed strongly that no taxpayer money should be funding these specially designated caucuses. It was not until 1981 that the CBC itself achieved the status of legislative service organization, but it also had to end this designation in 1995. Today the CHC functions as a forum for congressional members to coalesce around a collective legislative agenda and monitor more closely judicial and executive branch actions on their priority issues. Interestingly, both the CBC and the CHC have had members from both parties over the years, but in 2003 five Republican members of the CHC decided to establish their own caucus, the Congressional Hispanic Conference. Today both Hispanic caucuses continue to operate along party lines.

During Congressman Stokes's time as chair of the CBC Health Braintrust, which ended in 1999, the CBC and CHC generally worked independently of each other. It took some time before they started working closely on crosscutting priorities. This was not because there were any real problems between them. It was more a case of each caucus trying to establish its own identity first. During the late 1990s, the CBC Health Braintrust and the Congressional Hispanic Caucus Health Task Force along with the Congressional Asian Pacific American Caucus (CAPAC), which was established a few years before in 1994, began to share ideas, information, and strategies around educational, economic, health, housing, transportation, and civil rights issues affecting their mutual constituents.[29]

Congresswoman Eddie Bernice Johnson (D-TX), who chaired the Congressional Black Caucus from 2001 to 2003 during the 107th Congress, in conjunction with Congressman Sylvestre Reyes (D-TX), who chaired the Congressional Hispanic Caucus, and Congressman David Wu of Oregon, who chaired the Congressional Asian Pacific American Caucus, were instrumental in getting their independent caucuses to coalesce and collaborate as a united Tri-Caucus.[30] Each chair recognized the critical health policy issues impacting their respective communities and acknowledged that they could be so much more effective if they worked together to address them legislatively. As a result, for the first time, each caucus's health task force or brain trust started sharing information and strategizing about how best to move forward with one voice. With the increased number of racial and ethnic minority policy makers at the federal level demanding that more attention be paid to the minority health and health disparities crisis, there were more targeted policy efforts to address this problem.

The Birth of a New Movement: From Minority Health and Health Disparities to Health Equity

Health care is the civil rights issue of the twenty-first century.—*Congresswoman Donna M. Christensen*

After the civil rights movement, which was instrumental in quashing overt racism and discrimination in health care, a new movement arose focused on addressing the more subtle forms of inequities in health care. Thus began the health equity movement to ensure the development and implementation of laws, policies, and programs focused on achieving health equity and reducing disparities in health and behavioral health (which entails mental health and substance use) status and care. The movement also sought to cultivate and sustain a robust health equity leadership and advocacy enterprise and strengthen the evidence base for informing health laws and policies. These health equity advocates realized that addressing the multifaceted health and behavioral health needs of the US population is a complex issue that warranted attention from researchers, scientists, health care providers, behavioral health professionals, public health professionals, and policy makers. These stakeholders collectively offered unique perspectives and strategies to improve the health status and access to effective health services of vulnerable and increasingly diverse populations.

Although much had been done legislatively, administratively, and judicially to advance minority health and end blatant discrimination, it was not until the early 1980s that the federal government began to more directly address the issue of racial and ethnic health disparities. Reports from external groups, including the Institute of Medicine (IOM), now known as the National Academy of Medicine, and the Association of Minority Health Professions Schools highlighted the terrible impact that disparities in health care and lack of diversity among health care providers were having on racial and ethnic minority populations.[31] Dr. Louis Sullivan, founding dean and president of Morehouse School of Medicine; Dr. David Satcher, president of Meharry Medical College; Dr. Walter Bowie, dean of Tuskegee

University; and Dr. M. Alfred Haynes, dean of Charles R. Drew University of Medicine and Science, shared the findings from the AMHPS report with Margaret Heckler, who was the secretary of health and human services under the Reagan administration.

Congressman Louis Stokes, who had worked with Secretary Heckler when she was a representative in the House, continued to work with Heckler in her new capacity and urged her to address the minority health crisis. Together, Stokes, Sullivan, Haynes, and Satcher hoped that she would do something about it, which she did. Heckler, who was sensitive to this issue, realized that, while the overall health of the nation had steadily improved over the last several decades, the health status of African Americans, Latinos, Asian Americans, and American Indians was alarming. She recognized that substantial health disparities remained for these racial and ethnic groups and decided to investigate further.

Consequently, in April 1984 Secretary Heckler established the Task Force on Black and Minority Health to address this issue, which at that time was a brave act—one that was politically unpopular at the time and put her job at risk. Even her own staff tried to dissuade her from doing anything about the minority health gap issue. Health disparities issues made many policy makers uncomfortable. For years, minority health advocates had urged the government to address this issue in a comprehensive and thoughtful manner, but these pleas often fell on deaf ears because of the lack of research on health disparities. Health equity advocates needed to obtain accurate and appropriate data to establish the extent and root causes of health disparities. As a result, they urged the secretary to continue pushing forward with a comprehensive examination of this issue.

Ignoring political pressure, in 1985 Secretary Heckler's task force released the groundbreaking *Report of the Secretary's Task Force on Black and Minority Health*, which documented the existence of disparities in key health indicators for minorities. Although there were earlier publications underscoring minority health issues by African American leaders such as W. E. B. Du Bois in 1906 and Booker T. Washington in 1914, this was the first federal government report comprehensively examining the issue and calling for action. The *Heckler Report* affirmed what previous external reports had concluded. It analyzed existing health status information and national mortality data, and found that sixty thousand excess deaths occurred each year in minority populations.

The task force noted in the report, "It was evident that to bring the health of minorities to the level of all Americans, efforts of monumental proportions were needed."[32] As a result, it made several recommendations to the secretary, including an outreach campaign for minority populations, increasing patient education, bringing health professionals to minority communities, and improving communication and coordination among federal agencies. In 1986 as a result of the report, the Office of Minority Health (OMH) was created in the Department of Health and Human Services, but by that time Heckler had assumed a new position as ambassador to Ireland and never got to direct the implementation of the OMH.

Realizing the rare opportunity that the *Heckler Report* presented for legislative fixes to the minority health crisis and the health disparities problem, health equity champions in Congress and outside of Congress were determined to develop appropriate legislation. This was easier said than done and took tremendous time and effort. In fact, it took four years to convince lawmakers in the Senate and five years to convince lawmakers in the House to convene hearings on the health status of minorities and the disparities in health across racial and ethnic groups. Congressman Stokes and other Tri-Caucus leaders were concerned that although HHS had established an Office of Minority Health and had implemented some of the recommendations in the report, unless they were codified into law, they could easily be dismantled.

Working closely with the Bush administration, in particular, Dr. Louis Sullivan, who had recently become the secretary of health and human services, congressional members developed a bill titled Disadvantaged Minority Health Improvement Act of 1990, which was a direct result of Secretary Heckler's efforts. Stokes and others realized that if the OMH was going to endure, it had to be authorized and given enough funding to do its job. In 1986 Congressman Ed Towns (D-NY) and other members of the Tri-Caucus introduced a bill that was the precursor to the Disadvantaged Minority Health Improvement Act of 1990. In 1987, Senator Arlen Specter introduced a bill that was intended to congressionally authorize the OMH, and he introduced the bill again in the following Congress in 1989.

In 1988, Congressman Stokes, working closely with Senator Kennedy, introduced companion bills in their respective houses titled Disadvantaged Minority Health Improvement Act of 1990, on September 11, 1989, and September 12, 1989, respectively. Senator Kennedy, as chair of the Labor and Human Resources Committee, held the first hearing on the bill on September 11, 1989, the same day Stokes formally introduced his bill. The Senate committee invited Secretary Louis Sullivan, Congressman Louis

Stokes, Congressman Bill Richardson (D-NM), Dr. Herbert Nickens of the Association of American Medical Colleges, and Dr. Jane Delgado of the National Coalition of Hispanic Health and Human Services Organizations to present. Congressman Jaime B. Fuster (D-PR), who was chair of the Congressional Hispanic Caucus at that time, sent a letter urging Senator Kennedy to continue to use his influence to address this issue.

Almost a year after the Senate hearing on the bill, the House Energy and Commerce's Subcommittee on Health and the Environment, which was chaired by Congressman Henry Waxman (D-CA), convened a hearing June 8, 1990. Tensions were high at this hearing and Waxman was upset that, five years after the *Heckler Report*, no strategy had been developed to sustain and strengthen the OMH. The CHC was upset that Latinos were underrepresented in federal programs designed to increase the diversity of the health care workforce since the majority of funding at that time was being targeted to African American communities. The CHC, while supportive of the Stokes bill, pushed for support of a stand-alone bill on Hispanic health parity, while CBC and congressional Asian and Pacific Islander American members were urging support for a larger and more inclusive bill. During the House hearing, Congressman Stokes stated:

> I will just close saying this, that the legislation which I have introduced in the House, as you know, has been sponsored in the Senate by Senator Ted Kennedy. On the Senate side, they have passed this legislation. We are now awaiting action in the House. They are ready to go to conference if and when the House takes some substantive action. I have great confidence in you and the members of this subcommittee. I have worked closely with Mr. Rowland; I have worked with Mr. Towns; I have worked with Mr. Richardson on matters related to that for which we are here today, and I have great confidence that this committee is going to do what is right in terms of this legislation.[33]

The Disadvantaged Minority Health Improvement Act of 1990 had three primary objectives: increase support for health promotion and disease activities designed to reduce the occurrence of illnesses prevalent among minorities, authorize the Office of Minority Health with the funding and authority commensurate with its responsibility and mandate, and establish scholarships and loans to increase the supply of minority health professionals in the United States. During his testimony, Congressman Stokes elaborated on the tripartite objectives:

The health promotion and disease prevention aspects of the bill were designed to ameliorate many of the risk factors for the excessive causes of death among minorities—many of which are preventable or potentially modifiable through behavior. The increased funding for the Office of Minority Health would enable it to implement a comprehensive and integrated Federal approach to minority health problems. This office was established in 1986 to do just that, and those who have directed this office must be applauded for the outstanding job done thus far. However, it has not been authorized in statute and is poorly funded. Thus, the efforts of our Nation to deal with the problems have been woefully constrained. Let me point out that my own State of Ohio has an Office of Minority Health with the same level of funding as the HHS office which serves the entire Nation. Funding for minority students to pursue careers in the health professions and thus accelerate the rate of participation of minorities in the health field is a further provision of this bill. This stipulation directly addresses the Secretary's Task Force report which found that minorities are grossly underrepresented in the health professions, and that we are in need of more minority health professionals to help combat the health crisis facing minorities. H.R. 3240 also includes a loan repayment program that would increase the number of minority health faculty and researchers at health professions institutions. *This legislation is by no means a totally comprehensive solution to the problem.* The Disadvantaged Minority Health Improvement Act is a first step in raising the level of national commitment to improving health care for the minority community, and all Americans. It is clear that we cannot afford to neglect the development and expansion of unified strategies to meet this health crisis.[34]

Three months after the House hearing on this bill, a bipartisan group of members in both the House and Senate continued discussions and decided to craft a new bill that they thought would be easier to pass in Congress—one that addressed not only minority health but the health of individuals of lower socioeconomic status as well. Interestingly, just like the Freedmen's Bureau legislation, Congress could not garner the support that was needed to pass a bill intended to solely address minority health issues. Instead, the framers of this law had to include disadvantaged nonminority populations in order to gain support for its passage. On September 24, 1990, a new bill with the same title was introduced in the House (H.R. 5702). This bill was fast-tracked in both the House and Senate. On October 10, 1990, the House passed the new bill, and, almost one week later, the Senate passed it by unanimous consent on October 16,

1990. After passage of H.R. 5702, Senator Kennedy gave the following remarks:

> This legislation addresses a growing crisis in the health status of disadvantaged minorities. H.R. 5702 is the successor to S. 1606, the Disadvantaged Minority Health Improvement Act of 1989, which passed the Senate last November. The House companion bill to S. 1606, H.R. 3240, was introduced by Congressman Stokes, a leader on minority health issues. The new bill has been crafted through bipartisan discussions among members of the relevant House and Senate committees and the administration. Representatives Waxman, Stokes, and Madigan have been diligent in pursuing legislation to improve the health of disadvantaged minorities, and should also be commended. I especially want to thank Members of the Senate, particularly those who cosponsored S. 1606 and participated in developing some of the programs in H.R. 5702, including Senators Inouye, Hatch, Metzenbaum, Dodd, Simon, and Specter.[35]

Three weeks after H.R. 5702 was successfully passed by Congress, the White House agreed to sign it into law on November 6, 1990, on the urging of health equity champions in the Bush administration, including Dr. Louis Sullivan, who was appointed secretary of health and human services—the second African American to hold this post.

Substantive Federal Investments in Minority Health

Further strides in the government's involvement in minority health took place in the 1990s. The limited research funded by the government or private philanthropy initially focused on examining minority health, but then it shifted to acknowledging the existence of a gap between the health of whites and minorities and finally to an interest in closing that gap. Clear evidence of disparities was found everywhere: in access to health care, treatments, and health outcomes, as well as in government programs such as Medicare and Medicaid. Secretary Sullivan believed that health disparities was a serious issue that deserved more attention—more research to determine the root causes and develop culturally appropriate interventions.

Under the Bush administration, in 1990, there were significant advancements and investments in the health equity movement. The Office of Research on Minority Health was established by the NIH, evolving from the Office of Minority Programs.[36] Unlike the Office of Minority Health at HHS, which focused on policy and programs, the Office of Minority

Minority Health Policy Timeline

Major laws related to health care reform appear in bold.

PRE-20th CENTURY

1865 - The Freedmen's Bureau Act was signed into law.

1869 - Congress failed to reauthorize Freedmen's Bureau.

1872 - Freedmen's Bureau officially closed.

1875 - Civil Rights Act of 1875 was signed into law.

1883 - Civil Rights Act of 1875 ruled unconstitutional by the US Supreme Court.

1896 - *Plessy v. Ferguson* decided by the US Supreme Court promoting separate-but-equal doctrine.

1910s

1915 - National Negro Health Week established.

1930s

1932 - USPHS opened the Office of Negro Health Work.

1940s

1946 - President Harry S. Truman signed the Hospital Survey and Construction Act, also referred to as the Hill-Burton Act.

1950s

1956 - *Eaton v. Board of Managers of the James Walker Memorial Hospital* initiated by NAACP to challenge the separate-but-equal doctrine supported by the Hill-Burton Act.

1960s

1962 - *Simkins v. Moses H. Cone Memorial Hospital* initiated by the NAACP to challenge the separate-but-equal doctrine in health care privileges.

1964 - Civil Rights Act of 1964 signed into law.

1970s

1971 - Congressional Black Caucus established.

1976 - Congressional Hispanic Caucus established.

1978 - Congressional Black Caucus Health Braintrust established.

1979 - First *Hearing on Minority Health* held in the United States Senate by Sen. Edward Kennedy.

1979 - Patricia Roberts Harris appointed first African American US Secretary of Health, Education, and Welfare.

1980s

1983 - External groups presented reports on minority health and health disparities to Secretary Margaret Heckler.

1983 - Secretary Heckler realized significant gaps in minority health.

1984 - Secretary Heckler established the Task Force on Black and Minority Health.

1985 - The Emergency Medical Treatment and Active Labor Act was signed into law.

1985 - Secretary's Task Force on Black and Minority Health released landmark *Report of the Secretary's Task Force on Black and Minority Health*.

1986 - Office of Minority Health created at HHS.

1989 - Minority Health Bill introduced by Rep. Louis Stokes and Sen. Ted Kennedy.

1990s

1990 - *Healthy People 2000* released prioritizing "reduction of health disparities."

1990 - Congress passed the Disadvantaged Minority Health Improvement Act of 1990 and appropriated $1 million to support health disparities research the following year.

1990 - The Office of Research on Minority Health was established.

1991 - Congress appropriated $1 million to support health disparities research.

1992 - The Minority Health Initiative was launched and allocated $45 million for programs geared to addressing health disparities.

1994 - Congressional Asian Pacific American Caucus established.

1998 - Minority HIV/AIDS Initiative began with $156 million in funding from Congress.

1999 - The REACH program was created at the Centers for Disease Control and Prevention.

2000s

2000 - *Healthy People 2010* released prioritizing "elimination of health disparities."

2000 - Congress passed the Minority Health and Health Disparities Research & Education Act.

2001 - Institute of Medicine released report *Crossing the Quality*

Minority Health Policy Timeline

Chasm: A New Health System for the 21st Century.

2001 - Surgeon General released major report titled *Mental Health: Culture, Race and Ethnicity.*

2002 - IOM released report titled *Unequal Treatment: Confronting Racial and Ethnic Disparities in Health Care.*

2003 - AHRQ released the first *National Healthcare Disparities Report.*

2003 - The NIH *Strategic Research Plan and Budget to Reduce and Ultimately Eliminate Health Disparities* was issued.

2009 - President Barack Obama signed the American Recovery and Reinvestment Act.

2009 - National Working Group on Health Disparities and Health Reform.

2009 - President Obama and the Tri-Caucus declared support for addressing health disparities in a comprehensive health reform package.

2009 - The Joint Center released landmark report titled *The Economic Burden of Health Disparities in the United States.*

2010s

2010 - President Obama signed the Patient Protection and Affordable Care Act (ACA) into law, the first comprehensive health reform enacted into law.

2010 - *Healthy People 2020* released prioritizing achievement of health equity, elimination of

disparities, and improvement in the health of all groups.

2015 - President Obama signed into law the Medicare Access and CHIP Reauthorization Act, which extended many of the health reform programs from the ACA and expanded delivery and payment reforms.

Programs at NIH focused on bolstering health disparities research. The Ryan White Comprehensive AIDS Resources Emergency Act was enacted in 1990, and it was the single largest federal safety net program specifically for people with HIV/AIDS.[37] The following year, Congress authorized its first significant investment of $1 million to support health disparities research at the Centers for Disease Control and Prevention, and in 1992 the NIH established the Minority Health Initiative with the largest investment ever made by the federal government to address health disparities, $45 million. The same year, the CDC established its own Office of Minority Health, and the Advisory Committee on Research on Minority Health was established to provide advice and recommendations to the directors of ORMH and NIH on research and training relative to minority health.

For the first time ever, federal policy included as one of its key priorities the reduction of health disparities in the nation's public health agenda, in its HHS report, *Healthy People 2000*.[38] Healthy People is a federal initiative charged with tracking the health of the nation over the subsequent ten years and employing strategies to tackle the nation's most pressing public health problems. *Healthy People 2000* recognized that to improve the health of the nation it was necessary to address the problem of health disparities. Subsequent administrations, including the Clinton and Obama administrations, would go even further.

When health reform negotiations moved forward in 1993 under the Clinton administration, so did the introduction of bills targeting minority health and health disparities. However, when Clinton's health reform negotiations ceased during his first term, so did the introduction of bills addressing minority health and health disparities. After Clinton's reelection and the election of dedicated health equity champions such as Congresswoman Donna M. Christensen, the first female physician elected to Congress, there was a sharp rise in the introduction of health equity-focused bills.

Four years after enactment of the Disadvantaged Minority Health Improvement Act of 1990 and twenty-three years after the CBC was established, the Congressional Asian Pacific American Caucus was founded in 1994 to ensure that the public policy needs of Asian Americans and Pacific Islanders were properly addressed by the federal government. Former congressman Norman Y. Mineta (D-CA) helped to found this youngest of the three racial and ethnic congressional caucuses in the Tri-Caucus and was its first chair.[39] Unlike the CBC and CHC, however, the CAPAC has

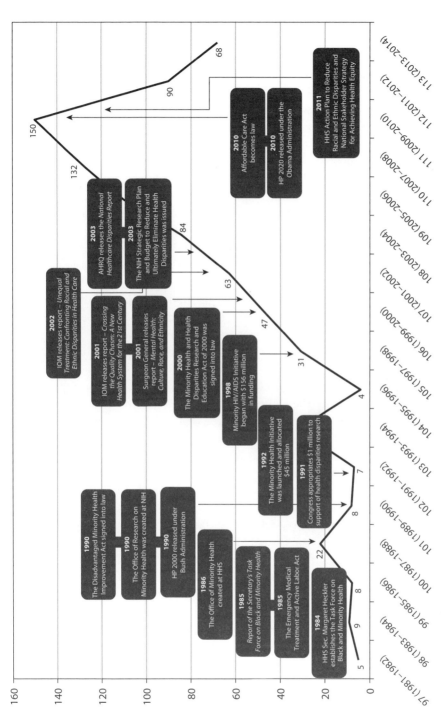

Figure 2.1. The incidence of bills introduced in Congress involving minority health and corresponding significant health policy milestones advancing a health equity agenda

always operated as a bicameral group, due largely in part to the participation of former Democratic senators Daniel Inouye and Daniel Akaka of Hawaii.

Senator Inouye ensured that appropriations legislation funded critical health equity programs, especially while leading the Senate Appropriations Committee from 2009 to 2012. Under his leadership as chair of the appropriations committee, health equity programs all received significant increases in funding. In fact, these programs were funded at higher levels than in previous years. These included Health Careers Opportunity Program (HCOP) and Area Health Education Centers (AHEC), which were designed to increase diversity in the health professions and the Office of Minority Health, as well as the Minority Fellowship Program, Indians into Psychology, and the Racial and Ethnic Approaches to Community Health (REACH) program. Senator Akaka also used his influence as a leader on authorizing committees to ensure that legislation prioritized health equity, and he sponsored the comprehensive health equity bill in the Senate several times. CAPAC's establishment and collaboration with the CBC and CHC certainly helped to bolster legislation addressing minority health and health disparities issues.

CAPAC is charged with the five following actions: (1) ensuring that legislation passed by the United States Congress, to the greatest extent possible, provides for the full participation of Asian Americans and Pacific Islanders and reflects the concerns and needs of the Asian American and Pacific Islander communities; (2) educating other members of Congress about the history, contributions, and concerns of Asian Americans and Pacific Islanders; (3) protecting and advancing the civil and constitutional rights of all Americans; (4) establishing policies relating to persons of Asian or Pacific Islands ancestry who are citizens or nationals of, residents of, or immigrants to, the United States, its territories, and possessions; and (5) providing a structure to coordinate the efforts, and enhance the ability, of the Asian American and Pacific Islander members of Congress to accomplish those goals.

Separate and Unequal Standards for Minorities

In early 1998, Secretary of Health and Human Services Donna Shalala and Dr. David Satcher, who was recently appointed US surgeon general, held a press briefing to unveil new initiatives to eliminate health disparities, which were part of the President's Initiative on Race at the time. They discussed the Clinton administration's intention to eliminate racial

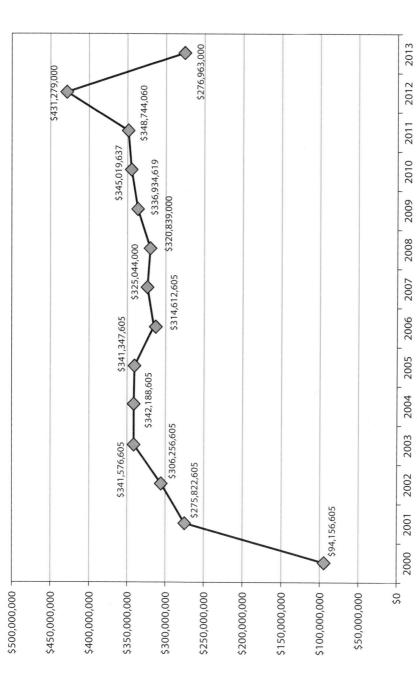

Figure 2.2. Total appropriations for selected health equity programs. Figures obtained from the US Department of Health and Human Services, Government Accountability Office, Office of Management and Budget, and the United States Statutes at Large for the following programs: AHEC, HCOP, NIMHD, OMH, and REACH.

and ethnic health disparities by the year 2010, which meant that for "the first time in its history the federal government will set universal national health goals, ending the practice of setting separate, lower goals for minority communities." According to Secretary Shalala, in the past when the federal government set certain health goals, it "had one set of goals for the racial and ethnic communities in the United States and another set of goals for the rest of the country."[40]

Shalala was referring to the federal government's *Healthy People 2000* report, which created "specific targets to narrow the gap between the total population and those population groups that now experience above average incidences of death, disease, and disability."[41] For example, although the goal for overall infant mortality was no more than 7 deaths per 1,000 live births, the goal for African Americans was 11 per 1,000 live births, for Native Americans 8.5 per 1,000 live births, and for Latinos 8 per 1,000 live births.[42] Proponents argued that because minorities were so far behind in health status compared to the rest of the population, this separate standard was necessary to help them catch up in a relatively reasonable time. Opponents, however, were troubled by this separate and unequal standard. The Clinton administration believed this double standard was unconscionable and decided to end the disparate health goals for each group. Under Surgeon General David Satcher's tireless leadership, the White House was convinced that no separate or lower goals should be set for different population groups unless clinical evidence warranted it.

Like health equity leaders before him, Dr. Satcher used every opportunity to address inequities in health status and health care in public policy. He led the Clinton administration's efforts in 1998 to address racial and ethnic health disparities and launched the national Racial and Ethnic Health Disparities Initiative. He boldly moved the policy discussion from reducing to eliminating health disparities as a national goal in *Healthy People 2010*. Later on the Obama administration would go on to raise the bar even higher, including as a key priority in the *Healthy People 2020* agenda not only the elimination of health disparities but the achievement of health equity and the improvement of health for all communities.

After deciding that something must be done, the Clinton administration elected to develop one set of goals and focus on eliminating health disparities in six specific areas: infant mortality, cancer screening and management, cardiovascular disease, diabetes, HIV/AIDS infection rates, and child and adult immunizations. Working with Grantmakers in Health, a major membership organization of leading foundations, Surgeon General

Satcher was charged with conducting a nationwide campaign to spread the word and organize the country to reduce disparities in all of these six areas. He communicated with and listened to communities throughout this country, identified successful models that could be scaled, and developed and implemented evidence-based strategies to reach vulnerable communities. While this effort was taking place, in October 1998, the White House, the US Department of Health and Human Services, the Congressional Black Caucus, including leaders such as Congresswoman Maxine Waters and Congressman Donald Payne, and the Congressional Hispanic Caucus announced the launch of initiatives that would be geared at reducing the impact of HIV/AIDS on racial and ethnic minorities—the Minority HIV/AIDS Initiative.

Like Secretary Heckler before her, Secretary Shalala established a task force to monitor the Clinton administration's progress in eliminating disparities in the six areas. This was another major breakthrough for health equity champions and a significant undertaking for the Clinton administration, which wanted a measurable set of goals to improve the health of minorities. The administration intended to report its progress each year. In addition to the Clinton administration's efforts to eliminate health disparities in the late 1990s, Congress passed the Health Professions Education Partnerships Act of 1998, P.L. 105-392, as amended by the Minority Health and Health Disparities Research and Education Act of 2000, P.L. 106-525, which mandated the establishment of the HHS Office of Minority Health's Advisory Committee on Minority Health.[43]

Further Strides in the New Millennium

In 2000, there was a substantial increase in the attention paid to health disparities by scientists, health services researchers, health professionals, public health experts, and the government. During the previous decade, despite the increased legitimization of health disparities as a public health concern, very few legislative or regulatory proposals were introduced directly addressing them, and none was ever enacted into law, except for the Disadvantaged Minority Health Improvement Act of 1990, until President Clinton signed into law the Minority Health and Health Disparities Research and Education Act of 2000.[44] This was the second legislation enacted into law by the federal government focusing directly on and strengthening its commitment to health disparities and built upon President Clinton's Racial and Ethnic Health Disparities Initiative.

Interestingly, similar to what transpired after the Reagan administration established a task force on minority health, which produced policy recommendations that Congress acted upon by passing legislation, Congress reacted once again and seized the opportunity to step in and produce legislation to build upon Clinton's disparities initiative. The Minority Health and Health Disparities Research and Education Act of 2000 was explicitly developed to make the elimination of health disparities a higher priority across the country, and it enjoyed significant bipartisan support from Senators Bill Frist (R-TN), Edward Kennedy, Jim Jeffords (R-VT), Christopher Dodd (D-CT), Mike DeWine (R-OH), Barbara Mikulski (D-MD), Mike Enzi, Paul Wellstone (D-MN), Kay Bailey Hutchinson (R-TX), Patty Murray (D-WA), Susan Collins (R-ME), Daniel Akaka, Christopher "Kit" Bond (R-MO), Frank Lautenberg (D-NJ), Orrin Hatch (R-UT), Max Cleland (D-GA), and Jeff Sessions (R-AL).[45]

Its House companion bill, H.R. 3250, was introduced by Representative Bennie Thompson, a Democrat from Mississippi and a member of the CBC, along with eighty-six cosponsors on November 8, 1999. Congressman Robert Underwood (D-GU), chair of the Congressional Asian Pacific American Caucus, and Congresswoman Lucille Roybal-Allard (D-CA), the chair of the Congressional Hispanic Caucus Task Force, at the time played a significant role developing and garnering support for the bill. While the House bill had overwhelming support from Democrats, including Tri-Caucus members, the bill also received bipartisan support from notable Republican congressmen, including Charles Norwood of Georgia, J. C. Watts of Oklahoma, Fred Upton of Michigan, and Ray La-Hood of Illinois. The House held a hearing on H.R. 3250 on May 11, 2000, and heard testimony from members of Congress, the administration, and various associations and advocacy groups that worked in concert to advocate for the passage of this bill, including the National Medical Association, the Association of Black Cardiologists, and universities and colleges across the United States.

However, to pass this bill, health equity champions inside and outside of Congress had to employ a strategy similar to the one used during negotiations over the Bureau of Refugees, Freedmen and Abandoned Lands legislation, and the Disadvantaged Minority Health Improvement Act of 1990. Both congressional leaders and some officials in the Clinton administration felt uneasy supporting the Minority Health and Health Disparities Research and Education Act of 2000 if it solely benefitted minority health. So, after intense negotiations, all sides compromised and included language that was beneficial to whites of lower socioeconomic status. Consequently, while the bill focused on improving minority health and eliminating health disparities, it also addressed health disparities in poor white Americans.

The statute elevated the NIH's Office of Research on Minority Health to a center—establishing the National Center on Minority Health and Health Disparities (NCMHD) within the NIH to bring increased national attention to the problem.[46] The NCMHD, which was led by Dr. John Ruffin until 2014, was tasked with increasing investments in minority health and health disparities research and with fostering, coordinating, and assessing the progress of all NIH-sponsored research activities involving minority health and health disparities. Dr. Ruffin, who joined the NIH in 1990, was a driving force for prioritizing health equity research at the NIH. He first directed the Office of Research on Minority Health and then became the first Director of the National Center on Minority Health and Health Disparities in 2001. As a center, the NCMHD was often perceived in an unfavorable light—relegated to an inferior status in the eyes of its sister institutes at the NIH as well as outside individuals or policy makers who were not concerned about issues impacting minority health and health disparities.

The Minority Health and Health Disparities Research and Education Act mandated that the NCMHD establish several programs. The first was a loan repayment program, which would provide funding toward student loan repayment of students entering health disparities research. The program would thus help to attract top minds to the field. The second was the Centers of Excellence program, which would provide funding to universities and institutions to conduct research on enhancing the understanding of health disparities. The third was a research endowment program, which would allow institutions to create or expand their health disparities research and training opportunities in biomedical research.

The Minority Health and Health Disparities Research and Education Act also authorized the Institute of Medicine to create a report highlighting the extent of health disparities across the United States and tasked the Agency for Healthcare Research and Quality (AHRQ) to measure progress on the reduction of disparities and publish a national health care disparities report each year. Although the Healthcare Research and Quality Act of 1999 (P.L. 106-129), had previously directed the AHRQ to develop two annual reports—the *National Healthcare Quality Report* (*NHQR*) and the *National Healthcare Disparities Report*—one year later, lawmakers amended that section of the law when it passed the Minority Health and Health Disparities Research and Education Act.[47] The amendment to the original provision mandating an annual national health care disparities report essentially expanded the AHRQ's authority in researching and developing appropriate resources to tackle disparities in health care. The law codified the health disparities reduction campaign that was initiated by the Clinton administration earlier in 1998. Congressman Danny Davis (D-IL), a member of the CBC, when introducing the amendment calling for the AHRQ national health care disparities report, stated, "We need an annual report to measure whether we are making progress in ending racial disparities in health care and improving the quality of life for all Americans . . . and make sure that we have adequate and accurate information on which to base policy and budgetary decisions."[48]

In the late 1990s and early 2000s, several major reports were issued by the sixteenth US surgeon general, Dr. David Satcher, highlighting and addressing issues impacting mental health, oral health, and sexual health, including the 2001 *Mental Health: Culture, Race, and Ethnicity* report.[49] That report showed significant disparities in access to and availability of mental health services by race and ethnicity and a resulting disproportionately high disability burden from unmet mental health needs. Minorities showed higher levels of tobacco use and less access to necessary mental health services compared to white members of the population. The report emphasized the role that cultural factors play in mental health and showed the necessity of programs to deliver culturally, linguistically, and geographically accessible mental health services. This report proved highly impactful by laying the foundation for recommendations made two years later when the New Freedom Commission on Mental Health, which was established by President George W. Bush, released its report, *Achieving the Promise: Transforming Mental Health Care in America*. This 2003 comprehensive mental health report documented the disparities that were experienced by racial and ethnic minorities in the mental health system and made recommendations for addressing them effectively.

In 2002, the IOM released its comprehensive and authoritative report documenting health care disparities, *Unequal Treatment: Confronting Racial and Ethnic Disparities in Health Care*, which was mandated by the Minority Health and Health Disparities Research and Education Act.[50] Dr. Brian Smedley, one of the nation's foremost policy experts on health equity, led the development of this crucial report, which provided insight into the disparities minorities were experiencing in health services, treatments, and care. Interestingly, the IOM report, itself authorized by legislation, resulted in the development of another major piece of legislation one year later—the Healthcare Equality and Accountability Act.[51] This bill was introduced in the House by Elijah Cummings (D-MD) during the 108th Congress when he was chair of the Congressional Black Caucus and in the Senate by Tom Daschle (D-SD) when he was minority leader. It was the first comprehensive legislation solely intended to address disparities in health status and health care.

In 2003 the Agency for Healthcare Research and Quality released its congressionally mandated *National Healthcare Disparities Report* one month after the first comprehensive health equity bill was introduced by Representative Cummings and Senator Daschle. This report was the first comprehensive national effort to measure differences in quality of and access to health care services as well as the progress the nation was making in eliminating health disparities. However, the release of this report was shrouded in controversy, much like the *Heckler Report* when it was unveiled, and many health equity champions questioned the changes that were made to the original report before it was released to the public and lawmakers in Congress.[52] Policy makers were concerned about the dismal numbers and impression people would have once the facts about gaps in care and disparities in health were made public. It took almost six months for the US Department of Health and Human Services to finally release the report in December 2003, although it was required by law to be released publicly in September 2003. However, once released, Secretary of HHS Tommy Thompson underscored the department's commitment to eliminating health disparities: "communities of color suffer disproportionately from diabetes, heart disease, HIV/AIDS, cancer, stroke and infant mortality. Eliminating these and other health disparities is a priority of HHS."[53]

The report showed a broad array of striking differences in access, use, and patient experience of health care by racial, ethnic, socioeconomic, and geographic groups, and demonstrated that improvement was possible. It continues to be the only national report tracking the country's progress each year in improving health care quality and reducing health care disparities across a broad range of conditions, services, and population groups. In addition to the release of the AHRQ report, the NIH issued its *Strategic Research Plan and Budget to Reduce and Ultimately Eliminate Health Disparities* in 2003.

In 2004, Senator Bill Frist, a physician and the new majority leader in the Senate, refused to allow Democrats to continue scoring political points for addressing racial and ethnic health disparities and led efforts to address this issue in public policy. As a result, he introduced the second comprehensive health equity bill, which took into consideration issues and recommendations highlighted in the IOM and AHRQ reports. In every Congress thereafter, at least two comprehensive bills were introduced—one by the Democratic Tri-Caucus members and another by a bipartisan group of congressional members primarily in the Senate.

Because of these investments in researching and addressing racial and ethnic health disparities in the 1980s, 1990s, and early 2000s, more than six hundred articles were published from 1980 to 2005 documenting racial or ethnic variations in health care.[54] After 2005, more than six thousand additional scholarly articles were published in medical, public health, and legal journals. In fact, over the past decade, the number of scholarly journal articles that have been published has significantly increased every single year, bringing renewed focus to an issue that few wanted to appropriately tackle in earlier decades. This unprecedented attention also resulted in more legislation than ever before being introduced in subsequent Congresses to close the gaps in health care in addition to the pair of comprehensive health equity bills introduced each Congress by the Tri-Caucus and Senate champions:

> 2003—Healthcare Equality and Accountability Act (Sen. Tom Daschle and Rep. Elijah Cummings)
> 2004—Closing the Health Care Gap Act (Sen. Bill Frist)
> 2005—Healthcare Equality and Accountability Act (Sen. Daniel Akaka and Rep. Mike Honda)
> 2006—Minority Health Improvement and Health Disparity Elimination Act (Sen. Bill Frist, Edward Kennedy, Barack Obama, and Jeff Bingaman; Rep. Jesse Jackson Jr.)
> 2006—Health Equity and Justice Act (Del. Donna Christensen)
> 2007—Minority Health Improvement and Health Disparity Elimination Act (Sen. Bill Frist, Edward Kennedy, Barack Obama, and Jeff Bingaman; Rep. Jesse Jackson Jr.)
> 2007—Health Equity and Accountability Act (Rep. Hilda Solis)
> 2009—Health Equity and Accountability Act (Del. Donna Christensen)

Unfortunately, the case law addressing health disparities has mirrored the legislation that has been introduced. While a handful of cases have cited published reports documenting racial and ethnic health disparities to bolster their arguments relative to affirmative action, these reports for the most part have been cited in dissents.

During the George W. Bush administration, there continued to be support for eliminating racial and ethnic health disparities and an increase in public/private initiatives to address this issue. The Bush administration, which had inherited the Minority Health and Health Disparities Research and Education Act, ensured the successful implementation of this law and continued to demonstrate the bipartisan credibility of advancing a health equity agenda. Congress also continued to introduce several bills directly addressing issues impacting minority health and health disparities, which were later incorporated in health reform proposals. While the Tri-Caucus led efforts in Congress to advance health equity-focused legislation, the executive branch also had unsung heroes—champions leading efforts to advance health equity via regulations and other subregulatory means.

One health equity vanguard in the US Department of Health and Human Services during the Bush administration was Dr. Garth Graham, who was appointed deputy assistant secretary for minority health and director of the Office of Minority Health. Under his leadership, which continued through the Obama administration, the issue of health equity remained a priority at HHS in both federal policies and programs. In 2007, Dr. Graham convened an expert working group on reducing racial and ethnic disparities in health care along with the National Association of Public Hospitals and Health Systems and developed a blueprint of strategies and interventions for providers to address health care disparities.[55] This resource, titled *Assuring Healthcare Equity: A Healthcare Equity Blueprint*, was released in September 2008 and was used by health equity champions to highlight the need to dedicate more resources to communities to address health care disparities in the development of the Affordable Care Act.

Building on the successes of his predecessors at HHS who increased investments in research around racial and ethnic health disparities, produced seminal reports on key health equity issues, and elevated or established new programs to increase minority health, Dr. Graham recognized that for the nation to move closer to meaningfully eliminating health disparities, a national action plan was needed. Despite being confronted with internal and external challenges, he led the development of the first comprehensive federal government action plan and community stakeholder strategy to eliminate health disparities across the United States. He led the development of the first national set of data standards for disability, race or ethnicity, and primary language, and he also expanded the number of state Offices of Minority Health across the country.

As time passed, it was increasingly clear that there was a rigid dichotomy between the House and Senate relative to advancing health equity policy. Although House and Senate members were committed to elevating minority health and eliminating disparities in health status and care among minorities, there was some contention about how broad and comprehensive bills should be in addressing the minority health crisis. House champions wanted any bill directly addressing health inequities to be as comprehensive as possible, while Senate champions in general took more of a "something is better than nothing" approach.

The Tri-Caucus was also adamant that any bill that passed Congress relative to health disparities should be vetted and approved by them. This caused Senate staff some angst because they wanted to pass legislation building on the Minority Health and Health Disparities Research and Education Act of 2000 signed by President Clinton, but politics played a major role in preventing this from happening. Democrats, especially Tri-Caucus House members, were reluctant to give Republicans any points for passing a more narrow health equity package. As a result, the Minority Health and Health Disparities Research and Education Act of 2000 would remain the last ever passed by Congress specifically targeting health disparities until the opportunity arose to advance a health equity agenda during health reform negotiations in 2009.

Universal Health

I am not the first President to take up this cause, but I am determined to be the last.—*President Barack Obama, in a speech concerning health care reform to the Joint Houses of Congress*

The Genesis of Increasing Access in America

The first significant federal health care legislation introduced in the United States was the Act for Relief of Sick and Disabled Seamen that President John Adams signed into law in 1798. The act created the Marine Hospital Service and mandated that privately employed sailors purchase health insurance. Merchant marines often got injured or caught tropical diseases, leaving captains without enough sailors to operate, putting a strain on the nation's economy. Realizing that a healthy maritime workforce was essential to the ability of merchant ships to engage in foreign trade, Congress and the president resolved to do something about it.[56]

The Marine Hospital Service was a series of hospitals built and oper-ated by the federal government to treat privately employed sailors. This service was financed by a mandatory tax on each maritime sailor's income that was to be paid by the owner or captain of each vessel. This tax equated to twenty cents per sailor for each month of employment. Upon passage of the law, ships were no longer permitted to sail in and out of US ports unless the health care tax had been collected by ship owners and paid to the government. When sailors needed medical assistance, the government would confirm that their payments had been collected and then give them a voucher to be admitted to the treating hospital. The system was eventu-ally expanded to cover sailors working private vessels on the Mississippi and Ohio rivers. This program eventually became the Public Health Service.[57]

Early Attempts to Strengthen Public Health, Expand Health Insurance Coverage and Access to Care

The next president to take an interest in public health was Theo-dore Roosevelt, who sought to ensure social justice and economic oppor-tunity through government regulation. He did not seek to fundamentally alter American society; in fact, he stated that there must be reform in or-der to stave off socialism, and that if the government did not act, the people would turn to more extreme measures. In his 1907 State of the Union he said, "There is a constantly growing interest in this country in the ques-tion of the public health. At last the public mind is awake to the fact that many diseases, notably tuberculosis, are National scourges. The work of the State and city boards of health should be supplemented by a constantly increasing interest on the part of the National Government. The Congress has already provided a bureau of public health and has provided for a hy-gienic laboratory. There are other valuable laws relating to the public health connected with the various departments. This whole branch of the Gov-ernment should be strengthened and aided in every way."[58]

Roosevelt did not seek a third term in 1908, and he was succeeded by Republican William Howard Taft. Roosevelt, however, ran for office again in 1912 as a member of the Progressive Party, and he endorsed social in-surance, including health insurance, as part of his platform. Roosevelt fa-vored health insurance legislation but assumed that such legislation would come from the states rather than the federal government and would cover only the working classes. He lost the election to Woodrow Wilson. Though the Progressive movement's attempt at health reform was unsuccessful, the American Association for Labor Legislation created a proposal in 1915 for a system of compulsory health insurance to protect workers against lost wages and medical expenses. The bill was modeled on existing systems in Europe, and it stimulated much debate across the country before being introduced as legislation in several states. The bill's only success was in New York, where it passed the Senate but was then killed in committee by the Speaker of the House.[59]

The federal government once again dedicated public resources to address public health issues in 1921 with the passage of the Sheppard-Towner Maternity and Infancy Protection Act. This statute provided funding to states to establish and run prenatal and child health centers. In 1912, President William Taft had established the Children's Bureau, which began a nationwide investigation of maternal and infant mortality rates. The agency soon discovered that nearly 80 percent of US women did not receive proper prenatal care. Women had long been the leading voices of reform in regard to child and maternal health care, and they had recently gained the right to vote with the passage of the Nineteenth Amendment. President Warren G. Harding responded to this newly created constituency by actively supporting the passage of Sheppard-Towner. Unfortunately, the Sheppard-Towner Act expired in 1929 and was not reauthorized. Moving forward, President Calvin Coolidge established the Committee on the Cost of Medical Care in 1927 to investigate the health care system. The committee recommended that private insurance or taxes support health care, but, after the stock market crashed in 1929, the idea was abandoned.[60]

The Right to Health Care

Franklin Delano Roosevelt was elected to the presidency during the Great Depression and had the task of rescuing the United States from the worst financial collapse in its history. During his election campaign, he had endorsed universal health insurance and sweeping changes to the health care system. However, because of the continued effects of the Great Depression and focus on economic recovery, universal health insurance and other health reforms were placed on hold.[61]

As governor of New York, FDR enacted a law to provide old-age pensions and sought to extend it nationally. By executive order, he created the Committee on Economic Security, and their recommendations provided the basis for Congress's 1935 Social Security Act. The act had long been a goal of liberals but had been stalled in Congress until FDR declared it vital legislation. Roosevelt intended to develop and implement a national health insurance program as part of the Social Security Act but realized that opposition to universal health care could effectually undermine the whole act, and so he decided to change course.[62]

The Social Security Act was ultimately approved by Congress and signed into law by President Roosevelt in 1935, despite the perception of some that the bill was rushed through Congress and was not given thoughtful consideration. The statute was one of the most significant and sweeping health laws ever passed in the United States. The act included Old Age Assistance (Title I), Old Age Insurance (Title II), Unemployment Insurance (Title III), Aid to Dependent Children (Title IV), and Aid to the Blind (Title V). It also included grants for maternal and child health, thus restoring many of the programs that the Sheppard-Towner Act of 1921 had established. The programs were financed through deductions from workers' incomes. In his public statement on the day of the bill's signing, Roosevelt said, "We can never insure one hundred percent of the population against one hundred percent of the hazards and vicissitudes of life, but we have tried to frame a law which will give some measure of protection to the average citizen and to his family against the loss of a job and against poverty-ridden old age."[63]

Roosevelt's achievement, however, was overshadowed by the opposition from not only some Republicans but groups representing minorities and women who were upset with the intentional exclusion of agricultural and domestic workers. These jobs were held largely by women and minorities, so the concern was that this policy would effectively leave out almost half of the working population. The NAACP decried the policy as exclusive and discriminatory and likened it to "a sieve with holes just big enough for the majority of Negroes to fall through."[64] Later on in 1936, Roosevelt established the Interdepartmental Committee to Coordinate Health and Welfare Activities by executive order to assess the health care needs of the people. This was devised as another means to push for health insurance reform.

Shortly after enactment of the Social Security Act, cases were filed challenging the statute on constitutional grounds. However, in one very narrow 5-4 decision and another 7-2 decision the Supreme Court upheld the law in 1937, stating that the government was exercising its taxation powers.[65] Then, in 1940 he enacted the Lanham Act, which provided federal funding to communities impacted by the defense industry so that they could improve their infrastructure, including health care facilities. The Lanham Act set a precedent for providing government aid to private hospitals. In his 1944 State of the Union address, FDR argued for "an economic bill of rights," including "the right to adequate medical care and the opportunity to achieve and enjoy good health." With this proposal Roosevelt became the first president to state outright that Americans had a right to health care and that the federal government should address it.[66]

Increasing the Government's Role in Health Care

President Roosevelt was succeeded by Harry Truman, and for the first time health care moved up as a major political issue. Truman was the first president to openly advocate for a national health care program. During a special address to Congress on November 19, 1945, only seven months into his presidency, President Truman argued that the federal government should play a role in health care: "Millions of our citizens do not now have a full measure of opportunity to achieve and enjoy good health. Millions do not now have protection or security against the economic effects of sickness. The time has arrived for action to help them attain that opportunity and that protection." Truman described the many problems with the delivery of health care, including high costs and loss of earnings during illness or injury. He proposed a solution, which would provide federal funding to attract doctors to rural or otherwise low-income areas, as he saw that "the earning capacity of the people in some communities makes it difficult if not impossible for doctors who practice there to make a living." He also sought to provide federal funding for the construction of new hospitals and to create new national standards for hospitals and other health centers.[67]

Truman's proposed plan would create a national health insurance fund under the jurisdiction of the Social Security program that would allow Americans to voluntarily participate. The Social Security payroll tax would be increased by 4 percent to finance the program. Eventually, President Truman's health care proposal was included as a revised, separate expansion of the Murray-Wagner-Dingell health insurance bill. The bill had first been introduced in 1943 by Senators James Murray (D-MT) and Robert Wagner (D-NY), as well as Congressman John Dingell Sr. (D-MI). It was the first national health insurance bill, and though President Roosevelt had not formally endorsed it, he had been supportive of it. The Murray-Wagner-Dingell bill died in committee, overshadowed by the war and Roosevelt's lack of endorsement.[68]

After Truman's address, the Murray-Wagner-Dingell bill authors redrafted their legislation to include President Truman's health care proposal. The bill had two parts: Title I focused on public health services and maternal and child health care, and Title II created universal health insurance. The bill had many adversaries. Although both chambers of Congress held a Democratic majority, the political sentiment at the time was conservative. The public had turned against the New Deal because of high taxes, and southern Democrats feared that federal involvement in health care might lead to federal action against segregation. Most significantly, the American Medical Association (AMA) was opposed to national health insurance.

The AMA, one of the most powerful lobbying groups in the United States, had supported compulsory health insurance legislation in 1915 but changed course and remained opposed to it. Members of the AMA believed that compulsory health care would limit physician autonomy and income. The AMA, therefore, launched a National Education Campaign with a dual purpose: to block passage of Truman's health care plan and to endorse and promote private health insurance.[69] The AMA, joined by the American Hospital Association, instead pushed for another bill, one that had bipartisan support, cosponsored by Senator Lister Hill (D-AL) and Senator George Aiken (R-VT). The Hill-Aiken bill authorized federal funding to states that provided subsidies to the poor to offset private health insurance premiums. Republicans also introduced proposals that promoted means testing or a private health insurance system. Truman, however, would not agree to any of these proposals, and although he enjoyed a relatively cordial relationship with Senator Hill, the two would not come together around universal health reform because of their stances on civil rights; Truman favored expanding civil rights protections whereas Hill did not.

During the congressional hearings for the Murray-Wagner-Dingell bill, the AMA presented a counterproposal that promoted private insurance options. Debates on the bill continued in the Senate Committee on Education and Labor, with little being accomplished. Afterward, Republicans gained the majority in both houses in the 1946 midterm election, and further action on this landmark legislation stalled.

Though his efforts at a national health care system were unsuccessful, Truman's administration was able to enact new programs to improve mental health, the health of mothers and children, and hospital construction. The Hospital Survey and Construction Act, also referred to as the Hill-Burton Act, was introduced by Senators Lister Hill (D-AL) and Harold Burton (R-OH) and was enacted on August 13, 1946. FDR's surgeon general, Thomas Parran, had been an important proponent of federal aid for hospital construction and was instrumental in the enactment of this law. The Hill-Burton Act provided federal aid to the states for hospitals and other health facilities. To be granted funds, states were required to survey existing facilities and assess the need for new construction. The law was designed to reduce inequities in access to hospital care, and it ensured that the poorer states would receive more federal aid. The Hill-Burton Act, as mentioned earlier, included a Community Service Assurance provision, requiring facilities to provide services to residents of their area without discrimination on the basis of race, national origin, or creed.

President Truman made national health insurance a central theme in his 1948 reelection campaign. After his election victory, Truman repeated his appeal for national health insurance. In his 1948 State of the Union address, he said, "We are rightly proud of the high standards of medical care we know how to provide in the United States. The fact is, however, that most of our people cannot afford to pay for the care they need." He went on to advocate for a "national system of payment for medical care based on well-tried insurance principles. This great Nation cannot afford to allow its citizens to suffer needlessly from the lack of proper medical care. Our ultimate aim must be a comprehensive insurance system to protect all our people equally against insecurity and ill health."[70]

At the start of his second term, President Truman again urged Congress to act on universal health insurance. Soon after, Democrats presented a proposal to Congress, but it met with strong opposition from many corners. Conservatives in Congress opposed the bill and formed a coalition with anti-Truman conservative southern Democrats. Republicans and southern Democrats controlled the committees through which health legislation had to pass, and they opposed any program that would allow federal intervention in the South's segregated health care system. They used the fact that unions were in favor of a health insurance bill to claim it was an effort by Democrats to socialize medicine. However, trade unions, which might have been expected to heavily promote a national health insurance campaign, instead focused on attaining private health insurance benefits for their union members in employment contracts.[71]

The most powerful opponent of the health insurance bill, however, was once again the American Medical Association. Having successfully helped block the Murray-Wagner-Dingell bill in 1946, the AMA immediately went on the offensive when the bill was reintroduced in 1949. The AMA was able to shape political will in the 1940s by leveraging its vast economic resources, thus stimulating and creating opposition by organizing other like-minded groups into a coalition to further spread the message. The AMA had a structure and resources that enabled it to effectively organize a grassroots campaign in nearly every city and small town across America. It distributed posters, leaflets, cartoons, and other materials, all with the goal of increasing and sustaining hostility toward national health insurance. The American Medical Association capitalized on the public's fear of communism and called White House staffers "followers of the Moscow party line." It obtained endorsements from more than 1,800 other national organizations, including the American Bar Association and the American Farm Bureau Federation. The AMA spent more than $4 million on its campaign against national health insurance—the largest lobbying effort in American history at that time.[72]

The strong opposition from organized medicine and conservatives, combined with a series of unpopular labor strikes, a pervasive public fear of socialism and communism, and the outbreak of the Korean War, collectively and effectively kept the Truman health care proposal from proceeding. The bill was never reported out of committee. Truman was able, however, to enact the Social Security Amendments, which provided federal funds to states for vendor payments for the provision of medical care to older adults of lower socioeconomic status. The program was called Old-Age Assistance, and it became the precursor to and the foundation for the Medicare program.[73]

The Rise of Private Insurance

Reform of the nation's health care system remained off the political agenda throughout the 1950s under President Dwight D. Eisenhower, who had taken a stance against national health insurance in his presidential campaign. During the 1940s, the private health insurance industry had risen to prominence and became the primary payer of health care for Americans. In fact, this trend continued throughout the years. Whereas in 1940 fewer than six million people had any kind of insurance, by 1950 more than seventy-five million Americans had private health insurance.[74] Though Eisenhower opposed compulsory national health insurance, he did support the notion of a government reinsurance program under which the federal government would subsidize partial payment of premiums for low-income individuals. The plan never materialized because it could not make it out of committee in the House.

In his 1956 State of the Union address, President Eisenhower continued to acknowledge the rising costs of health care and the need for some

Universal Health Policy Timeline

Major laws related to health care reform appear in bold.

PRE-20th CENTURY

1798 - President John Adams signed into law the Act for Relief of Sick and Disabled Seamen.

1910s

1912 - President Theodore Roosevelt endorsed social insurance as part of his platform, including health insurance but lost election.

1912 - President William Howard Taft established the Children's Bureau, which began a nationwide investigation of maternal and infant mortality rates.

1920s

1921 - President Warren G. Harding signed the Sheppard-Towner Maternity and Infancy Protection Act, which provided funding to states to establish and run prenatal and child health centers. It expired eight years later in 1929 and was not reauthorized.

1927 - President Calvin Coolidge established the Committee on the Cost of Medical Care to investigate the health care system, but recommendations from this committee were put on hold.

1930s

1935 - President Franklin D. Roosevelt signed the Social Security Act but abandoned the inclusion of national health insurance coverage because of the strong opposition.

1936 - FDR established by executive order the Interdepartmental Committee to Coordinate Health and Welfare Activities to assess the health care needs of the people.

1940s

1940 - FDR enacted the Lanham Act, which provided federal funding to communities so that they could improve their infrastructure, including health care facilities.

1945 - President Truman argued that the federal government should play a role in health care. After his speech the Murray-Wagner-Dingell bill was redrafted to include health care.

1950s

1956 - President Eisenhower argued for federal reinsurance under which the federal government would subsidize partial payment of premiums for low-income individuals.

1960s

1960 - President-elect John F. Kennedy appointed the presidential Task Force on Health and Social Security for the American People, which recommended private health insurance for older adults.

1965 - President Lyndon B. Johnson signed the Medicare and Medicaid legislation into law.

1970s

1971 - Senator Ted Kennedy introduced a health insurance reform statute, which was countered by a proposal from President Richard Nixon a few months after titled National Health Insurance Partnership Act.

1973 - President Nixon signed into law the Health Maintenance Organization Act.

1974 - President Gerald Ford prioritized universal health insurance and set a goal of passing the Kennedy-Mills plan that year.

1979 - President Jimmy Carter developed a national health insurance plan and delivered it to Congress.

1980s

1989 - President George H. W. Bush developed a comprehensive health insurance proposal, but it was set aside because of pressing international issues.

1990s

1993 - President Clinton convened the White House Task Force on Health Reform, a group of more than 500 policy experts, physicians, and other health professionals and appointed First Lady Hillary Clinton as chair.

1993 - Democratic Sen. George Mitchell introduced a 1,370-page bipartisan bill with 29 cosponsors entitled the Health Security Act, which was the embodiment of the Clinton Plan. That same day, Republican Sen. John Chafee introduced the bipartisan Health Equity and Access Reform Today Act of 1993 with 20 cosponsors. The Clinton plan was defeated in 1994.

2000s

2007 - President George W. Bush proposed a plan to address health insurance coverage, but it was never acted upon by Congress.

2009 - **President Barack Obama signed the American Recovery and Reinvestment Act, also referred to as the stimulus law, laying the foundation for health reform.**

2010s

2010 - **President Obama signed the Patient Protection and Affordable Care Act into law, the first time comprehensive health reform was enacted.**

2015 - **President Obama signed into law the Medicare Access and CHIP Reauthorization Act, which extended many of the health reform programs from the ACA and expanded delivery and payment reforms.**

sort of reform: "We must aid in cushioning the heavy and rising costs of illness and hospitalization to individuals and families. Provision should be made, by Federal reinsurance or otherwise, to foster extension of voluntary health insurance coverage to many more persons, especially older persons and those in rural areas. Plans should be evolved to improve protection against the costs of prolonged or severe illness. These measures will help reduce the dollar barrier between many Americans and the benefits of modern medical care."[75]

Government-financed health care returned to the political stage in the 1960 presidential campaign. Republican nominee Richard Nixon proposed a health care plan in which Americans age sixty-five and older could choose between government insurance or private insurance. Democratic nominee John F. Kennedy endorsed a compulsory health insurance law for older Social Security beneficiaries that would pay for most medical expenses, financed by increasing the Social Security payroll tax. However, health care proposals that were raised during the election would soon be overshadowed by foreign policy and other domestic policy issues.[76]

Medicare, Medicaid and the Government's Role in Public Welfare

Soon after winning the election, President-elect John F. Kennedy appointed the presidential Task Force on Health and Social Security for the American People. The following year, the task force recommended a program that would provide health insurance for older Americans through the Social Security system. This would later become known as Medicare. In his 1961 State of the Union address, Kennedy said, "Medical research has achieved new wonders—but these wonders are too often beyond the reach of too many people, owing to a lack of income (particularly among the aged), a lack of hospital beds, a lack of nursing homes and a lack of doctors and dentists. Measures to provide healthcare for the aged under Social Security, and to increase the supply of both facilities and personnel, must be undertaken."[77]

Perhaps trying to counter arguments by President Franklin Pierce over a hundred years ago and by others throughout the decades that there is no constitutional authority for government involvement in health services, welfare, and other human services, President Kennedy in a widely watched speech in 1962 advocating Medicare said, "This bill serves the public interest. It involves the government because it involves the public welfare."[78] President Kennedy made the passage of Medicare one of the priorities of his administration, but he died before achieving this objective.

After Kennedy's assassination, President Lyndon B. Johnson made the passage of Medicare his top legislative priority. During the 1964 presidential campaign, Johnson emphasized his vision of the Great Society, of which the enactment of Medicare was a key component. To avoid the appearance of socializing medicine, President Johnson emphasized that Medicare was a program that would cover many health care costs borne by consumers, but not all costs. The outpouring of civil rights demonstrations and advocacy activities at the time encouraged politicians to support Medicare as part of Johnson's War on Poverty. It did not hurt that this time major unions and civil rights organizations strongly endorsed the legislation.[79]

In the summer of 1965, advocates succeeded in their campaign, and Medicare and Medicaid were enacted as Title XVIII and Title XIX of the Social Security Act. On July 30, President Johnson traveled to the Harry S. Truman Presidential Library in Independence, Missouri, to sign the bill into law in the presence of former president Truman, saying he wanted to recognize Truman as the "daddy of Medicare." Johnson declared, when signing the bill, "No longer will older Americans be denied the healing miracle of modern medicine. No longer will illness crush and destroy the savings that they have so carefully put away over a lifetime so that they might enjoy dignity in their later years. No longer will young families see their own incomes, and their own hopes, eaten away simply because they are carrying out their deep moral obligations to their parents, and to their uncles, and their aunts. And no longer will this Nation refuse the hand of justice to those who have given a lifetime of service and wisdom and labor to the progress of this progressive country." Medicare Part A would pay for hospital care and limited skilled nursing and home health care for individuals ages sixty-five and over. Optional Medicare Part B would help pay for physician care. Roughly nineteen million older adults enrolled in Medicare when the program began on July 1, 1966.[80]

Further Attempts at National Health Insurance

Richard Nixon won the presidential election in 1968, and government-financed health care was not a concern for his administration, although national health insurance returned to the political stage in 1968, when Walter Reuther, president of the United Auto Workers, made a speech before the American Public Health Association. Reuther asserted that it was the only way to remove economic barriers to care and contain costs. Reuther organized the Committee of 100 for National Health Insurance, a team that included Senator Edward Kennedy. The team developed a plan called Health Security, under which the federal government would pay for all health services. Senator Kennedy introduced the Health Security Act in 1971, which would provide federal payment of nearly all health care costs for all US citizens. However, because of the Vietnam War, the OPEC oil crisis, and the absence of grassroots support, the Health Security Act failed to move forward in Congress in 1972.[81]

A few months after Kennedy introduced the Health Security Act, President Nixon announced the National Health Insurance Partnership Act. Nixon expressed concern over the rising costs of health care and favored using federal funds to stimulate the creation of health maintenance organizations, or HMOs. In an HMO, members receive health services through privately prepaid group insurance. Nixon's proposal would provide a government-prescribed minimum amount of medical and hospital insurance coverage financed by mandatory employer and employee payment of premiums, with a government subsidy in specific situations. The act would also provide government-paid benefits for families earning less than $5,000 per year.[82]

Although Nixon's plan eventually lost favor internally at the White House, it was embraced by several influential congressional Republicans, including Senator Jacob K. Javits of New York, and a prominent Democratic physician, Representative William R. Roy of Kansas. Working with several key Democrats, they adopted Nixon's plan. After three years of legislative effort and external advocacy, Nixon signed into law the Health Maintenance Organization Act, which allocated $375 million to fund and expand these health maintenance organizations. The act helped to broaden the presence of and increase consumer participation in health maintenance organizations. It created an experimental program to underwrite HMO development and became a forerunner to the debate over whether to increase HMOs during the 1990s. Nixon also signed into law in the early 1970s the Social Security Amendments of 1972, the first major adjustment to Medicare since its enactment. The amendments allowed people under age sixty-five with long-term disabilities and end-stage renal disease to qualify for Medicare coverage. Two million individuals were thus newly entitled to Medicare.[83]

In 1974, as the Watergate scandal was escalating, President Nixon announced a new national health insurance plan in his State of the Union address. The health insurance plan, which centered on private insurance, was perceivably announced as a way to distract from Watergate and to forestall a more comprehensive and sweeping proposal from Senator Ted Kennedy.[84] Senator Kennedy and Ways and Means Committee chair Wilbur Mills (D-AR) in conjunction with Congressman Andrew Young had been developing a health plan. Like the Health Security Act, the Kennedy-Mills plan would replace the current system with a single national health insurance program. Unlike Health Security however, the Kennedy-Mills legislation would preserve many aspects of the existing system, by including copayments and deductibles, allowing private insurers to act as fiscal intermediaries, and allowing for supplementary benefits.

When Gerald Ford became president after Nixon's forced resignation, he prioritized universal health insurance and set a goal of passing the Kennedy-Mills plan that year. However, like prior attempts at health insurance reform legislation, the Kennedy-Mills plan was bombarded with opposition. Insurance industry lobbyists and the American Medical Association immediately swooped down on Congress and worked heavily against the legislation. The AMA criticized the plan as socialist, and the National Federation of Independent Business called it "nothing more than a first step towards socialized medicine." Trade unions were also against the plan, protesting the major role it gave to the health insurance industry. The plan's opponents were successful. Congressman Mills announced that health insurance reform would be set aside and that the bill would be removed from consideration.[85]

Undeterred, President Ford continued to advocate for some kind of health reform, and in his 1976 State of the Union he proposed expanding Medicare, though he acknowledged that a national health insurance plan was not feasible:

> Hospital and medical services in America are among the best in the world, but the cost of a serious and extended illness can quickly wipe out a family's lifetime savings. Increasing health costs are of deep concern to all and a powerful force pushing up the cost of living. The burden of catastrophic illness can be borne by very few in our society. We must eliminate this fear from every family.
>
> I propose catastrophic health insurance for everybody covered by Medicare. To finance this added protection, fees for short-term care will go up somewhat, but nobody after reaching age 65 will have to pay more than $500 a year for covered hospital or nursing home care, nor more than $250 for 1 year's doctor bills.

We cannot realistically afford federally dictated national health insurance pro-
viding full coverage for all 215 million Americans. The experience of other countries raises questions about the quality as well as the cost of such plans. But I
do envision the day when we may use the private health insurance system
to offer more middle-income families high quality health services at prices
they can afford and shield them also from their catastrophic illnesses.

Using resources now available, I propose improving the Medicare and
other Federal health programs to help those who really need protection—
older people and the poor. To help States and local governments give better
health care to the poor, I propose that we combine 16 existing Federal programs, including Medicaid, into a single $10 billion Federal grant.[86]

President Ford later found this to be quite a challenge and was never successful in achieving health reform.

"Universal and Mandatory": Another Health Insurance Proposal

The election of Jimmy Carter, the first Democratic president in ten
years, reopened the issue of health care reform as a political issue. Carter
had made health care a priority in his 1976 campaign, promising "universal and mandatory" health insurance, which would provide comprehensive coverage and be funded by income taxes. Despite his best efforts to
move forward, his health reform priorities were overshadowed in the
first years of his term by other pressing issues, such as economic stimulus, energy conservation, the Panama Canal treaties, and budgetary and tax
reform. His administration did eventually develop a health insurance plan
in the Department of Health, Education, and Welfare, and in 1979 delivered
the National Health Plan to Congress. The plan included catastrophic coverage for Americans, financed by requiring employers to purchase insurance
for employees, with subsidized premiums for small businesses and public
insurance for the unemployed. Prenatal, delivery, and infant care would
be provided without deductibles, and coverage would be extended to children under six years old. The threshold for low-income coverage would
be lowered to 55 percent of the poverty line, and Medicare and Medicaid
would be combined under one federal program.[87]

President Carter did not promise a comprehensive health reform plan
with his proposal but instead stated in a message to Congress that the plan
he offered created "both the framework and momentum for a universal,
comprehensive national health plan." The plan was publicly condemned

by Senator Kennedy, who firmly believed it fell short of providing truly comprehensive coverage. He pointed out that, under the plan, doctors would be paid less for attending older adults and individuals of lower socioeconomic status than insured workers, and that catastrophic coverage with fixed benefits meant that the wealthy would pay a lower percentage of income for health care. Furthermore, the National Health Plan proposal was stalled by conservatives in Congress in 1980. The Senate Finance Committee dropped the maternal and infant benefits and federal control of Medicaid or catastrophic care. Hearings continued with no progress, and, by the fall of 1980, it became apparent that President Carter's health legislation would not make it out of committee before the upcoming presidential election.[88]

President Carter's unsuccessful attempt to pass health reform legislation in a Congress controlled by Democrats was due to several factors. By taking months to develop his proposal, he lost the momentum of the "honeymoon period" of his first few months of the presidency.[89] In addition, while progress was delayed, health costs were rising, making the health plan more expensive. In addition, once midterm elections and primaries took place, Carter lost support from his liberal base. The legislation also suffered from a lack of cooperation within the Carter administration, as various cabinet departments were working separately on the same goal. By the time the proposal made it to Congress, there was not enough time to get legislation enacted. In the end, Carter's commitment to mental health reform outshined his commitment to national health reform, so while he was able to pass his Mental Health Systems Act, his health reform legislation suffered as a result.

Austerity in the 1980s: Cutting Health Care Costs

Ronald Reagan's election to the presidency in 1981 ushered in an era of limited social welfare. President Reagan's perspective on America's values and identity stressed individualism, the free market, and limited government. He immediately launched an effort to reorganize the federal health care system, announcing plans to consolidate all twenty-six health services programs into two block grants: one for health services and the other for preventive health. During Reagan's eight years in office, many changes were made to Medicare and Medicaid. This was done primarily through annual budget reconciliation legislation. For example, the Omnibus Budget Reconciliation Act of 1981 reduced funding for all health services programs, collapsed funding for many grant programs into block grants to states, and increased local and state governance over remaining programs. The act changed Medicare by creating a new prospective payment system for inpatient hospital services, risk contracts for HMOs, and new Peer Review Organizations to improve the quality of health care.[90]

Though President Reagan's primary goal with health care was lowering or cutting costs, in 1986 he proposed expanding Medicare to cover the cost of catastrophic illness. However, he made it clear that he would not support any proposal unless it was entirely voluntary, self-funded, and not intrusive on the private market. A plan was sent to Congress in February of 1987. It was not opposed by the American Medical Association, as long as the fee-for-service system remained unaffected. The insurance industry also did not oppose the proposal. In 1988, Congress passed the Medicare Catastrophic Coverage Act with large bipartisan majorities in both the House and the Senate. Reagan signed this bill into law. In addition to extending Medicare to cover the costs of catastrophic illness, it improved hospital and skilled nursing facility benefits, outpatient prescription drug benefits, and put a cap on beneficiary cost-sharing liability. The act was the largest expansion of Medicare since its enactment.[91]

By the time the Bush administration began its tenure, the Medicare Catastrophic Coverage Act proved hugely unpopular among senior citizens, who descended on Congress, demanding that the program be repealed or changed. This came as quite a surprise to both members of Congress and officials in the White House in the Bush administration, especially to Dr. Louis Sullivan, the newly confirmed secretary of health and human services at the time. Benefits were financed by beneficiaries through new premiums and an income tax surcharge. Part B premiums increased from $122 a year to $511, and higher-income Medicare beneficiaries had to pay a surcharge up to $800 for a single person and $1,600 for a couple. Higher-income seniors did not want to pay for the new benefits, since they were already receiving similar benefits through their employer-provided health insurance. After months of protests, the law was repealed in 1989, before most of it had taken effect.[92]

George H. W. Bush had an approach to health care similar to Reagan's. Toward the end of his term, however, he acknowledged the need for health reform and developed a proposal. Secretary Louis Sullivan, working in conjunction with William Toby Jr., the acting Centers for Medicare and Medicaid Services (CMS) administrator; Dr. Gail Wilensky, who served in the White House as a senior health and welfare advisor to the president; and others, were charged with developing this plan. Sullivan formed a health care reform task force at the US Department of Health and Human Services, and the White House formed another task force that included the US Department of Labor, the Attorney General's Office, and other key stakeholders. Together these health reform task forces worked with external groups, including the Heritage Foundation and the American Enterprise Institute, to develop a comprehensive proposal, which included recommendations such as requiring individuals to purchase health insurance (individual mandate), group purchasing for small businesses to afford health insurance coverage and spread the risk, and tax credits to low-income families.

When Saddam Hussein invaded Kuwait in the summer of 1990, the Bush administration had to focus its attention on this issue—working diligently with the United Nations to pass resolutions, building an international coalition to support an offensive strategy, and launching a military campaign against Saddam Hussein's forces. After forcing the Iraqi military out of Kuwait, President Bush enjoyed skyrocketing approval ratings. However, the country was experiencing a recession, and Bush's popularity began to fall. His senior advisors did not want to tackle any volatile policy issues that would upset his standing further.

Health reform was certainly an issue that Bush's advisors thought would be too controversial, so they put a hold on introducing the plan that Dr. Sullivan and other health policy experts in the administration had developed internally and externally. They thought it would be best to wait until after the election before releasing the proposal. Interestingly, those White House officials who had opposed the release of the Bush health reform plan changed their mind when Richard "Dick" Thornburgh lost a special Senate race in Pennsylvania to Harris Wofford, a Democrat who had campaigned strongly for health care reform. Thornburgh, who had been serving as attorney general, had resigned to run for the Senate seat that became vacant when Senator John Heinz (R-PA) was killed in a plane crash. When Thornburgh lost the race, the Bush administration decided it could not afford to hold off on introducing its health reform proposal any longer. Likewise, during the presidential campaign, Bush's opponent, Bill Clinton, called for sweeping health reform. To trump the Democrats on this issue, President Bush unveiled his health reform plan.

In making his case, in 1992 President Bush identified two options: implementing a national health care system, which he opposed, or providing insurance security for everyone while preserving choice. To accomplish this, he proposed the Comprehensive Health Reform Program, which featured tax credits and vouchers. His plan would make basic health insurance affordable for all low-income persons who were not currently covered or who changed jobs or experienced medical crises by providing a health insurance tax credit of up to $3,750 for each family. Bush described his plan to the nation in his 1992 State of the Union:

> We must reform our health care system. For this, too, bears on whether or not we can compete in the world. American health costs have been exploding. This year America will spend over $800 billion on health, and that is expected to grow to 1.6 trillion by the end of the decade. We simply cannot afford this. . . .
>
> Really, there are only two options. And we can move toward a nationalized system, a system which will restrict patient choice in picking a doctor and force the Government to ration services arbitrarily. And what we'll get is patients in long lines, indifferent service, and a huge new tax burden. Or we can reform our own private health care system, which still gives us, for all its flaws, the best quality health care in the world.
>
> Well, let's build on our strengths. My plan provides insurance security for all Americans while preserving and increasing the idea of choice. We make basic health insurance affordable for all low-income people not now covered, and we do it by providing a health insurance tax credit of up to $3,750 for each low-income family. And the middle class gets help, too. And by reforming the health insurance market, my plan assures that Americans will have access to basic health insurance even if they change jobs or develop serious health problems.[93]

Disappointed and Defeated

President Bush, however, did not take action on his proposal, and in November he lost the presidential election. President Bill Clinton returned the health care issue to the fore of national politics. He had campaigned heavily on a platform of reforming the nation's health care system, advocating a staunchly liberal proposal for universal coverage. After winning the election, Clinton vowed to have a health reform bill before Congress within his first one hundred days. A crisis in Somalia and a battle over the North American Free Trade Agreement, however, delayed his health reform plans for most of the year.

Within his first week in office, President Clinton convened the White House Task Force on Health Reform, a group of more than five hundred policy experts, physicians, and other health professionals, and he appointed

First Lady Hillary Rodham Clinton as chair. Their work resulted in the Health Security Act, which promoted universal health coverage but also sought to save health care costs, preserve consumer choice, maintain and enhance a high quality of health care, and reduce the complexity and high administrative costs of the existing system. The plan would guarantee universal coverage through an employer mandate, while containing inflation through purchasing alliances and a national health budget. The health insurance industry's antitrust exemption under the McCarran-Ferguson Act would be repealed, thus subjecting insurers to federal antitrust provisions and consumer protection requirements. The act endorsed "managed competition" as the way to provide universal coverage while also containing costs. This approach was a compromise between those who believed that the market is the best method for efficient distribution and those who believed that health care is a service that is not amenable to market forces.[94]

President Clinton unveiled his proposal to the nation in a speech to Congress on September 22, 1993, saying that the First Lady had consulted with government leaders of both parties. He proposed a concept first conveyed by Republican president Richard Nixon: that every employer and every individual would be asked to contribute to national health care. According to President Clinton, "Our families will never be secure, our businesses will never be strong, and our Government will never again be fully solvent until we tackle the health care crisis. We must do it this year." He vowed to deliver to Congress "a comprehensive plan for health care reform that finally will bring costs under control and provide security to all of our families, so that no one will be denied the coverage they need but so that our economic future will not be compromised either."[95] On November 22, 1993, Senator George Mitchell (D-ME) introduced the Health Security Act, a 1,370-page bipartisan bill with twenty-nine cosponsors, which was the embodiment of the Clinton plan. That same day, Senator John Chafee (R-RI) introduced the bipartisan Health Equity and Access Reform Today Act of 1993 with twenty cosponsors.[96]

Not surprisingly, the Clinton plan met with a great deal of opposition from many sides. The most vehement opponent of the Health Security bill was the Health Insurance Association of America, which spent more than $15 million on an advertising campaign against the measure. The popular "Harry and Louise" television advertisements showed a couple at home discussing various attributes of the proposed plan, such as forcing people to buy insurance through health alliances. These advertisements were singled out as undermining congressional support for the plan. They zeroed in on people's fears about how the act would affect their existing insurance coverage and invoked the belief that it would create a vast, inefficient government bureaucracy. The insurance industry also set up an 800 number to enlist grassroots supporters and formed teams of supporters to write letters and lobby lawmakers.[97]

Small business owners also became one of the most vocal and effective lobbies against Clinton's plan, ultimately forcing the US Chamber of Commerce to withdraw its support. Special interest groups had appealed to it using the prospective costs of the employer mandate. The National Federation of Independent Business mobilized its own grassroots effort against the Health Security bill and sent faxes and action alerts from its Washington, DC, office to tens of thousands of small business owners. It organized groups of activists who attended local meetings when congressional representatives visited their home districts and used radio talk shows to further foment opposition from the public.

By contrast, the American Medical Association was uncharacteristically quiet about any opposition to the Clinton plan, especially in comparison to its previous campaigns against national health care plans. This may have been because a large and growing number of physicians no longer worked in fee-for-service settings, and they were frustrated at the amount of paperwork required to get reimbursement from third-party payers. The AMA was also divided with regard to the plan; some physician organizations endorsed the basic features of Health Security, while others opposed them.[98]

Republicans criticized the plan as too complicated, including Senator Robert Dole (R-KS) in his speech following the 1994 State of the Union address. This situation was also not helped by the perceived untimely and ineffective explanation of the bill's provisions to the public, despite full text publication. Some have argued that potential supporters such as advocacy groups felt alienated since the bill was drafted without their input, with the White House turning to them for support only after it was already written. Advocates became frustrated because oftentimes deals cut late into the evening one day would then unravel the very next morning. Advocates on one side of a coalition built to tackle a particular issue frequently found themselves having to join a competing coalition on another issue the next day. This was so because with a bill so large and information difficult to attain at each stage of the negotiations, entities usually had multiple, incongruent priorities to advocate for, and eventually coalitions organized around these priorities clashed. For many advocates during this time, it seemed to be a constant battle.

And the plan itself was found unsatisfactory by potential supporters, who argued that the complex system would increase the power of private insurers and move further away from the goal of universal health coverage. The administration assembled town hall meetings and developed local groups to press for congressional support, but its opponents came out on top, and by 1994 the bill had been defeated. It was simply no match for the "Republican Revolution" that took place in the midterm elections and resulted in Republicans now controlling both the House and Senate. In his 1995 State of the Union address, President Clinton stated, "Last year we almost came to blows over healthcare, but we didn't do anything. . . . Let's do whatever we have to do to get something done. Let's at least pass meaningful insurance reform."[99] At this point, the Clinton administration, though aspiring to comprehensive health reform, was willing to settle for health insurance reform.

After the demise of the Health Security Act, health policy focused on improving the private health insurance system through regulations. In 1996, President Clinton signed into law the Health Insurance Portability and Accountability Act, which restricted use of preexisting conditions in health insurance coverage determinations, set standards for medical records privacy, and established tax-favored treatment of long-term care insurance. He also created the State Children's Health Insurance Program, which extended health insurance coverage to children in families with incomes too high for Medicaid but not high enough to afford private insurance. The same year, Clinton enacted the Balanced Budget Act of 1997, which made several changes to Medicaid and Medicare. The law revised limits on Medicaid payments to disproportionate share hospitals, which are those hospitals that serve a disproportionate number of uninsured patients, and established new Medicaid and Medicare managed care options. It also expanded Medicare information and education for beneficiaries, expanded preventive benefits, provided beneficiary protections, and slowed the rate of growth in Medicare spending.

The White House went back to Republican leadership in 2001, with the election of George W. Bush. Privatization of health care was a hallmark of his domestic policy, and he proposed private health insurance through tax and other incentives. In his 2005 State of the Union, Bush urged Congress "to move forward on a comprehensive healthcare agenda with tax credits to help low-income workers buy insurance, a community health center in every poor county, improved information technology, association health plans for small businesses and their employees, expanded health savings accounts, and medical liability reform that will reduce healthcare costs and make sure patients have the doctors and care they need."[100] In 2007, he announced a health reform plan that would replace the current tax preference for employer-sponsored insurance with a standard health care deduction. The proposal was not acted upon by Congress.

Comprehensive Health Reform: The Law of the Land
In this great future, you can't forget your past.—*Robert N. Marley*

Recognizing that the future is nothing without the past, lawmakers in the 111th Congress took lessons from history and successfully traversed the political minefield that had long deterred prior health reform attempts. As a result, two years after he was elected, President Barack Obama and congressional Democrats succeeded in passing and enacting the most comprehensive health reform statute in the history of the United States. One of the most remarkable aspects of the Obama administration's achievement was that it succeeded in bringing together early on the independent successive campaigns around mental health, minority health, and universal health insurance, as well as other priorities under one umbrella— the Patient Protection and Affordable Care Act and the Health Care and Education Reconciliation Act. By intentionally converging separate advocacy campaigns, health equity champions crafted a more effective, inclusive, and organic strategy, solving a problem that had challenged lawmakers for decades.

This evolution of a new and bolder strategy of including all of these groups' priorities under one bill was brilliant, since everyone would have a stake in its success. In some respects this strategy was also dangerous: it could have eventually led to the bill's demise if proponents of health reform had failed to keep the majority of interested stakeholders engaged. The development and passage of President Obama's health care law was far from static and will be explored at length in subsequent chapters. However, it is useful at this point to contrast Obama's success with the efforts of prior administrations and to note how every successive attempt at health reform allowed champions to test various approaches and develop more effective strategies for passing comprehensive health reform. Health reform champions in government and outside of government were able to avoid past mistakes or mishaps, which were necessary in laying the groundwork for ObamaCare.

First, President Obama acted with speed. Presidents Jimmy Carter, George H. W. Bush, and Bill Clinton all suffered from the long delays in getting their health bills before Congress and so lost the advantage of the "honeymoon period" of the earliest years of their presidencies. In contrast, President Obama pressed the need to get reform passed as soon as possible. Clinton had the benefit of Democratic majorities in the House and Senate but lost them during the Republican Revolution in 1994. Like Clinton, Obama also lost Democratic majorities during his first term, although the Senate remained in Democratic hands, but by that time his health reform legislation had already been enacted.

Second, despite arguments that President Obama was not transparent or inclusive enough during the health reform negotiations, his efforts were certainly more transparent than those of previous presidents. Perhaps Obama was successful in part because of the former Clinton administration officials who were now working in his administration and had a second bite at the apple. Similarly, Presidents George H. W. Bush and Jimmy Carter left the task of drafting a proposal primarily to their HHS officials instead of working closely with Congress to develop the legislation. Remembering past strategies that had failed, the Obama administration moved and reacted differently. Clinton and his administration drafted their health reform bill in White House task force meetings behind closed doors and later delivered the completed proposal to Congress. Many lawmakers complained that they never got to see the Clinton health reform bill and were not sure what it contained because the task force members kept it close to their chest.[101] Obama, in contrast, presented the broad principles of what he wanted in a health care bill and let Congress fill in the details in committee drafting sessions.

Third, President Obama persisted through crisis. Whereas prior presidents shelved or postponed their health reform plans when other pressing issues arose, President Obama insisted on pushing ahead with his plans despite the economic crisis of 2008. It probably helped that advocates for health reform were determined to achieve success this time around and kept the pressure on the president and members of Congress to finally pass a comprehensive health reform law. They realized that if lost, this opportunity to pass health reform would not present itself again for decades. The urgency to get this bill passed was furthered by the notion that the US Supreme Court during that time had not demonstrated sensitivities toward past civil rights and health care issues and was chipping away protections that were included in key federal statutes.

It is also interesting to note how similar the Affordable Care Act is to earlier proposals like the bipartisan Hill-Aiken bill, including Republican proposals, such as Senator John Chafee's 1993 health reform bill, the Health Equity and Access Reform Today Act of 1993 and President George W. Bush's 2005 proposal involving tax credits. It seems that a Democratic administration must push closer to the right to hope for success, and vice versa. Proposals may start out strongly leaning liberal or conservative, but eventually after negotiation and compromise, they all seem to adopt a middle-ground approach. In addition, although the health care law is not identical to past bills, it is, nonetheless, a combination of many organized parts—sections or provisions—that over the decades had been carefully vetted in a bipartisan manner. So while the final bill itself ultimately did not enjoy bipartisan support, its individual parts had always enjoyed bipartisan support through the years.

Finally, it is significant that much of the advocacy highlighted in this chapter involved efforts to block or bring down health reform proposals, for example, the campaigns against President Truman's national insurance plans and President Clinton's comprehensive health reform plan. In these cases, advocates against a particular measure managed to be louder and more effective. With President Obama's health plan, the reverse was finally true, as will be highlighted in the next chapter.

NOTES

1. "The Bundle of Sticks," *Aesop's Fables.*

2. John F. Kennedy, inaugural address.

3. Manning, "Tragedy of the Ten-Million-Acre Bill," 44.

4. Cong. Globe, 31st Cong., 2d sess., February 11, 1851, p. 507; Manning, "Tragedy of the Ten-Million-Acre Bill," 45–46.

5. Pierce, "Veto Message."

6. Grob, "Public Policy and Mental Illnesses," 426; "American Presidents and Health Reform."

7. Kemp, *Mental Health in America.*

8. Grob, "Public Policy and Mental Illnesses," 425–426, 430.

9. Ibid., 442, 445.

10. Carter, "Mental Health Systems Legislation Message"; Carter, "Mental Health Systems Act Remarks on Signing"; Grob, "Public Policy and Mental Illnesses," 445. The correct title of the statute that President Kennedy signed

into law is the Mental Retardation Facilities and Community Mental Health Centers Construction Act of 1963.

11. *Sutton v. United Air Lines*; *Toyota Motor Manufacturing v. Williams.*

12. Edward M. Kennedy, "Role of the Federal Government in Eliminating Health Disparities," 453.

13. Rice, *Public Policy and the Black Hospital*, 5.

14. Ibid., 6.

15. The National Medical Association is the nation's oldest and largest organization representing African American physicians and health professionals in the United States. It was founded in 1895 during the Jim Crow era when black physicians were excluded from various professional associations, including the American Medical Association.

The National Dental Association, the nation's oldest and largest organization representing African American dentists and other health professionals in the United States, followed in 1900, likewise in response to the Jim Crow-era exclusion of black dentists from various professional associations, including the American Dental Association.

16. Northington Gamble and Stone, "U.S. Policy on Health Inequities."

17. The education cases included *Meyer v. Nebraska* (1923), *Missouri ex rel. Gaines v. Canada* (1938), *Sweatt v. Painter* and *McLaurin v. Oklahoma State Regents* (1950), and *Brown v. Board of Education* (1955). Interestingly, a year before, in 1955, Congress decided to create a federal agency that would provide health services to tribal members. In 1955, the Indian Health Service was established to provide comprehensive and culturally competent health services to American Indians and Alaska Natives.

18. Passed March 1, 1875, this legislation was titled An Act to Protect All Citizens in Their Civil and Legal Rights. 18 Stat. 335.

19. *The Civil Rights Cases*. The lone dissenting Justice in this case was Justice Harlan, who was also the only judge to dissent from the Court's holding in *Plessy v. Ferguson*. The Court reasoned that the Constitution "does not invest Congress with power to legislate upon subjects which are within the domain of State legislation; but to provide modes of relief against State legislation, or State action, of the kind referred to. It does not authorize Congress to create a code of municipal law for the regulation of private rights; but to provide modes of redress against the operation of State laws, and the action of State officers, executive or judicial, when these are subversive of the fundamental rights specified in the amendment." The Court further reasoned:

> An inspection of the law shows that it makes no reference whatever to any supposed or apprehended violation of the Fourteenth Amendment on the part of the states. It is not predicated on any such view. It proceeds *ex directo* to declare that certain acts committed by individuals shall be

deemed offenses, and shall be prosecuted and punished by proceedings in the courts of the United States. It does not profess to be corrective of any constitutional wrong committed by the States; it does not make its operation to depend upon any such wrong committed. It applies equally to cases arising in states which have the justest laws respecting the personal rights of citizens, and whose authorities are ever ready to enforce such laws as to those which arise in States that may have violated the prohibition of the amendment. In other words, it steps into the domain of local jurisprudence, and lays down rules for the conduct of individuals in society towards each other, and imposes sanctions for the enforcement of those rules, without referring in any manner to any supposed action of the state or its authorities.

The Court also reasoned that it was

proper to state that civil rights, such as are guaranteed by the Constitution against State aggression, cannot be impaired by the wrongful acts of individuals, unsupported by State authority in the shape of laws, customs, or judicial or executive proceedings. The wrongful act of an individual, unsupported by any such authority, is simply a private wrong, or a crime of that individual; an invasion of the rights of the injured party, it is true, whether they affect his person, his property, or his reputation; but if not sanctioned in some way by the State, or not done under State authority, his rights remain in full force, and may presumably be vindicated by resort to the laws of the State for redress.

20. Hasnain-Wynia and Beal, "The Path to Equitable Health Care."

21. Shirley Chisholm (D-NY), William L. Clay (D-MO), George W. Collins (D-IL), John Conyers (D-MI), Ronald Dellums (D-CA), Charles Diggs (D-MI), Augustus F. Hawkins (D-CA), Ralph Metcalfe (D-IL), Parren Mitchell (D-MD), Robert Nix Sr. (D-PA), Charles B. Rangel (D-NY), Louis Stokes (D-OH), and Washington, DC, delegate Walter Fauntroy.

22. Crayton, "Changing Face of the Congressional Black Caucus"; "Stokes, Louis," History, Art & Archives, U.S. House of Representatives; Congressional Black Caucus website; "Creation and Evolution of the Congressional Black Caucus," *History, Art & Archives United States House of Representatives.*

23. Crayton, "Changing Face of the Congressional Black Caucus."

24. Brain trusts that were established early on in the late 1970s included Arts & Humanities, Aging, Communications, Criminal Justice, Education, Employment/Inflation, Foreign Affairs, Housing, Minority Enterprise, Voter Participation, and Science & Technology.

25. Ways and Means had jurisdiction over taxes, Medicare, and Medicaid; Energy and Commerce had jurisdiction over major health policy issues.

26. Invited speakers included the leaders of the National Black Nurses Association, National Dental Association, National Medical Association, and the National Society of Allied Health.

27. Representative Louis Stokes's Health Braintrust directors included Yvette Hutchinson, Millicent Gorham, Jacqueline Bowens, Leslie Atkinson, Fredette West, and Angela Blount. Under Congresswoman Christensen's leadership, the Health Braintrust staff included Aranthan Jones and Britt Weinstock.

28. Herman Badillo (D-NY), Baltasar Corrada del Río (NPP-PR), Kika de la Garza (D-TX), Henry B. Gonzalez (D-TX), and Edward R. Roybal (D-CA).

29. Although the Native American Caucus was not officially a member of this group, the Tri-Caucus made it its duty to ensure that issues impacting American Indians, Alaska Natives, and Native Hawaiians were addressed. The Native American Caucus believed its issues were unique, and since it was a bipartisan caucus with Republican leadership the two caucuses' objectives did not always align.

30. The term was formally embraced by each of the racial/ethnic congressional caucuses in the early 2000s and first appeared in the congressional record on May 11, 2004, when Congresswoman Hilda Solis mentioned all three caucuses as the Tri-Caucus.

31. Institute of Medicine, *Health Care in a Context of Civil Rights*; Association of Minority Health Professions Schools, *Blacks and the Health Professions in the 1980s*.

32. US Department of Health and Human Services, *Report of the Secretary's Task Force on Black and Minority Health*, 2.

33. *Health Status and Needs of Minorities in the 1990s*.

34. Ibid. (testimony of Louis Stokes, emphasis added).

35. Cong. Rec. S31182 (October 19, 1990).

36. It was codified into law three years later by the National Institutes of Health Revitalization Act of 1993 (P.L. 103-43). This law also established an Office of Research on Women's Health and required the director of NIH to ensure the inclusion of women and minorities in clinical research.

37. The Ryan White CARE Act provided these individuals and families with care and support services, filling in the gaps in care for those with no other source of coverage or who faced coverage limits.

38. US Department of Health and Human Services, *Healthy People 2000*.

39. The Honorable Norman Mineta later went on to serve as secretary of commerce in the Clinton administration, making him the first Asian American to serve in a presidential cabinet post, as well as secretary of transportation in the George W. Bush administration.

40. Clinton, "Press Briefing by Secretary of H.H.S. Donna Shalala and Surgeon General Dr. David Satcher."

41. Friedman, "Separate and Unequal."

42. US Department of Health and Human Services, *Healthy People 2000.*

43. Not to be confused with the Advisory Committee on Research on Minority Health established for the Office of Research on Minority Health at NIH.

44. Initially this bill (S. 1880) was called the Health Care Fairness Act of 1999 when it was introduced by Senator Kennedy, but an amendment by Senator Bill Frist to completely substitute the bill almost a year after it was introduced changed the title to Minority Health and Health Disparities Research and Education Act of 2000 and tweaked certain sections in the original bill. This bill also included elements of the National Center for Domestic Health Disparities Act, which was sponsored by the following bipartisan group of congressional members: Donna Christensen, Jesse Jackson Jr., and Charlie Norwood.

45. The Health Care Fairness Act was originally introduced by Senators Edward Kennedy, Daniel Akaka, Daniel Inouye, Blanche Lincoln, and Paul Wellstone, but after almost a year of negotiations by advocates and congressional champions, Republican leaders also joined and supported the bill.

46. The Office of Research on Minority Health was codified and elevated into a center at NIH, now called the NCMHD.

47. The agency was created in December 1989 as the Agency for Health Care Policy and Research and reauthorized by the Healthcare Research and Quality Act of 1999 ten years later on December 6, 1999, as the Agency for Healthcare Research and Quality. The AHRQ had been created in response to emerging research showing significant variations in Medicare spending in different regions of the country, and that people living in the regions showing higher spending did not have better health outcomes. US Department of Health and Human Services, "Agency for Healthcare Research and Quality," in *Guidelines.* In March 2015, AHRQ combined these two reports into one single report in order to show the nexus between quality and health equity.

48. Agency for Healthcare Research and Quality, *National Healthcare Disparities Report, 2003.*

49. This report was a supplement to the 1999 report issued by Dr. David Satcher, *Mental Health: A Report of the Surgeon General,* which also included some information about racial and ethnic disparities, diversity, and cultural competence.

50. Institute of Medicine, *Unequal Treatment.*

51. The Healthcare Equality and Accountability Act would eventually be referred to as the Tri-Caucus health disparities bill.

52. 150 Cong. Rec. H487-05 (February 11, 2004) WL 251901. According to Rep. McDermott:

Let me give my colleagues an example. The first sentence of the original health disparities report circulated last June said, and I quote, "Inequalities in health care that affect some racial, ethnic, socioeconomic and geographic subpopulations in the United States ultimately affect every American." The alteration was, "The overall health of Americans has improved dramatically over the last century." One would hardly think they were talking about the same subject. It is a whitewash. It is a blatant disregard for the American people and an insult to every person of color. This was a study we commissioned to find out about the health disparities between groups in this country. Congress asked for science, and the administration's spin doctors buried it. They hid it from view and substituted their own version of the country. In the June original document, the Department's scientists found "significant inequality" in health care. The last one, the doctored one, became "national problems." The scientists emphasized that these disparities are "pervasive in our health care system." The whitewash omitted those conclusions. Text describing data tables inside the paper was altered. In the key findings section, the whitewash omitted 28 of the 30 references to disparity. Everything was done to hide the real facts from people of color, from every citizen in America.

53. Agency for Healthcare Research and Quality, *National Healthcare Disparities Report, 2003.*

54. Edward M. Kennedy, "Role of the Federal Government in Eliminating Health Disparities."

55. The National Association of Public Hospitals and Health Systems is now known as America's Essential Hospitals.

56. Hoenisch, "Health Care Policy of the Republican Party"; Ungar, "Congress Passes Socialized Medicine and Mandates Health Insurance—in 1798."

57. Ungar, "Congress Passes Socialized Medicine and Mandates Health Insurance—in 1798."

58. Theodore Roosevelt, "Seventh Annual Message."

59. Centers for Medicare and Medicaid Services, *Tracing the History of CMS Programs*; Hoffman, "Health Care Reform and Social Movements in the United States," 76.

60. Social Security Administration, "Chronology of Significant Events Leading to Enactment of Medicare," *Social Security History*; Heisdorffer, "Timeline."

61. Heisdorffer, "Timeline," 1.

62. Igel, "History of Health Care as a Campaign Issue," 13; Miller Center of Public Affairs, "Franklin D. Roosevelt"; Heisdorffer, "Timeline."

63. Franklin D. Roosevelt, "Statement on Signing the Social Security Act"; Miller Center of Public Affairs, "Franklin D. Roosevelt."

64. Coates, "Case for Reparations."

65. *Steward Machine Company v. Davis* upheld the Social Security Act in a 5-4 vote and another case that was decided on the same day challenging the Social Security Act, *Helvering v. Davis*, upheld the statute in a 7-2 decision.

66. Hospitals & Health Networks, "American Presidents and Health Reform."

67. Truman, "Special Message to the Congress Recommending a Comprehensive Health Program"; Igel, "History of Health Care as a Campaign Issue," 12; Schremmer and Knapp, "Harry Truman and Health Care Reform," 399.

68. Wolfensberger, "Health Care Reform and the Medicare Analogy," 2.

69. Quadagno, "Why the United States Has No National Health Insurance."

70. Truman, "Annual Message to the Congress on the State of the Union"; Morone, "Presidents and Health Reform," 1097.

71. Quadagno, "Why the United States Has No National Health Insurance."

72. Ibid.; Schremmer and Knapp, "Harry Truman and Health Care Reform."

73. Igel, "History of Health Care as a Campaign Issue," 13; Hoenisch, "Health Care Policy of the Republican Party."

74. Quadagno, "Why the United States Has No National Health Insurance."

75. Eisenhower, "Annual Message to the Congress on the State of the Union."

76. Wolfensberger, "Health Care Reform and the Medicare Analogy," 5.

77. John F. Kennedy, "Annual Message to the Congress on the State of the Union."

78. John F. Kennedy, "Address at a New York Rally in Support of the President's Program of Medical Care for the Aged."

79. Igel, "History of Health Care as a Campaign Issue," 14; Hoffman, "Health Care Reform and Social Movements in the United States," 78.

80. Centers for Medicare and Medicaid Services, *Tracing the History of CMS Programs*; Johnson, "Remarks with President Truman at the Signing in Independence of the Medicare Bill"; Centers for Medicare and Medicaid Services, *Tracing the History of CMS Programs*.

81. Quadagno, "Why the United States Has No National Health Insurance," 31.

82. Ibid., 33.

83. Heisdorffer, "Timeline," 2; Igel, "History of Health Care as a Campaign Issue," 14; Centers for Medicare and Medicaid Services, *Tracing the History of CMS Programs*.

84. Quadagno, "Why the United States Has No National Health Insurance," 34.

85. Ibid.

86. Ford, "Address before a Joint Session of the Congress Reporting on the State of the Union" (emphasis added).

87. Finbow, "Presidential Leadership or Structural Complaints?," 172, 178.

88. Ibid.

89. Ibid.

90. Hoenisch, "Health Care Policy of the Republican Party"; Morone, "Presidents and Health Reform," 1098.

91. Quadagno, "Why the United States Has No National Health Insurance," 35.

92. Centers for Medicare and Medicaid Services, *Tracing the History of CMS Programs.*

93. George H. W. Bush, "Address before a Joint Session of the Congress on the State of the Union."

94. Caplan, "Clinton's Health Care Reforms," 813.

95. Clinton, "Address before a Joint Session of Congress on Administration Goals."

96. Two Democrats cosponsored the bill.

97. Lefebrvre, "Health Reform in the United States," 319. The Health Insurance Association of America is now known as America's Health Insurance Plans.

98. Quadagno, "Why the United States Has No National Health Insurance," 38; Caplan, "Clinton's Health Care Reforms," 813.

99. Clinton, "Address before a Joint Session of the Congress on the State of the Union."

100. Bush, George W. "Address before a Joint Session of the Congress on the State of the Union."

101. Bacon, "Clinton Presents Plan for Universal Coverage"; Brooks, "Vince Lombardi Politics"; Nather, "How the Clinton White House Bungled Health Care Reform."

BIBLIOGRAPHY

Agency for Healthcare Research and Quality. *National Healthcare Disparities Report, 2003.* Rockville, MD, 2004. http://archive.ahrq.gov/qual/nhdr03/nhdrsum03.htm.

Association of Minority Health Professions Schools. *Blacks and the Health Professions in the 1980s: A National Crisis and a Time for Action,* June 1983.

Bacon, Perry, Jr. "Clinton Presents Plan for Universal Coverage." *Washington Post,* September 18, 2007. http://www.washingtonpost.com/wp-dyn/content/article/2007/09/17/AR2007091701026_2.html.

Braithwaite, Ronald L., Sandra E. Taylor, and Henrie M. Treadwell, eds. *Health Issues in the Black Community.* 3rd ed. San Francisco: Jossey-Bass, 2010.

Brooks, David. "Vince Lombardi Politics." *New York Times,* June 30, 2009. http://www.nytimes.com/2009/06/30/opinion/30brooks.html?_r.

Brown v. Board of Education, 349 U.S. 294 (1955).

"The Bundle of Sticks," *Aesop's Fables.* http://www.umass.edu/aesop/content.php?n=4&i=1.

Bush, George H. W. "Address before a Joint Session of the Congress on the State of the Union," January 28, 1992. Online by Gerhard Peters and John T. Woolley, *The American Presidency Project.* http://www.presidency.ucsb.edu/ws/index.php?pid=20544#axzz1itPInr00.

Bush, George W. "Address before a Joint Session of the Congress on the State of the Union," February 2, 2005. Online by Gerhard Peters and John T. Woolley, *The American Presidency Project*. http://www.presidency.ucsb.edu /ws/index.php?pid=58746#axzz1itPInr00.

Caplan, Art. "Clinton's Health Care Reforms: An Unstoppable Momentum for Change." *British Medical Journal* 307, no. 6908 (October 2, 1993): 813-814.

Carter, Jimmy. "Mental Health Systems Act Remarks on Signing S. 1177 into Law," October 7, 1980. Online by Gerhard Peters and John T. Woolley, *The American Presidency Project*. http://www.presidency.ucsb.edu/ws/?pid=45228.

———. "Mental Health Systems Legislation Message to the Congress Transmitting the Proposed Legislation," May 15, 1979. Online by Gerhard Peters and John T. Woolley, *The American Presidency Project*. http://www.presidency .ucsb.edu/ws/?pid=32339.

Centers for Medicare and Medicaid Services. *Tracing the History of CMS Programs: From President Theodore Roosevelt to President George W. Bush*. Baltimore, October 29, 2013. http://www.cms.gov/About-CMS/Agency-Information /History/Downloads/PresidentCMSMilestones.pdf.

The Civil Rights Cases, 109 U.S. 3 (1883).

Clinton, William J. "Address before a Joint Session of Congress on Administration Goals," February 17, 1993. Online by Gerhard Peters and John T. Woolley, *The American Presidency Project*. http://www.presidency.ucsb.edu /ws/index.php?pid=47232.

———. "Address before a Joint Session of the Congress on the State of the Union," January 24, 1995. Online by Gerhard Peters and John T. Woolley, *The American Presidency Project*. http://www.presidency.ucsb.edu/ws/index .php?pid=51634#axzz1itPInr00.

———. "Press Briefing by Secretary of H.H.S. Donna Shalala and Surgeon General Dr. David Satcher," February 21, 1998. Online by Gerhard Peters and John T. Woolley, *The American Presidency Project*. http://www.presidency .ucsb.edu/ws/?pid=48378.

Coates, Ta-Nehisi. "The Case for Reparations." *Atlantic*, June 2014. http://www .theatlantic.com/features/archive/2014/05/the-case-for-reparations/361631/.

Colorado State University. "A Brief History of Legislation." *Resources for Disabled Students*. http://rds.colostate.edu/history-of-legislation.

Congressional Black Caucus website. http://cbc-butterfield.house.gov/.

Congressional Globe. 31st Cong., 2d sess. February 11, 1851.

Congressional Record. H487-05 (February 11, 2004) WL 251901.

Congressional Record. S31182. October 19, 1990.

Crayton, Kareem. "The Changing Face of the Congressional Black Caucus." *Southern California Interdisciplinary Law Journal* 19 (2010): 473-500.

"Creation and Evolution of the Congressional Black Caucus," *History, Art & Archives, U.S. House of Representatives*. Washington, DC: US Government

Printing Office, 2008. http://history.house.gov/Exhibitions-and-Publications
/BAIC/Historical-Essays/Permanent-Interest/Congressional-Black-Caucus/.

Eisenhower, Dwight D. "Annual Message to the Congress on the State of the
Union," January 5, 1956. Online by Gerhard Peters and John T. Woolley, *The
American Presidency Project.* http://www.presidency.ucsb.edu/ws/index.php
?pid=10593#axzz1jvpiDND6.

Finbow, Robert. "Presidential Leadership or Structural Constraints? The Failure
of President Carter's Health Insurance Proposals." *Presidential Studies
Quarterly* 28, no. 1 (Winter 1998): 169–186.

Ford, Gerald. "Address before a Joint Session of the Congress Reporting on the
State of the Union," January 19, 1976. http://www.ford.utexas.edu/library
/speeches/760019.asp.

Friedman, Emily. "Separate and Unequal." *Health Forum Journal* (September
2002). http://www.emilyfriedman.com/columns/2002-09-separate-and
-unequal.html.

Grob, Gerald, N. "Public Policy and Mental Illnesses: Jimmy Carter's Presidential
Commission on Mental Health." *Milbank Quarterly* 83, no. 3 (2005): 425–456.

Hasnain-Wynia, Romana, and Anne C. Beal. "The Path to Equitable Health
Care." *Health Services Research* 47, no. 4 (2012): 1411–1417. http://www.ncbi
.nlm.nih.gov/pmc/articles/PMC3401391/.

*Health Status and Needs of Minorities in the 1990s: Hearing before the Subcommittee
on Health and the Environment of the Committee on Energy and Commerce, House
of Representatives.* 101st Congress. Second session, June 8, 1990.

Heisdorffer, Allison. "Timeline: Presidential Influence on Health Care Reform
throughout the 20th Century." *Columbia Missourian*, March 23, 2010.
http://www.columbiamissourian.com/a/124341/timeline-presidential
-influence-on-health-care-reform-throughout-20th-century/.

Helvering v. Davis, 301 U.S. 619 (1937).

Hoenisch, Steve. "Health Care Policy of the Republican Party." *The Encyclopedia
of the American Democratic and Republican Parties.* Last updated on July 29,
2004. http://www.criticism.com/policy/republicans-health-care-policy.php.

Hoffman, Beatrix. "Health Care Reform and Social Movements in the United
States." *American Journal of Public Health* 93, no. 1 (January 2003), 75–85.

Hospitals & Health Networks, "American Presidents and Health Reform: A
Chronology," *H&HN Magazine*, February 2009.

Igel, Lee. "The History of Health Care as a Campaign Issue." *Physician Executive*
(May 2008): 12–15.

Iglehart, John. "Health Policy Report: The American Health System—
Introduction." *New England Journal of Medicine* 326, no. 14 (April 2, 1992):
962–967.

Institute of Medicine. *Health Care in a Context of Civil Rights.* Washington, DC:
National Academy of Sciences Press, 1981.

———. *How Far Have We Come in Reducing Health Disparities? Progress since 2000; Workshop Summary*. Washington, DC: National Academies Press, 2012.

———. *Unequal Treatment: Confronting Racial and Ethnic Disparities in Health Care*. Washington, DC: National Academies Press, 2012.

Johnson, Lyndon B. "Remarks with President Truman at the Signing in Independence of the Medicare Bill," July 30, 1965. http://www.lbjlib.utexas.edu /johnson/archives.hom/speeches.hom/650730.asp.

Kemp, Donna R. *Mental Health in America: A Reference Handbook*: Santa Barbara, CA: ABC-CLIO, 2007.

Kennedy, Edward M. "The Role of the Federal Government in Eliminating Health Disparities." *Health Affairs* 24, no. 2 (March 2005): 452–458.

Kennedy, John F. "Address at a New York Rally in Support of the President's Program of Medical Care for the Aged," May 20, 1962. http://www.jfklibrary .org/Asset-Viewer/Archives/JFKWHA-096.aspx.

———. "Annual Message to the Congress on the State of the Union," January 30, 1961. Online by Gerhard Peters and John T. Woolley, *The American Presidency Project*. http://www.presidency.ucsb.edu/ws/index.php?pid =8045#axzz1itPInr00.

———. Inaugural address, January 20, 1961. John F. Kennedy Presidential Library and Museum. http://www.jfklibrary.org/Research/Research-Aids /Ready-Reference/JFK-Quotations/Inaugural-Address.aspx.

Lefebrvre, R. Craig. "Health Reform in the United States: A Social Marketing Perspective." *Journal of Public Policy & Marketing* 13, no. 2 (Fall 1994): 319–320.

Manning, Seaton W. "The Tragedy of the Ten-Million-Acre Bill." *Social Service Review* 36, no. 1 (March 1962): 44–50.

McLaurin v. Oklahoma State Regents, 339 U.S. 637 (1950).

McRoberts, Robert. "U.S. Presidents and Health Care Reform: The History of Public Health Politics in America." *Suite*, September 10, 2009. https://suite.io /robert-mcroberts/27xv2z5.

Meyer v. Nebraska, 262 U.S. 390 (1923).

Miller Center of Public Affairs, University of Virginia. "Franklin D. Roosevelt: Domestic Affairs." *American President*. Accessed July 28, 2015. http:// millercenter.org/president/biography/fdroosevelt-domestic-affairs.

———. "Theodore Roosevelt: Domestic Affairs." Accessed July 28, 2015. *American President*. http://millercenter.org/president/biography/roosevelt-domestic -affairs.

Missouri ex rel. Gaines v. Canada, 305 U.S. 337 (1938).

Morone, James A. "Presidents and Health Reform: From Franklin D. Roosevelt to Barack Obama." *Health Affairs* 29, no. 6 (2010): 1096–1100.

Nather, David. "How the Clinton White House Bungled Health Care Reform." *Politico*, February 28, 2014. http://www.politico.com/story/2014/02/bill -hillary-clinton-health-care-reform-104109.html.

Northington Gamble, Vanessa, and Deborah Stone. "U.S. Policy on Health Inequities: The Interplay of Politics and Research," *Journal of Health Politics, Policy and Law* 31 (February 2006): 93-122. http://academic.udayton.edu /health/11disparities/Disparities07.htm.

Pierce, Franklin. "Veto Message," May 3, 1854. Online by Gerhard Peters and John T. Woolley, *The American Presidency Project*. http://www.presidency .ucsb.edu/ws/?pid=67850.

Quadagno, Jill. "Why the United States Has No National Health Insurance: Stakeholder Mobilization against the Welfare State." In "Health and Health Care in the United States: Origins and Dynamics," special issue, *Journal of Health and Social Behavior* 45 (2004): 25-44.

Quinn, Sandra C., and Stephen B. Thomas. "The National Negro Health Week, 1915 to 1951: A Descriptive Account." *Minority Health Today* 2, no. 3 (March/ April 2001): 44-49.

Rice, Mitchell. *Public Policy and the Black Hospital: From Slavery to Segregation to Integration*. Westport, CT: Greenwood, 1994.

Roosevelt, Franklin D. "Statement on Signing the Social Security Act," August 14, 1935. Online by Gerhard Peters and John T. Woolley, *The American Presidency Project*. http://www.presidency.ucsb.edu/ws/?pid=14916.

Roosevelt, Theodore. "Seventh Annual Message," December 3, 1907. Online by Gerhard Peters and John T. Woolley, *The American Presidency Project*. http://www.presidency.ucsb.edu/ws/?pid=29548.

Schremmer, Robert D., and Jane F. Knapp. "Harry Truman and Health Care Reform: The Debate Started Here." *Pediatrics* 127, no. 3 (March 2011): 399-401.

Smith, Susan L. "Teaching the History of Public Health and Health Reform." *OAH Magazine of History* 19, no. 5 (September 2005): 27-29.

Social Security Administration. "Chronology of Significant Events Leading to Enactment of Medicare." *Social Security History*, appendix A. http://www.ssa .gov/history/cornignappa.html.

State of the Union and Healthcare: 100 Years of Good Intentions. http://www .medscape.com/features/slideshow/sotu.

Steward Machine Company v. Davis, 301 U.S. 548 (1937).

"Stokes, Louis." *History, Art & Archives, U.S. House of Representatives*. Accessed November 26, 2014. http://history.house.gov/People/Detail/22311.

Sutton v. United Air Lines, Inc., 527 U.S. 471 (1999).

Sweatt v. Painter, 339 U.S. 629 (1950).

"This Day in Truman History—November 19, 1945: President Truman's Proposed Health Program." *Harry S. Truman Library & Museum*. http://www .trumanlibrary.org/anniversaries/healthprogram.htm.

Toyota Motor Manufacturing, Kentucky, Inc., v. Williams, 534 U.S. 184 (2002).

Truman, Harry. "Annual Message to the Congress on the State of the Union." January 7, 1948. Online by Gerhard Peters and John T. Woolley, *The*

American Presidency Project. http://www.presidency.ucsb.edu/ws/index.php?pid=13005#axzzlic2XE7I4.

———. "Special Message to the Congress Recommending a Comprehensive Health Program," November 19, 1945. Online by Gerhard Peters and John T. Woolley, *The American Presidency Project.* http://www.presidency.ucsb.edu/ws/index.php?pid=12288&st=&stl.

US Department of Health and Human Services. "Agency for Healthcare Research and Quality." In *Guidelines for Ensuring the Quality of Information Disseminated to the Public.* Last revised December 13, 2006. http://aspe.hhs.gov/infoquality/Guidelines/AHRQinfo.shtml.

———. *Healthy People 2000.* Washington, DC: US Department of Health and Human Services, 1990.

———. *Mental Health: Culture, Race, and Ethnicity—A Supplement to Mental Health: A Report of the Surgeon General.* Rockville, MD: US Department of Health and Human Services, 2001.

———. *Report of the Secretary's Task Force on Black and Minority Health.* Washington, DC: US Department of Health and Human Services, 1985.

Ungar, Rick. "Congress Passes Socialized Medicine and Mandates Health Insurance—in 1798." *Forbes,* January 17, 2011. http://www.forbes.com/sites/rickungar/2011/01/17/congress-passes-socialized-medicine-and-mandates-health-insurance-in-1798/.

Wolfensberger, Don. "Health Care Reform and the Medicare Analogy: An Introductory Essay." Paper presented at the Seminar on Universal Health Care at the Woodrow Wilson International Center for Scholars, Washington, DC, September 21, 2009.

3

Pulling Back the Curtain
The Advocacy for Health Reform and Health Equity

A good president or a new Congress is only going to be as good as the citizens outside demanding it. —*Marian Wright Edelman, President of the Children's Defense Fund*

The Beginning of Change

The year 2008 was an exhilarating time to be involved in health equity advocacy. Presidential elections were taking place in November, and health reform was proving to be a major campaign issue. Republican candidate John McCain proposed improving the quality of health insurance through competition. McCain's plan would provide individuals with tax credits to purchase insurance and loosen state rules governing the sale of insurance by allowing people to buy policies across state lines. Though he opposed federally mandated universal coverage, McCain was the first candidate to endorse the use of universal tax credits to provide access to private health insurance.[1] Republican candidate Mitt Romney also endorsed a system of tax deductions to help individuals buy insurance. Romney, despite having enacted universal coverage in Massachusetts while governor of that state, disavowed mandated coverage on a national level. He proposed allowing states to devise their own insurance plans and providing states with financial incentives to deregulate their health insurance markets.

The Republican primaries were short lived, with John McCain securing the nomination by March 2008. By contrast, the Democratic primary contest ran well into the summer. The final two candidates, Barack Obama and Hillary Clinton, both listed health reform as a major priority and endorsed proposals seeking to make health insurance affordable for all Americans. Unlike the Republican proposals, which emphasized using market competition to control health care costs, the Democratic candidates sought to increase the government's involvement in the health care system. Both candidates' proposals provided for government-offered insurance plans; however, while Clinton's plan would require that everyone have insurance, Obama's plan did not.

Both candidates also would prevent private insurers from denying health insurance on the basis of preexisting conditions—an issue that resonated with millions of Americans. In fact, this particular issue hit close to home for many families who struggled to get affordable health coverage. Even independent insurance agents who had been selling health insurance for years were not immune to exclusion from coverage on the basis of their preexisting conditions. Whether McCain or one of the two remaining Democratic candidates won the election, it was clear that some kind of health reform package was possible with the next administration. Past failures at passing health reform did not mean it was impossible to achieve this feat. This was the atmosphere of the time, of potentially sweeping reform, and we knew major changes were ahead.

The possibility of health reform became especially evident when the Senate Finance Committee on May 6, 2008, under the leadership of Max Baucus (D-MT), held the first in a series of hearings on health reform during the second session of the 110th Congress, titled *Seizing the New Opportunity for Health Reform*. The hearings would take place over the next year, when the 111th Congress would more than likely be tackling these issues. Their purpose was to lay the foundation for developing policy and building consensus "on how to provide access to affordable high-quality health care for all Americans." Unlike in 1993, when the Senate Finance Committee chair Daniel Patrick Moynihan (D-NY) was not particularly enthusiastic about health reform, Senator Baucus expressed his confidence that, this time around, he and his colleagues would succeed in passing a health reform bill.

During the hearings Baucus underscored that the issues impacting the health care system had become unmanageable, the incremental or piecemeal solutions Congress employed to date were simply inadequate, and the problems would only get worse before they got better unless Congress meaningfully addressed them. From his standpoint, the moral and economic argument for health reform had never been stronger, and the health reform proposals that had been developed by both Democrats and Republicans over the decades showed striking similarities and shared principles, including universal health coverage and greater protections for consumers and providers, value-based purchasing, comparative effectiveness research, and greater use of health information technology and electronic health records.

In addition, Baucus believed that the opportunity was ripe, since it was increasingly evident there was unprecedented eagerness to work together to fix these problems in our health care and public health systems "among major health care stakeholders, interest groups, coalitions, and even presidential candidates." He did, however, recognize the challenges that were ahead despite these significant gains in consensus. The committee would have to resolve key issues such as whether to mandate health insurance coverage, how to finance universal health insurance coverage, and what roles the federal government, state governments, employers, and families should play.

Senator Chuck Grassley (R-IA) of Iowa, the ranking member of the committee, also acknowledged the growing and costly problem of uninsurance in our country—how difficult it was for many Americans to access affordable coverage. Just like Baucus, Grassley recognized that the incremental solutions Congress had initiated to date were not effective in curbing health care costs. He believed that private market solutions were the best route and issued a warning to the committee about not repeating past mistakes or disrupting the system too much:

> It makes the most sense to build on the private health insurance system. As you all know, people are used to their employer providing health benefits. They like their employers' work and they do not want us to disturb that. They like that their employers take care of their billing, and by and large they are satisfied. We learned 14 years ago during the Clinton health plan debate that, even in the midst of call for change, many people like what they have. So health reform should not up-end the system and do harm while trying to help folks without insurance. I also think we need to be prudent in taking on new obligations through government.[2]

Senator Grassley warned that any health reform package must be bipartisan and should have broad support among the American people. He stated that although these were "tough policy problems," he was "encouraged that the issue is back on the table."[3]

At the hearing ideas were solicited from two former secretaries of health and human services, Donna Shalala from the Clinton administration and Tommy Thompson from the Bush administration. Shalala emphasized the areas of consensus between both sides that Senator Baucus had outlined earlier, which included addressing the health workforce issue. She echoed Senator Grassley's warning about being extremely careful when developing a bill that would impact virtually everyone—a lesson she had learned in 1993. Shalala also urged the committee to reach consensus on not only the problem but the solutions.

Secretary Thompson also used his time to emphasize the need for health reform to reduce costs and to accomplish this in a bipartisan manner. Like Senator Baucus, he recognized that all three presidential candidates had elevated health reform in their campaigns and urged the next president of the United States to convene a commission with an equal number of Republicans and Democrats to offer recommendations for health reform. Interestingly, Thompson was the first in the hearing to emphasize the need to address wellness and prevention of chronic disease in a health reform bill—moving from a disease system to a wellness system. He was also the first person to mention the urgent need to address racial and ethnic health disparities, stating, "But there are ways in which we can get information out on nutrition, which we really have to do, especially with minorities. Being overweight leads into diabetes, which is an epidemic in Native Americans, Latinos, and African Americans. *We have to do something about it.*"[4]

After this hearing, House and Senate committee chairs and their staff who had jurisdiction over health care issues convened informal discussions and strategic planning around health reform. When it became apparent that these discussions were taking place, health equity advocates knew this was an opportunity of a lifetime we had to seize immediately. Taking Thompson's words to heart, we were convinced it was time to take action to inform lawmakers about the health policy issues impacting vulnerable and underserved communities in the United States.

Around this period, it was announced that Senator Edward M. Kennedy, who chaired the Senate Health, Education, Labor and Pensions Committee, had been diagnosed with a malignant brain tumor and required aggressive treatments. Kennedy had dedicated much of his career to ensuring that all Americans had access to high-quality, affordable health care, and in speaking of health reform in *Newsweek*, he said, "This is the cause of my life." In 1971, he became the chair of the Senate health subcommittee and began his campaign for national health insurance. Among the many landmark laws enacted under his leadership and sponsorship over the years were the Protection and Advocacy for Mentally Ill Individuals Act of 1986, the Americans with Disabilities Act of 1990, the Ryan White

Comprehensive AIDS Resources Emergency Act of 1990, the National Institutes of Health Revitalization Act of 1993, the Health Insurance Portability and Accountability Act of 1996, the Mental Health Parity Act of 1996, and the creation of the State Children's Health Insurance Program in 1997. Despite his illness, Kennedy declared his commitment to realizing health reform once and for all: "I am resolved to see to it this year that we create a system to ensure that someday, when there is a cure for the disease I now have, no American who needs it will be denied it."[5]

In the midst of this upheaval in the health policy arena, a major news story broke that brought the issue of health disparities to light in a tragic way. Esmin Green was a forty-nine-year-old African American woman who had been brought to the emergency room of a local hospital on the morning of June 18, 2008. Hospital records stated that she was exhibiting agitation and psychosis and was involuntarily admitted after refusing treatment. During the first week of July, major news media outlets aired a video showing Green sitting in a waiting room at a hospital in New York for nearly twenty-four hours and then collapsing from her chair. Once she collapsed, neither fellow patients nor the hospital's staff moved to help her, even as she writhed on the floor trying to get up. Two security guards and a member of the hospital's medical staff could be seen on the video, briefly stopping to look at Green before walking away. She stopped moving roughly thirty minutes after falling and was dead when a nurse finally examined her another thirty minutes after that. According to the medical examiner, she had died after developing blood clots in her legs from the long period of physical inactivity.[6] The widespread outcry from the public spurred health equity advocates into action and provided a vivid and tragic example of the results of health disparities.

Despite the major media attention around disparate treatment at the time and the broad health reform principles that both the Democratic and Republican candidates had promulgated, addressing health disparities did not seem to be "a priority issue in the 2008 election." However, it is interesting to note that unlike Senator John McCain's (R-AZ) proposal, which included provisions that would implicitly address health disparities, Senator Barack Obama's (D-IL) proposal did explicitly aim to address their "root causes." Obama's proposal included language that would prioritize data collection on disparate populations' access to quality care, increasing the diversity of the health workforce, ensuring cultural competence, and improving the capacity of safety-net institutions.[7] Whichever candidate won the presidential election, we knew Secretary Thompson was right—

we had to do something to address health disparities and prioritize health equity when health reform negotiations picked up full speed in the new year.

The Turning Point: Laying the Foundation for ObamaCare

In November of 2008, Senator Barack Obama was elected the forty-fourth president of the United States. Health reform had been a major part of his campaign platform, and he proposed a significant overhaul of the health care system. Among many other changes, his Plan for a Healthy America would create a new federal health plan or "public option" for the uninsured, providing benefits comparable to those offered to federal employees, and establish a national health insurance exchange where individuals would be able to select the public plan or an approved private plan.[8] Premiums would be subsidized for low-income and middle-class individuals and families. Insurance companies would be prohibited from denying coverage on the basis of illness or preexisting conditions, and insurance coverage would be mandated for children. Prevention and public health as well as the adoption and use of health information technology were also a cornerstone of his health reform proposal.

Although President Obama produced and promulgated an outline of his health reform priorities, Congress was charged with building upon those priorities and determining the scope of the health reform package. The Senate Finance Committee operated with lightning speed, and only eight days after the presidential election, on November 12, 2008, produced a white paper—*Call to Action: Health Reform 2009*—which served as a blueprint for comprehensive health reform. In the paper, the chair of the Senate Finance Committee, Max Baucus, stated, "It is the duty of the next Congress to reform America's health care system."[9] This helped to lay the foundation for major changes to the health care system under the Obama administration.

Once the Obama-Biden transition team was set in place, numerous organizations and health care stakeholders began to share their ideas for health reform, which helped White House officials get a better sense of what external advocacy groups wanted to see in a health reform bill. Health equity champions from various organizations also voiced their concerns and shared their policy recommendations during the transition period. Some even shared their hopes and concerns for health reform publicly, including Congresswoman Hilda Solis (D-CA) and Dr. Brian Smedley, who participated in a Kaiser Family Foundation webcast in December 2008.[10] They voiced their hope that health reform would prioritize health equity, as President Obama had promised when he was campaigning.

In addition to the historic election of the nation's first African American president, the House of Representatives had selected its first woman Speaker of the House, Nancy Pelosi (D-CA), during the previous Congress. Pelosi had long championed efforts to increase access to health care and worked closely with Senator Harry Reid (D-NV) and the congressional Tri-Caucus to address health disparities. She once revealed that health reform was one of the pillars of who she was and later admitted, "I knew I came [to Congress] to vote for health care for all Americans."[11] She wasted no time naming the new chairs for the various committees in the House. Once those names were revealed, health reform advocates were hopeful that a comprehensive health reform bill was possible, one that would be broad and inclusive of a health equity agenda.

In a speech to a joint session of Congress on February 24, 2009, President Obama urged lawmakers to move forward with health reform: "The cost of health care has weighed down our economy and our conscience long enough. So let there be no doubt, health care reform cannot wait, it must not wait and it will not wait another year."[12] As he did during his election campaign, the president underscored the increasing number of uninsured Americans and rapidly rising premiums, pledging to make changes that would both bring down costs and save lives. That month, serious negotiations over several health reform proposals were taking place in key committees of the House and Senate, namely the Senate Health, Education, Labor and Pensions Committee led by Edward Kennedy, the Senate Finance Committee led by Max Baucus, the House Energy and Commerce Committee led by Henry Waxman, the House Ways and Means Committee led by Charles Rangel, and the House Education and Labor Committee led by George Miller (D-CA). It became clear that health reform was going to take place, and soon. The leaders were showing unprecedented unity and an eagerness to cooperate in order to realize the ultimate goal that had escaped Congresses and White House administrations through the decades.

Health equity advocates realized that this was another rare opportunity to advance a health equity agenda and address health disparities once and for all in a more comprehensive manner. However, health equity advocacy coalitions and organizations were not well-coordinated, collaborative, or consistent in their legislative requests. Some advocates were focused only on health care quality improvement, some were focused primarily on data collection and reporting, and others were focused primarily on health workforce development, prevention and wellness, or language access. The disorganization among health equity advocates weakened the argument for including robust health equity provisions in the legislation.

The drafters of the health reform legislative proposals were uncertain where to seek counsel and whose priorities to include. They wanted assurance that any language submitted by advocates had been properly vetted and agreed upon by the majority of stakeholders. And with the community disorganized and focused on competing goals, drafters were hesitant to proceed in helping us. Consequently, the need to unite and mobilize, as well as streamline efforts, and create a one-stop shop for information sharing and collaboration, became increasingly important if health equity advocates wanted to be effective in realizing our goals.

The likelihood of health reform coming to fruition became even more clear to advocates during the first week of March, when President Obama announced the appointment of Kathleen Sebelius as Department of Health and Human Services secretary and Nancy-Ann DeParle as director of the White House Office of Health Reform. In remarks given on March 2, 2009, President Obama publicly recognized the success his administration had already achieved by advancing health reform via the American Recovery and Reinvestment Act, noting "we have done more to advance the cause of Health Care Reform in the last month than we have in the last decade."[13]

The stimulus law, which the act is often called, did, in fact, include provisions that laid the foundation for comprehensive health reform. It included investments in comparative effectiveness research, health workforce development, public health, and incentivizing providers to adopt and meaningfully use health information technology, most of which President Obama had championed during his campaign.[14] The president could have stopped there and argued that he did, in fact, fulfill his campaign promise, but he did not. He went on to urge the passage of a comprehensive bill that included critical health insurance reforms, delivery system reforms, and payment system reforms.

Three days after this announcement, on March 5, 2009, the White House convened a special four-hour summit on health care reform, inviting approximately 150 congressional and executive branch officials and other health policy experts to start serious deliberations on the issue. More than fifty members of Congress attended the event, including Speaker Nancy Pelosi, Del. Donna Christensen, Rep. Jan Schakowsky, Rep. Allyson Schwartz, Senator Max Baucus, Senator Ted Kennedy, Senator Tom Harkin, Senator Sheldon Whitehouse, Senator Orrin Hatch, Senator Mike Enzi, Rep. Eric Cantor, and Senator Mitch McConnell.

A wide range of stakeholders and community leaders were also in attendance, including representatives from AARP, the American Medical Association, the American Heart Association, the American Hospital Association, Planned Parenthood, the National Medical Association, the American Cancer Society, the National Minority AIDS Council, the Service Employees International Union, and the US Chamber of Commerce. Interestingly, many of the same people and organizations that had waged an aggressive campaign against health reform attempts under the Clinton administration were in attendance professing their interest in achieving health reform this time around. Physicians groups, nurses groups, hospital groups, labor unions, small and big businesses, and health insurance groups all echoed their readiness to be active and constructive participants in the process.

Opening the summit in the East Room, Melody Barnes, the White House's director of the Domestic Policy Council, introduced a firefighter who had heeded the president's call to organize a community discussion about health care back in December 2008. He presented a compilation of information, suggestions, and feedback from this effort. During the program, the president also gave remarks, declaring, "Our goal will be to enact comprehensive health reform by the end of this year."[15] In breakout sessions afterward, both Republican and Democratic lawmakers repeatedly stated that Congress needed to put politics aside and get health reform done as well as expressed their optimism that this Congress could succeed.

While attending the special forum, Congresswoman Donna Christensen and one advocate, Fredette West, who had served as an advisor to Congressman Stokes and was leading a coalition around health disparities, urged the president to ensure that the elimination of racial and ethnic health disparities was prioritized in health reform. President Obama agreed that this was a serious issue that should be addressed in health reform, and, for the first time since becoming president, Obama publicly acknowledged support for including a health equity agenda in the law. At the same time the White House was doing its part to advance ideas around health reform, negotiations were getting more serious in the Senate. Following the lead of the White House, the Senate HELP Committee held a stakeholders meeting on March 12 to provide updates on health reform efforts and continue the momentum initiated by the administration.

Seizing the Opportunity: Creating a Drumbeat across America

Without that outside drumbeat and outside mobilization, it is impossible for us to do the inside maneuvering to get the votes out to pass a bill.—*House Speaker Nancy Pelosi to advocates for health reform*

While these activities were ramping up in the White House and the Senate, health reform advocates were proceeding with their advocacy efforts. After Rosalynn Carter's annual mental health symposium in Atlanta, Georgia, on November 20, 2008, that year titled *Unclaimed Children Revisited: Fostering a Climate to Improve Children's Mental Health,* a landmark report was released concerning the children's mental health system. Dr. Janice Cooper and Dr. Jane Knitzer of the National Center for Children in Poverty at Columbia University coauthored the report, which showed that the needs of children and youth with mental health conditions were not being adequately addressed. The report provided guidance and impetus for improving mental health policies on a national level.[16]

Former First Lady Carter, along with Jane Knitzer, Janice Cooper, other mental health champions, and me, believed that this was a great opportunity to push forward mental health priorities for children, and so we convened an ad hoc group to discuss the issue and strategize about how best to proceed. Our group thought an appropriate strategy should include outreach to the Congressional Children's Caucus. So we drafted and sent a letter to Congresswoman Sheila Jackson Lee, who was chairing the caucus at the time, urging her support for improving the children's mental health system and providing specific policy recommendations for developing a comprehensive public health framework for children and adolescent mental health.

We had started our advocacy in isolation, focusing primarily on children's mental and behavioral health issues, but we soon realized that we could be more effective if we joined with other groups that shared our larger goal of advancing a health equity agenda. While we were strategizing, the National Health Equity Coalition, under the leadership of Lark Galloway-Gilliam, who was based in Los Angeles, was in preliminary

March 11, 2009

The Honorable Sheila Jackson Lee
Congressional Children's Caucus
2160 Rayburn House Office Building
Washington, DC 20515

Dear Representative Jackson Lee:

As you and your colleagues begin to address health care reform, the undersigned organizations would like to urge your support for improving and enhancing the children's mental health system. Over 25 years ago Jane Knitzer, Ed.D., in the report *Unclaimed Children: The Failure of Public Responsibility to Children in Need of Mental Health Services*, documented policy and program disconnects that meant children and youth with mental health needs and their families did not get the services they needed.

Last year, a follow-up report by Janice Cooper, Ph.D., titled *Unclaimed Children Revisited* illustrated how states are still struggling to respond appropriately to the needs of children and youth with mental health conditions, HIV/AIDS, and other disabilities. It also underscored the critical need to address the needs of children and youth at risk for those conditions. While it is clear that some progress has been made, the needs of children, youth, and families will not adequately be addressed without a comprehensive set of children's mental health policies at the national level, and a focused strategy for attaining the same.

The report's overarching goal is to provide guidance that will offer policy recommendations to move current care-delivery systems toward the vision of a comprehensive public health framework for children and adolescents' mental health.

The undersigned organizations recommend:

Family-centered Infant and Early Childhood Mental Health Services. There is an explosion of knowledge that calls attention to the importance of early relationships in setting the stage for a child's social and emotional development and mental health. There is a need to support state efforts to infuse early childhood mental health services into early childhood settings, including child care and home visiting programs, as well as to address widespread parental depression that can have life long negative consequences for the children.

A Comprehensive Financing Strategy. Develop and implement a comprehensive financing strategy that supports a public health focus to mental health. Place empirically-supported family-based treatment and supports at the center of financing children's mental health care.

Applying a Public Health Approach to Children's Mental Health. Incorporate a public health approach to children's mental health services, which provide age and developmentally

appropriate comprehensive services and on-going supports, and incorporate strategies of prevention, early intervention, and positive behavioral interventions and supports.

Enhancing Service Delivery to Transition Age Youth. Transition youth with serious mental illness (SMI) encounter numerous obstacles as they transition from school and child welfare systems to their adult lives. Efforts to address the needs of this population require the provision of crucial programming to prepare them to address their own housing and independent living needs, increased collaboration across systems providing services to these young adults to facilitate access, and access to health insurance and social services for youth with mental health conditions up to age 25.

Eliminating Disparities in Mental Health Status and Mental Health Care. Overall, mental health services meet the needs of only 13 percent of minority children. Despite the fact that minorities are less likely to receive mental health services, when they do access services, those services tend to be ineffective and of low quality. Eliminating disparities in mental health status and mental health care and increasing the cultural competence of service programs and providers is essential to improving mental health services to racial and ethnic minority children because when a program is developed with consideration of the culture of the community being served, there is an increase in service utilization and decrease in early termination of treatment.

Investing in Health Professions Training and Education. Increase and enhance mental and behavioral health workforce education and training. As documented in the report of the Annapolis Coalition on the Behavioral Health Workforce (2007): There is substantial and alarming evidence that the current workforce lacks adequate support to function effectively and is largely unable to deliver care of proven effectiveness in partnership with the people who need services. The improvement of care and the transformation of systems of care depend entirely on a workforce that is adequate in size and effectively trained and supported.

Too few resources have been expended to develop and implement a comprehensive framework for addressing the needs of children and youth with mental health conditions, HIV/AIDS, and other disabilities. We have an opportunity to improve the trajectory of children's mental health policy, and improve the overall health, education, and future employability of children and adolescents in our country. Thank you for your thoughtful consideration and continued efforts on this important issue.

In closing, we would like to thank you for your consideration of this serious matter and to offer our assistance in addressing these critical issues impacting children and adolescents with mental health conditions, HIV/AIDS, and other disabilities. Please contact Daniel E. Dawes, J.D., at the American Psychological Association's Public Interest Government Relations Office at ***.**** or ***@***, if you would like any additional information.

Figure 3.1. First health reform letter, before the formation of the National Working Group

discussions with almost fifty organizations about creating a national campaign to interject the elimination of health disparities into national policy. Some individuals, however, were concerned about the use of the term "campaign" since they argued it sounded "more short-term" or narrowly focused or implied that the goals of their effort had already been established. They were concerned that other organizations that were interested in joining them would perceive that they would not have a say over shaping the activities of the group. Others argued for establishing a coalition to bring organizations together and create unity around a common cause.

While the National Health Equity Coalition was strategizing, one major health reform advocacy group, Health Care for America Now, was also forming a health disparities working group, and another organization, Community Catalyst, was interested in forming a similar group as well. Other groups representing disability advocates, LGBT advocates, women's advocates, rural advocates, and advocates of older adults were also forming their own coalitions to address disparities in health status among their respective populations. Various advocates among them started worrying that these efforts would actually undermine the overall goal of igniting a push for health equity in the health reform negotiations. They were concerned about being overwhelmed with meetings and argued for better coordination of these groups since their agendas, missions, and goals seemed remarkably similar. Congressional staff, once again, worried about the impact these independent, competing campaigns would have or how effective they would be.

It was clear that a single umbrella group needed to serve as a point of contact to health reformers in Congress and the White House on health equity priorities. This was necessary to resolve conflicts, steer the strategy, initiate actions, build consensus, and develop vetted legislative language for inclusion in health reform bills. While all of these groups were creating coalitions or discussing how best to proceed, one thing was for sure: advocates recognized that health equity and the elimination of health disparities were not being addressed at all during health reform negotiations. So, a few weeks later, our children's mental health ad hoc group decided to broaden the scope of its advocacy to focus more broadly on health equity among all vulnerable populations. Working closely with incredible health equity vanguards such as Sherice Perry, Mara Youdelman, Debbie Reid, James Albino, Liliana Ranon, Carlos Jackson, Dr. Marjorie Innocent, Deeana Jang, and Kali Lindsey, we agreed to form a working group whose primary purpose would be to spearhead and coordinate advocacy to include robust health equity provisions in health reform proposals. That way we would not disrupt newly formed coalitions but instead serve as a convener or collaborative for all of these organizations.

This idea came out of prior lessons learned while working on the Mental Health Parity Act and the Americans with Disabilities Act Amendments Act on the Senate HELP Committee in 2007. Together with my colleague Day Al-Mohamed, Esq., who helped to spearhead efforts, we invited all of these coalitions and other health equity stakeholders and convened our first meeting. Executives at the American Psychological Association, Dr. Norman Anderson, Dr. Gwen Keita, Annie Toro, Esq., and Dr. Ellen Garrison generously allowed us to leverage the organization's resources for this initiative. On April 1, 2009, we invited people representing various health care stakeholders from mental and behavioral health, civil rights, women's rights, faith-based, disability, rural, providers, consumers, and LGBT organizations to join us in a serious dialogue on ensuring the prioritization of health equity in reform legislation.

The turnout on the day of the meeting was bigger than we expected, and far more diverse. Instead of mainly groups or individuals focused on racial and ethnic issues, there were attendees from prominent groups with a broader health focus, such as the American Academy of Pediatrics, American Hospital Association, National Association of Public Hospitals and Health Systems (now known as America's Essential Hospitals), American Association of Marriage and Family Therapists, American Cancer Society Cancer Action Network, Families USA, America's Health Insurance Plans, American Public Health Association, Asian & Pacific Islander American Health Forum, National Association of Social Workers, the American Dental Association, the National Black Nurses Association, National Dental Association, the National Medical Association, National Hispanic Medical Association, National Immigration Law Center, AIDS Action, Child Welfare League of America, First Focus, National Association of Community Health Centers, National Urban League, NAACP, National Health Law Program, National Partnership for Women and Families, Japanese American Citizens League, National Alliance for Hispanic Health, National Coalition for LGBT Health, Hispanic Federation, and Society for Public Health Education. We were excited to see not only organizations but coalitions coming together to share information and strategies to advance the discussion.

During the meeting, we explained the purpose of the anticipated group, which was to coordinate health equity efforts, develop one voice, and le-

April 16, 2009

The Honorable Fortney Stark
Chairman
Subcommittee on Health
House Ways and Means Committee
1102 Longworth House Office Building
Washington, DC 20515

The Honorable Wally Herger
Ranking Member
Subcommittee on Health
House Ways and Means Committee
1102 Longworth House Office Building
Washington, DC 20515

Dear Chairman Stark and Ranking Member Herger:

As you and your colleagues continue to work on health reform, the over one hundred undersigned coalitions, groups, and organizations urge your support for addressing health inequities among underserved communities and populations, and ensuring the safety and quality of health services for all. We respectfully request a hearing to discuss opportunities within health reform to ameliorate and eliminate the grave disparities in health status and health services.

Striking disparities in health status exist among various communities and populations throughout the United States, which include shorter life expectancy, higher rates of chronic health conditions, and disability. According to the Agency for Healthcare Research and Quality (AHRQ), disparities are also observed in most aspects of health care, including care for chronic conditions such as mental health disorders and substance use, HIV/AIDS, cancer, diabetes, heart disease, stroke, oral health conditions, infant mortality and morbidity, respiratory disease, and end stage renal disease.

The undersigned organizations recognize that comprehensive health reform is essential to improving the safety and quality of health services, and will help to improve the health of everyone in our country. As the United States continues to struggle with how to improve health equity and ensure that all have access to culturally and linguistically appropriate health services, we urge you to seriously address this issue in health reform and convene a hearing.

We would like to thank you for your thoughtful consideration of this request and offer our assistance in addressing this critical issue. Please contact Daniel E. Dawes, J.D., at (202) ***-**** or ***@***, if you would like any additional information.

Sincerely,

Figure 3.2. First National Working Group health reform letter

verage resources. Our newly formed group agreed to draft a letter that would highlight specific language and recommendations for health disparities as a part of comprehensive health care reform. The goal was to represent the priorities of as many organizations and coalitions as possible. We also decided to develop a "master list" of coalitions and organizations to better facilitate information dissemination and shared actions. And, finally, we decided to send a sign-on letter to key committees requesting a hearing on health disparities, to ensure congressional responsiveness to the issue. The letter, which was sent on April 16, 2009, was the first to come from this diverse group of advocates for disparate populations.

The result of this mobilization became formally known as the National Working Group on Health Disparities and Health Reform, a group of initially thirty-five organizations, associations, and coalitions that quickly grew and banded together to make health disparities elimination a priority during the health reform debates. Our group agreed to several overarching objectives to advance a health equity agenda in health reform, including (1) developing a robust advocacy strategy, (2) drafting model legislative language to incorporate in health reform proposals, (3) monitoring and analyzing any legislative proposals to ensure that they included health equity provisions, and (4) monitoring the implementation of these provisions.

Members of the working group convened weekly internal strategy meetings and external meetings with key congressional and administration officials. In the 111th Congress, Congresswoman Barbara Lee (D-CA) became chair of the forty-two-member Congressional Black Caucus, and several members were elevated to key positions leading the House Judiciary, Homeland Security, and Ways and Means Committees. Representative James Clyburn (D-SC) became the majority whip.

Our group worked closely not only with these champions for health reform but also with the Congressional Black Caucus Health Braintrust under the leadership of Congresswoman Donna M. Christensen (D-VI); as well as with the Congressional Hispanic Caucus Health Care Task Force, under the leadership of Congresswoman Lucille Roybal-Allard; and the Congressional Asian Pacific American Caucus, under the leadership of Congressman Mike Honda (D-CA). The Tri-Caucus has proven to be a guardian of health equity and has long been a promoter and defender of policies in Congress intended to elevate the health of all communities.

The National Working Group also worked closely with the Congressional Native American Caucus, the White House, and key health policy-focused committees in Congress, including Energy and Commerce, Ways and Means, and Education and Labor. In one of the most contentious struggles over the chairmanship of the Energy and Commerce Committee, Congressman Henry Waxman in a secret ballot vote in the Cannon Caucus Room won the leadership position in a vote of 137-122. Democrats in the House, essentially, ratified an earlier decision by the Steering and Policy Committee to replace Congressman John Dingell Jr. (D-MI), the Dean of the House of Representatives.

Waxman and his team had launched their challenge for this position the day after the November 2008 elections. Dingell and his team immediately launched a counteroffensive against Waxman and his supporters, but they ultimately lost to the Waxman machine, which had been lobbying behind the scenes to persuade other Democratic House members to support his bid and defy the seniority system that had long been in place. Some thought the eighty-two-year-old was too old and that Waxman, who was sixty-nine, would be better able to handle the intense and brutal negotiations over health reform that were expected. Nevertheless, Congressman Waxman, after winning the position, appointed Dingell "chairman emeritus" of the committee and allowed him to keep his office suite in the Capitol building.

During the negotiations around health reform, both Waxman and his staff and Dingell and his staff worked cooperatively and closely on the health reform package in their committee. Although we worked closely with Congressman Charles Rangel's staff on the Ways and Means Committee and Congressman George Miller's staff on the Education and Labor Committee, we spent more of our time working with both Waxman and Dingell's staff to develop their bill before it was merged with the other two committees to become the Tri-Committee health reform bill. Waxman's team, most notably Naomi Seiler, Anne Morris, Camille Sealy, and Julia Elam, as well as Dingell's team, most notably Virgil Miller and Rebekah Caruthers worked closely with us to understand and champion our priorities during internal committee negotiations over what provisions should be included in the bill. During our meetings with congressional members and staff, we emphasized the fact that it had been almost ten years since President Bill Clinton signed into law the Minority Health and Health Disparities Research and Education Act of 2000, a critical but limited law on health disparities research, and that the United States could not afford to wait another ten years to get more comprehensive legislation around health equity passed.

By the end of April 2009, our group had grown in the space of a month from 35 to more than 250 organizations, associations, and coalitions across the country. We were pleasantly surprised by the tremendous growth and interest in this group—word of mouth about our efforts was spreading like wildfire across the United States. People were calling and writing us, wanting to participate and to lend their voices to this cause. We represented diverse stakeholders, including consumers, racial and ethnic minorities, rural populations, people with disabilities, children, women, LGBT individuals, community health centers, hospitals and other health care entities, health professionals, insurers, and businesses. Our goal was to urge lawmakers and the Obama administration to ensure that any final comprehensive health reform legislation included provisions to address health inequities and to reduce and eliminate health care disparities. Like President Obama, we too had an outline of issues we wanted included in health reform:

1. *High-quality, affordable health care coverage must be available to everyone, particularly populations and communities that have traditionally suffered health disparities and barriers to coverage.* Coverage must include prevention, wellness, chronic disease management, behavioral health, and support services, such as social work and language services.

2. Health insurance coverage alone does not ensure access to health services. *A full range of culturally and linguistically appropriate health care and public health services must be available in every community and accessible to all.* A greater investment is necessary to expand grants and demonstration projects to support community-based programs designed to reduce health disparities and barriers to health services through education and outreach, health promotion and disease prevention activities, and health literacy education and services. In addition, reimbursement for Medicaid, the State Children's Health Insurance Program, or any other subsidized public insurance plans must be adequate to ensure a sufficient pool of providers willing to treat beneficiaries.

3. *Every community must have the health workforce and infrastructure necessary to provide a full range of health care and public health services.* A greater investment must be made in programs under Title VII and VIII of the Public Health Service Act, the National Health Service Corps, AIDS Education and Training Centers, the Minority Fellowship Program, and Graduate Medical Education programs to strengthen the recruitment, retention, training, and continuing education of primary care, behavioral health, public health, and other health professionals, as well as to increase their diversity, distribution, cultural competence, and knowledge of treating the

unique needs of different populations. Support must also be provided to sustain and expand institutions, such as community health centers and public hospitals, that have traditionally served populations that suffer from health disparities.

4. *All efforts to reduce health disparities and barriers to quality health services require better data.* Federal, state, and local governments and health care and public health providers must be required to support the collection and accurate reporting of standardized demographic data on patients and the community, and they must be provided the resources to do so. Data and findings should be disseminated to inform policy decisions and assist in efforts to eliminate health disparities.

5. *Recognition of diversity is critical to improving health care quality.* Quality improvement and pay-for-performance policies must take into account the needs and challenges of populations that have traditionally suffered health disparities and barriers to health services, and they must reward efforts that reduce them. Resources should be provided to design and implement evidence-based quality improvement strategies, such as the medical/health home model, to eliminate disparities and barriers to health care delivery. Studies must be done to ensure that efforts to improve quality of care for the general population do not inadvertently exacerbate health disparities.

Growing Pains: More Progress, More Problems

During the expansion of the National Working Group several key events occurred. On April 8, 2009, President Obama signed an executive order reemphasizing health reform as a key goal of his administration and establishing the White House Office of Health Reform and the US Department of Health and Human Services Office of Health Reform. Both offices were ordered to coordinate closely with each other.[17] Over in the Senate, we saw increased cooperation between the Senate Finance and HELP Committees on health reform. On April 20, 2009, Senator Kennedy (chair of HELP) and Senator Baucus (chair of Finance) sent a letter to President Obama stating their mutual commitment to passing comprehensive health reform and marking up legislation in early June.

> Since our committees share jurisdiction over health care reform legislation in the Senate, we have jointly laid out an aggressive schedule to accomplish our goal. . . . Our intention is for that legislation to be very similar, and to reflect

a shared approach to reform, so that the measures that our two committees report can be quickly merged into a single bill for consideration on the Senate floor.

We have a moral duty to ensure that every American can get quality health care. We must act to contain the growth of health care costs to ensure our economic stability; to help American businesses deal with the health care challenge; and to make sure that we are getting our money's worth. With your continued leadership and commitment, and working together, we remain certain that our goal of enacting comprehensive health care reform can be accomplished with the urgency that the American people rightly demand.[18]

In previous attempts to pass health reform legislation, these committees had competed against each other instead of working together on a bill. This demonstration of unity signaled to health law and policy experts that health reform stood a serious chance of passing. The following day, Senator Baucus and Senator Chuck Grassley held the first of three roundtables bringing together health policy and industry experts to discuss the development of health care reform legislation.

One week after its joint letter to the president and it first roundtable, the Senate Finance Committee on April 28, 2009, released detailed policy options for reforming America's health care delivery system, which was the first of three sets of policy options released publicly for members of Congress and the public to review.[19] This was in keeping with the committee's track record of producing resources aimed at influencing the health reform agenda.

After the first set of policy options was released, the National Working Group attempted to meet with the Senate Finance Committee to discuss the inclusion of provisions aimed at increasing access to quality health care and public health services, research on health disparities, cultural competence, and more robust and accurate data collection and reporting. At first, the committee ignored our requests to meet. Fact sheets, issue briefs, and other materials we created to inform committee members were never acknowledged, nor was any language we offered for inclusion in the first policy paper accepted. We became troubled that the leading committee on health reform in the Senate seemingly failed to appreciate the seriousness of our issues. Members of our National Working Group then reached out to American Indian tribes in Montana since Senator Baucus represented that state and was the chair of the Senate Finance Committee, and discussed our concerns. Members of the Montana American Indian community made sure to voice their disapproval to the committee for failing to meet with us. After this occurred, members of our group were finally given an audience with senior staff on the Finance Committee.

From the Senate HELP Committee, we experienced quite a different reception. Senator Kennedy, who had long been a champion for addressing health disparities and had previously worked with Senator Frist to develop legislation tackling this issue, agreed that provisions directly addressing the problem should be included in any health reform proposal. His staff, most notably Caya Lewis, Dr. Kavita Patel, David Johns, and Dr. Craig Martinez, worked diligently to negotiate these priorities in committee along with senior staff from other senate offices, including Darrel Thompson, Priscilla Ross, Mayra Alvarez, and Mona Shah.[20] When seeking individual champions on the two committees of jurisdiction in the Senate over health policy, we encountered both supportive and unsupportive staff, and senators who either did not see the relevance of including our provisions or thought them too controversial. They deemed these health equity provisions deal killers for the larger bill, despite our best efforts to demonstrate how these priorities had long enjoyed bipartisan support.

One Democratic senator's staff, for instance, employed a tactic designed to keep health equity advocates thinking they stood a chance to have their issue addressed: the staff person, knowing full well no Republican was on board with health reform at that point, told us they would consider our legislative priorities if we secured a Republican cosponsor. Early on, when we knew Republicans were not going to support any health reform package, we decided to focus our attention on Democrats who were proponents of health reform and launch an educational and advocacy campaign to advance health equity. Senators Harry Reid, Ben Cardin (D-MD), Barbara Mikulski, Tom Harkin, Richard Durbin (D-IL), Daniel Inouye, Daniel Akaka, and Roland Burris (D-IL) became our primary champions in the Senate.[21]

At this point, while there was increasing unity among old congressional competitors, member groups were beginning to express dissatisfaction with the National Working Group, concerned that their priorities were not being addressed. Advocates from the disability community began to push back against other members of the National Working Group, complaining about insufficient language relating to the disability community in group letters. The LGBT community also was equally upset about not explicitly mentioning their issues. Likewise, advocates from the racial and ethnic minority community voiced concern about losing ground on this issue since health disparities had long been focused on them. All of these communities were informed that the larger group letters that we created were purposely designed to address health disparities broadly, and that it was up to each group to speak out for its respective population. Moreover, the National Working Group reminded them that we had not yet received any specific language, except on one or two occasions, to include in our material. Eventually, these disagreements faded and the diverse stakeholders continued to collaborate to push for health equity.

Turning the Tide

While communicating with congressional health reform champions, members of the National Working Group were also corresponding with the White House to prioritize health equity in the negotiations. The US Department of Health and Human Services and the White House Office of Health Reform expressed interest in mid-April in scheduling a meeting or event around health disparities. We remained persistent in pushing this issue, even as White House staffers were moving slowly in scheduling the meeting. The National Working Group continued forward with our efforts and on April 22 held our second meeting, which was attended by Caya Lewis of the Senate HELP committee. After the meeting, we sent out an e-mail summarizing our agenda and announcing our next meeting.

On April 29, 2009, the White House Office of National AIDS Policy, under the leadership of Jeffrey S. Crowley, a major champion for health equity and one of our greatest allies, convened a meeting with a select group of health reform stakeholders, which some members of the National Working Group attended. James Albino, who had helped to organize the National Working Group and was one of our exceptional leaders, worked tirelessly to secure this meeting. The objectives of the meeting were to (1) highlight the challenges of HIV/AIDS prevention, treatment, and care and the less than optimal response at the federal level; (2) identify not only the HIV/AIDS community's needs but highlight the responses that have been pursued; (3) facilitate involvement of the underserved community (e.g., regular meetings, conversations) in the development of a national AIDS strategy; (4) frame the issue as an example of a health disparity for underserved communities; and (5) encourage the inclusion of this and other health disparities in the overall national health reform conversation. Although we were pleased that the issue of health disparities was included in this

From: Dawes, Daniel <***@***>
Date: Fri, Apr 24, 2009 at 12:17 AM
Subject: Health Disparities Meeting Summary and Next Steps for Health Reform
To: "Dawes, Daniel" <***@***>

Greetings—

Thanks to all those who attended yesterday's meeting on strategies to advance health disparities reduction and elimination in health reform. For those who were not able to attend, Caya Lewis from the Senate HELP Committee updated the group about health reform efforts on their end and the next steps they are taking. She also discussed possible strategies, congressional targets, and next steps for us to take to ensure that health and health care disparities is given proper consideration. We'll briefly discuss those in the next meeting for the benefit of those who were not able to attend. The next meeting will be held next week Thursday, April 30 at 9:30 am at the American Psychological Association building in the 6th floor boardroom (750 First Street, NE) located next to Union Station.

Because of our efforts with the first letter requesting a hearing on health disparities, Congress is beginning to respond. The House is interested in holding a stakeholder meeting to discuss the issue of health disparities in health reform and listen to our concerns, ideas, and thoughts around this issue. I'll make sure to let you know when that is once they have determined an appropriate date and time to meet with us.

To further enhance cooperation between all the various coalitions, groups, and organizations and to better target our efforts on the Hill and with the Administration, it was agreed in the meeting that we would:

1. In response to Hill staff requests, draft a general letter that would ensure congressional and the Administration's responsiveness to the issue of health disparities, and send it to key congressional Members and Administration officials requesting the inclusion of health disparities as a part of comprehensive health care reform. (In addition to the larger group letter individual organizations and coalitions were encouraged to send their own letters that would better address their specific populations).

Please find the larger group sign-on letter attached for comments/feedback. Send any comments to Daniel Dawes at: ***@*** by Tuesday, April 28. Remember – this is just a draft. After this letter has been vetted by you all, we will send out a final copy right after sign-ons.

2. Finalize which Members of Congress we need to concentrate our efforts on and develop a schedule for Hill visits to ensure efforts are not being duplicated. Please find attached a draft list of congressional Members that have been identified as individuals we should reach out to for your consideration. During the next meeting we will discuss these congressional targets.

3. Because of the significant number of organizations and various coalitions working on health disparities initiatives and the increasing confusion and complexity involved in determining who's doing what, it was agreed that we needed to develop a "master list" of health disparities coalitions and groups to better facilitate information dissemination and shared actions. We also intend on sharing this list with White House and congressional staff working on health reform.

If you are interested in having your coalition, group, or organization included on this list, please forward the name and contact information to Van Nguyen at: ***@*** as soon as possible.

4. Develop a grassroots strategy in order to ensure that all of our resources and energy are used efficiently and effectively. It was agreed that we needed to ensure that this not only involved organizations and coalitions, but constituents. From the letters that we draft, Sherice Perry at: ***@*** we will also draft an action alert for everyone to use as a template.

Because of the speed in which Congress and the White House is moving, the next meeting for all interested parties, groups, and coalitions has been scheduled for Thursday, April 30 at 9:30 am at the American Psychological Association boardroom on the 6th floor. Please mark your calendars. Senate HELP Committee staff will update us about their efforts. We will continue to have updates from various officials during forthcoming meetings. Senate HELP staff have asked for a list of those who will be attending the April 30 meeting so if you plan on attending, please RSVP to ***@*** to let us know.

Please pass this missive on to any coalitions, groups or organizations involved in health disparities efforts so that they too can be included in these efforts.

Again, thanks to everyone for their cooperation and support to this effort. Please feel free to contact me if you have any questions.

Respectfully,
Daniel

Daniel E. Dawes, J.D. | Senior Legislative & Federal Affairs Officer, Public Interest Directorate American Psychological Association
750 First Street NE, Washington, DC 20002-4242
Tel: ***-**** | Fax: ***-****
email: ***@*** | www.apa.org

Figure 3.3. Grassroots e-mail to health equity advocates summarizing next steps and strategy during April

May 20, 2009

The Honorable Edward Kennedy
Chairman
Senate HELP Committee
428 Dirksen Senate Office Building
Washington, DC 20510

The Honorable Michael Enzi
Ranking Member
Senate HELP Committee
835 Hart Senate Office Building
Washington, DC 20510

Dear Chairman Kennedy and Ranking Member E

As you and your colleagues continue to work on h
coalitions, groups, and organizations urge you to e
equities and makes certain that health and health c
is prioritized. We envision health reform legislatio
and provides individuals with the ability to access
guistically appropriate health care and public heal
consistent with the rest of the population.

Striking disparities in health status exist among va
throughout the United States, which include short
chronic health conditions and disability. Accordin
and Quality (AHRQ), disparities are also observe
and treatment, including care for mental health dis
cancer, diabetes, heart disease, stroke, oral health
respiratory disease, and end stage renal disease.

Health reform legislation provides a unique oppo
and achieving many of the health equity recomme
(IOM) Unequal Treatment report and Healthy Peo
reduce health disparities not only along lines of ra
gender and geography and among other populatio

Comprehensive health reform is essential to impro
communities that have traditionally suffered healt
and public health services. We urge your support f
health reform legislation.

We would like to thank you for your thoughtful co
assistance in addressing this critical issue. Please
-* or ***@***, if you would like any add

Sincerely,

May 20, 2009

The Honorable Max Baucus
Chairman
Senate Finance Committee
219 Dirksen Senate Office Building
Washington, DC 20510

The Honorable Charles Grassley
Ranking Member
Senate Finance Committee
219 Dirksen Senate Office Building
Washington, DC 20510

Dear Chairman Baucus and Ranking Member Grassley:

As you and your colleagues continue to work on health reform legislation, the undersigned
coalitions, groups, and organizations urge you to ensure the legislation addresses health inequities and makes certain that health and health care disparities reduction and elimination
is prioritized. We envision health reform legislation that ensures equity and accountability,
and provides individuals with the ability to access comprehensive and culturally and linguistically appropriate health care and public health services and achieve health outcomes
consistent with the rest of the population.

Striking disparities in health status exist among various communities and populations
throughout the United States, which include shorter life expectancy and higher rates of
chronic health conditions and disability. According to the Agency for Healthcare Research
and Quality (AHRQ), disparities are also observed in most aspects of disease prevention
and treatment, including care for mental health disorders and substance use, HIV/AIDS,
cancer, diabetes, heart disease, stroke, oral health conditions, maternal and child health,
respiratory disease, and end stage renal disease.

Health reform legislation provides a unique opportunity for addressing critical disparities
and achieving many of the health equity recommendations from the Institute of Medicine's
(IOM) Unequal Treatment report and Healthy People 2010. These recommendations will
reduce health disparities not only along lines of race and ethnicity, but also along lines of
gender and geography and among other populations affected by health inequities.

Comprehensive health reform is essential to improving the health of populations and
communities that have traditionally suffered health disparities and barriers to health care
and public health services. We urge your support for including health equity provisions in
health reform legislation.

We would like to thank you for your thoughtful consideration of this request and offer our
assistance in addressing this critical issue. Please contact Daniel E. Dawes, J.D., at
-* or ***@***, if you would like any additional information.

Sincerely,

Figure 3.4. Second National Working Group health reform letter

discussion, members of the National Working Group took the opportunity
to ask for a follow up meeting with the White House Office of Health Reform dedicated to the issue of health disparities, specifically the inclusion
of health equity in health reform.

The following day, the third meeting of the National Working Group
took place. We finalized the second letter to be sent to key members of
Congress and administration officials requesting the inclusion of health
disparities as a part of comprehensive health reform. We continued devel-

oping a master list of coalitions, groups, and organizations committed to this cause. Our group coordinated congressional visits and began developing talking points on health disparities for these visits. The framework for the talking points would follow along the lines of categories delineated by the Senate HELP Committee: (1) coverage, (2) access, (3) quality, (4) service delivery, and (5) data collection. We also discussed developing a website that would highlight all submitted recommendations, principles, and documents on health disparities as an additional tool for congressional staff to incorporate stakeholder recommendations when crafting health reform legislation.

On May 11, 2009, the Senate Finance Committee published its second set of policy options, focused on expanding health care coverage. These options included an entire section on health equity, titled "Options to Address Health Disparities." This section was a direct result of the National Working Group's persistent advocacy efforts—our recommendations were instrumental in the final product. The proposed options would expand data collection measures, require health care quality data to be published by race, ethnicity, and gender, expand translation services for Medicaid beneficiaries, and allow states to waive the five-year waiting period for Medicaid coverage. Senate Finance Committee chair Max Baucus in the announcement stated, "Expanding health care coverage is not just a moral imperative—it's an economic necessity. . . . These policy options propose a uniquely American approach to provide affordable, quality coverage to all Americans through a mix of public and private solutions, and drive down health care costs for every American."[22]

Gaining Momentum for Health Equity

May was a particularly busy month for the National Working Group. It was a period of intense activity, and we worked long, grueling hours strategizing, responding to congressional requests, drafting model legislative language, and drafting letters and messages. We had to be careful with our language at all times, to avoid the risk of alienating members from any of the groups represented in the National Working Group. Our second letter, supporting the Senate Finance Committee's inclusion of health equity options and seeking to ensure that other committees also included health disparities provisions, was finalized and sent to members of Congress and the White House on May 6, 2009.

We created a group listserv to help with scheduling congressional meetings and sharing information between National Working Group members.

From: Dawes, Daniel ***@***
Date: Thu, May 21, 2009 at 12:52 AM
Subject: Health Disparities in Health Reform Update and Next Steps
To: "Dawes, Daniel" ***@***

Greetings—

Thanks to all those who attended last Friday's health disparities meeting. It was a great meeting. A lot was accomplished. Congressman Dingell's staff updated the group about their efforts around health reform and discussed the importance of our outside advocacy efforts to help advance health disparities reduction and elimination efforts in health reform legislation.

Because many individuals will be taking off early for the Memorial Day weekend, **there will not be a meeting this Friday.** Instead the **next meeting** will occur next Thursday, **May 28** at 9:30 am in the American Psychological Association 6th floor boardroom (750 First Street, NE) right next to Union Station.

Please find attached a final copy of the second letter with the list of signatories urging Congress and the Administration to ensure the inclusion of health disparities reduction and elimination efforts in health reform legislation for your records.

Please find attached the finalized health disparities talking points, which were developed by a diverse group of coalitions and organizations representing various populations groups affected by health disparities. These talking points were developed as a result of congressional staff requests. These talking points will be sent to congressional staff by next Wednesday, May 27. If you wish to be added to the list of signatories supporting these talking points, please contact me ASAP by noon Wednesday, May 27 at ***@***. Many thanks to Nicky Bassford from APHA for coordinating this effort.

Please find attached a copy of a list that was developed at the last meeting for congressional alliance building and community meetings. Hill visits will be made to these offices to let them know how much we appreciate their support and to discuss efforts to include health disparities in health reform. Meetings that have already been confirmed include: Meeting with Sen. Harkin June 2 at 1:00 p.m. Meeting with Rep. Waxman June 2 at 2:00 p.m. Meeting with Sen. Menendez June 2 at 3:00 p.m. We will discuss this list and future hill visits at the next health disparities meeting.

Because congressional staffers are requesting specific recommendations on health disparities, everyone agreed that it was a good idea to develop a website that would highlight all submitted recommendations, principles, and documents on health disparities as an additional tool for congressional staff to facilitate use of stakeholder recommendations when crafting health reform legislation. The website was unveiled during the meeting and is now live. It is being hosted by the National Health Law Program. The direct website address is: http://www.healthlaw.org/library/folder.250311Working_Group_on_Health_Disparities_and_Health_Reform

• There's also a link from NHeLP's homepage, www.healthlaw.org and then click on "Working Group on Health Disparities and Health Reform."

• If you'd like to add resources to the webpage, please send an email to Patti Ruppa, ***@*** and Mara Youdelman, ***@***.

• In addition, a listserv was developed to coordinate hill visits for those who are interested in participating. The address is disparities@healthlaw.org .... If you already signed up to participate, then you should already be in the system. If you wish to be added, please let me know at ***@***.

During the meeting, National Partnership for Women and Families discussed their draft comments to the latest Senate Finance Committee paper, which was done jointly with Brian Smedley from the Joint Center for Political and Economic Studies and encouraged coalitions, groups and organizations who were interested in signing on to let them know.

During the meeting, the Healthcare Equality Project discussed their upcoming event on June 24 to bring attention to health disparities issues in our country. It was agreed that individual organizations, groups and coalitions would lend support to this cause by spreading the word about this event to their respective members so that we have great attendance and media coverage. Please see attached for a save the date flyer. More information will be forthcoming.

During the meeting, Health Care for America Now (HCAN) also discussed their major initiative on June 25, which involves advocacy efforts on the hill and a rally. The rally will be held on June 25th at 11:45 am to 12:30 pm at the Senate side. It was agreed that it is critical to get as many people to the rally as we can to show Congress that there is major support for including health disparities in health reform. More information is forthcoming.

During the meeting, the idea of holding a briefing on health disparities was discussed. This idea will be discussed further in the next health disparities meeting.

Please mark your calendars! The next large group meeting on health disparities will be next Thursday, May 28 at the American Psychological Association building (750 First Street, NE) right next to Union Station. The meeting will begin at 9:30 am in the 6th floor boardroom. This will be a very important meeting as we discuss next steps.

Additional Announcement:

The Coalition on Human Needs is requesting sign-ons to a letter, which will be sent to the Finance Committee (view letter at: http://chn.org/pdf/2009/healthcoveragecomments.pdf). The letter thanks the Committee for its promising proposals, such as expanding Medicaid for low-income people and families, and offers suggestions on ways to remove barriers and strengthen coverage for vulnerable populations. **You can sign your organization's name here:** http://salsa.democracyinaction.org/o/125/petition.jsp?petition_KEY=1953. **The deadline for signing is Friday, May 22 at noon.**

If you have any questions, please let me know. Please pass this missive on to any coalitions, groups or organizations involved in health disparities efforts so that they too can be included in these efforts.

Again, thank you all for your cooperation and support to this effort.

Respectfully,
Daniel

Daniel E. Dawes, J.D. | Senior Legislative & Federal Affairs Officer.
Public Interest Directorate
American Psychological Association
750 First Street NE, Washington, DC 20002-4242
Tel: ***-**** | Fax: ***-****
email: ***@*** | www.apa.org

Figure 3.5. Grassroots e-mail to health equity advocates summarizing next steps and strategy during May

We also created advocacy packets containing information on various health equity issues and drafted and vetted a cover letter to include with them. Finally, we created and unveiled a website to house materials developed by group members, which served as a comprehensive database of information on health disparities accessible to policy makers.

The National Working Group continued on, and at our next meeting we hammered out our talking points, organized visits to Capitol Hill, and considered organizing a congressional briefing on health disparities. During this time the Congressional Black Caucus was alarmed by the inadequate attention being paid to racial and ethnic health disparities and started to pressure the Obama administration to increase its support for this issue in the health reform bills. Members of the CBC were particularly upset that the president had not included reference to addressing disparities in health care in his June 2, 2009, letter to Senators Edward Kennedy and Max Baucus.[23] President Obama's letter made the case for tackling health reform because of the escalating health care costs that were bankrupting families and straining health care delivery. He argued the need for various delivery system and payment system reforms such as accountable care organizations and for cuts to Medicare and Medicaid spending, and he expressed interest in their ideas around shared responsibility, but he did not mention the impact of health disparities and the tremendous economic burden this issue had on our nation.

Three days after the president sent his letter to the chairs of the two Senate committees that had jurisdiction over health policy issues, the CBC issued an advisory alerting the media of a health equity news conference they planned to convene June 9 at 10 a.m., and sent a letter to the president firmly urging him to ensure that health equity is an integral component of health reform. The caucus was troubled that some in the administration seemed to hold the belief that health insurance coverage alone would meaningfully tackle racial and ethnic health disparities. It wanted to make sure that the president kept his promise about addressing health disparities in health reform legislation that he made during his first health reform town hall at the White House. In the CBC letter, Barbara Lee, Donna Christensen, and Danny K. Davis strongly urged the president "to ensure that efforts to reform the nation's health care system integrate aggressive solutions to the nation's current plight with pervasive health disparities" and asserted that health reform efforts should "include provisions that address the root causes of all health inequities." They also stated, "We, like you, share a keen interest in ensuring that as we work together to reform the nation's health care system, that we do so in a manner that truly transforms it into one that serves all Americans appropriately, consistently, and equitably, regardless of their racial and ethnic background, gender, geography, language preference, or sexual orientation."[24]

As a result of the efforts by the Tri-Caucus, especially the CBC, and the National Working Group health equity advocates achieved a major breakthrough in June when the White House agreed to convene a stakeholder meeting on health disparities and health reform, confirming that these concerns were indeed being treated as a priority. On June 9 several health disparities experts, most of us members of the National Working Group, met with Secretary Kathleen Sebelius, Nancy-Ann DeParle, and Tina Tchen. We thought it was fitting that the meeting was held in the Indian Treaty Room at the Eisenhower Executive Office Building since it gave all of us a sense that the White House deemed this issue important enough to host it in a room that has long been associated with major announcements or events in our nation's history. Participants were given approximately two minutes each to discuss their priorities for health reform and how the health reform proposals could address health disparities.

During the meeting, we tried to reinforce our health equity priorities: that high-quality, affordable health care coverage must be available to everyone, particularly underresourced communities, and that every community must have the health workforce and infrastructure necessary to provide a full range of health care and public health services. We also emphasized that governments and health providers must be required to support the collection and accurate reporting of standardized demographic data on patients and the community and be provided the resources to do so. We recognized that without that data the disparities in health care among these marginalized groups cannot be accurately tracked. In addition, the US Department of Health and Human Services, during the meeting, released a report on health disparities titled *Health Disparities: A Case for Closing the Gap*.

June 9, 2009, was certainly a busy day for health equity advocates. In addition to the White House's stakeholder meeting on health disparities and health reform, the Senate Health, Education, Labor and Pensions Committee released a draft health reform bill that included health equity provisions—the Affordable Health Choices Act—and the Congressional Tri-Caucus released a draft of its comprehensive health equity bill—the Health Equity and Accountability Act of 2009—which was officially introduced on June 26, 2006, by Congresswoman Donna Christensen on the Energy and Commerce Committee.

The next day, on June 10, 2010, the Ways and Means Subcommittee on Health, under the leadership of Chair Fortney Pete Stark (D-CA) and ranking member Dave Camp (R-MI), held the first-ever hearing focused solely on health disparities for that committee, titled *Addressing Disparities in Health and Healthcare: Issues of Reform*. Both Representatives Stark and Camp recognized that although health insurance coverage would put "a dent in addressing disparities," that alone would not resolve the crisis.[25] For months, health equity champions had been pushing congressional leaders on both sides of the aisle to convene a hearing on this critical issue and were thrilled that once again our voices had been heard and our request for a hearing was granted.

Due in part to the incredible advocacy of Congressman Xavier Becerra (D-CA) and Congresswoman Stephanie Tubbs Jones (D-OH), the subcommittee decided to dedicate one hearing to addressing this issue and fleshing out priorities. Witnesses included three Tri-Caucus members: Congresswomen Donna M. Christensen, Hilda L. Solis, and Madeleine Z. Bordallo (D-GU). In addition, representatives from several organizations, including the Kaiser Family Foundation, the National Medical Association, the Asian & Pacific Islander American Health Forum, and the American Enterprise Institute were also invited to give testimony. Other groups that provided written submissions included the American Dental Education Association, America's Health Insurance Plans, American College of Physicians, American Hospital Association, National Council of Urban Indian Health, the National Black Nurses Association, and the Special Olympics International.

During what was arguably the busiest week for health equity advocacy during the entire negotiations around health reform in 2009, one other noteworthy event was convened. On Friday, June 12, 2009, the US Commission on Civil Rights, which is an independent, bipartisan agency established by Congress in 1957 charged with monitoring federal civil rights enforcement, held a public briefing to examine the reasons for persistent gaps between the health status of minorities and nonminorities in the United States.[26] Dr. Louis Sullivan, Dr. Garth Graham, Dr. Herman Taylor, Dr. Bruce Siegel, and others presented testimony highlighting the need to increase the diversity and cultural competence of the health professions workforce; address data collection gaps and challenges especially for subpopulation groups; address the multifactorial causes of disparities and the interplay among socioeconomic, environmental, individual and personal factors as well as other social determinants of health; improve the quality of care and address the need for culturally and linguistically appropriate care; and address unconscious bias in health care.

Dr. Sally Satel, a scholar with the American Enterprise Institute also testified that there were indeed disparities among minorities, but she argued that the causes of these disparities were debatable. She sought to discredit the *Unequal Treatment* report by outlining what she perceived to be some of its methodological problems. She concluded that "the elimination of health differentials is not feasible because we cannot eliminate the disparities, the social disparities, many of which take their most profound toll in terms of the habits of mind and view of the future. Such an agenda clearly transcends the work of public health and is best left to politicians, voters and social welfare experts."[27]

Throughout the negotiations we continued to hear others raise the points she had made, particularly that it is impossible to eliminate disparities because approximately 50 percent of the disparities in health result from social and physical determinants of health that are out of any provider's control. Some argued that providers have significant control over the 20 percent of input related to clinical care and shared control over 30 percent related to health behaviors, but when it comes to socioeconomic factors (40 percent) and physical environment (10 percent), hospitals and physicians have limited control and capabilities. Health equity advocates pushed back, however, and argued that many of these social and physical determinants of health transpired because of past practices and promulgation of policies that could be addressed through meaningful collaboration with community stakeholders and leaders.[28]

Two weeks after the White House's stakeholder meeting, health equity advocates mobilized and held a rally on the evening of June 24, 2009—Lighting the Night: Healthcare Equality '09—at Freedom Plaza in Washington, DC. This rally, which was sponsored by the Service Employees International Union Healthcare Equality Project and organized by Sinsi Hernández-Cancio, JD; Martine Apodaca; and Van Nguyen, brought hundreds of people from across the country to demand that health reform truly work for everyone. Participants at this rally believed that health care had to go beyond simply expanding coverage to all uninsured Americans; it had to put us on a path toward health care equality. Participants also believed that all people, no matter the color of their skin, deserve afford-

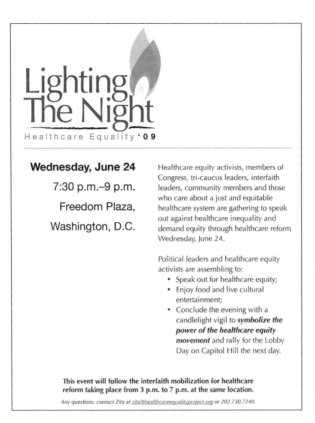

Lighting The Night

Healthcare Equality '09

Wednesday, June 24

7:30 p.m.–9 p.m.

Freedom Plaza,

Washington, D.C.

Healthcare equity activists, members of Congress, tri-caucus leaders, interfaith leaders, community members and those who care about a just and equitable healthcare system are gathering to speak out against healthcare inequality and demand equity through healthcare reform Wednesday, June 24.

Political leaders and healthcare equity activists are assembling to:

- Speak out for healthcare equity;
- Enjoy food and live cultural entertainment;
- Conclude the evening with a candlelight vigil to **symbolize the power of the healthcare equity movement** and rally for the Lobby Day on Capitol Hill the next day.

This event will follow the interfaith mobilization for healthcare reform taking place from 3 p.m. to 7 p.m. at the same location.

Any questions. contact Zita at zita@healthcareequalityproject.org or 202.730.7240.

Figure 3.6. Flier for Lighting the Night: Healthcare Equality '09 rally

able, accessible health care of the highest quality. The venue provided an opportunity for advocates to speak out to demand health care equity, enjoy cultural foods and live entertainment, culminate the evening with a candlelight vigil to symbolize the power of the health equity movement, and urge their members of Congress to fight for equitable reform. During the event, Congresswoman Lucille Roybal-Allard, chair of the Congressional Hispanic Caucus Health Task Force, joined the rally and urged health equity champions to continue their fight for health equity. She stated, "I stand with you in our shared commitment to achieve a nation free of health disparities, with quality health outcomes for all, regardless of ethnic, racial or cultural background. For we all know that the only way to improve the health of ALL Americans is to enhance the health of EVERY American."[29]

Advocacy Action Steps

Once health equity advocates formed the National Working Group on Health Disparities and Health Reform, which ultimately included more than three hundred national organizations, associations, and coalitions committed to health equity, we immediately went to work developing and implementing a flexible advocacy strategy around communications and media, grassroots, and outreach to Congress and the Obama administration, including Tri-Caucus members. This flexible approach allowed group members to sequentially and simultaneously develop and implement certain components of the advocacy strategy depending on various existing and emerging factors.

The first step in organizing the group and ensuring better facilitation of information dissemination among group members internally was to create a master list of all organizations, associations, and coalitions committed to the inclusion of health equity provisions in health reform. Each organization was urged to specify its areas of expertise around health disparities in regard to quality improvement, behavioral health, prevention and public health, research, and workforce development so that congressional members and staff could more easily identify experts when needed to give briefings or share information on specific health equity issues.

Our second action step was to identify and recruit external champions of health equity in Congress and the administration, as well as organizations that had not yet joined the group, including health care, behavioral health, and public health experts in Washington, DC, and around the country. The intent of this action step was to get health equity included in the larger health reform discussions that were taking place around prevention and wellness, quality improvement, workforce development, insurance expansion, and comparative effectiveness research. For many health equity advocates, addressing health disparities elimination as a singular issue was worrisome because it would not receive enough attention to get included in a larger health reform proposal. They were also concerned that even if it were included in a larger health reform proposal, opponents of health equity would be able to more easily strike the health equity provisions.

The third action step of the advocacy strategy was to collect and share stories about different populations that were experiencing inequities in health care and public health. One such story was that of Esmin Green, who died at a hospital after being ignored by guards and medical staff. Advocates used this story as a wake-up call to show that health care disparities are real and can have tragic consequences. The story also served to highlight the lack of compassion toward individuals with mental health problems and the need for more culturally competent health professionals. Stories such as Esmin Green's were effective in putting a face to the somewhat abstract problem of health disparities.

After collecting stories from across the country, health equity advocates then developed targeted messaging to the relevant congressional members and committees. In the fourth action step of the strategy, we initiated a postcard campaign and drafted letters to congressional leadership explaining the importance of addressing health disparities and urging them to support the inclusion of health equity provisions in health reform legislation. Each organization, association, or coalition lent its name as a signatory to these letters to bring attention to the issue of health disparities. One goal for these postcards and letters was to demonstrate the tremendous support for a health equity agenda that advocates had created and sustained so that they could not be ignored. A second goal was to provide leverage to congressional members and staff to move forward with a health equity agenda in health reform. Each letter had 250 to 300-plus national, regional, and local organizations, associations, and coalitions signed on, and thousands of postcards were delivered to health cham-

pions in Congress. In addition, groups like the American Hospital Association bought ads in major newspapers in DC emphasizing that "true reform should work for everyone—that means eliminating persistent disparities in care for racial and ethnic minorities."[1]

After the foundation had been laid by identifying and recruiting internal and external health equity champions, collecting compelling health equity stories to share with policy makers, and writing to Congress about the importance of including a health equity agenda in health reform, health equity advocates then executed our fifth action step, which involved developing health equity principles, talking points, legislative outlines, and legislative language to share with the key congressional committees charged with drafting the health reform bill. Once these items were vetted by members of the group, health equity advocates then proceeded to tirelessly advocate for their inclusion in congressional white papers and legislative proposals. The group also developed a simple website to house and categorize, by specific health disparity populations, all materials that were created to facilitate use of stakeholder recommendations and to serve as an additional resource for congressional staff when crafting health reform legislation.[2]

The sixth action step by the group involved holding congressional meetings and briefings to educate members of Congress about this critical issue and to serve as a reminder that health equity advocates were persistent and adamant about the inclusion of robust provisions in health reform to address health disparities. These meetings focused on reaching out to members of key committees in Congress, which had jurisdiction over the health reform bills. As these Hill visits were being organized, members of our group found it helpful to establish a listserv to communicate meetings that were secured, in case individual organizations were interested in meeting with a particular member of Congress or had members of their own organizations who were constituents of the representative or senator. We also sought the placement of health disparities experts on panels during congressional hearings and during meetings on health reform to ensure that this issue would continue to receive maximum attention.

Overall, the convening of the National Working Group on Health Disparities and Health Reform resulted in enhanced cooperation, as well as efficient and more targeted use of resources to overcome challenges and leverage opportunities. It led to the creation and execution of a more effective strategy to inform members of Congress and the Obama administration about health disparities and their impact on the health status and care of vulnerable populations as well as the cost burden to the United States.

Notes

1. AHA advertisement supported by more than twenty national associations.
2. Several of the materials have been archived on the National Health Law Program's website www.healthlaw.org and may be accessed by clicking on the tab "Issues" and then clicking on the tab "Health Disparities."

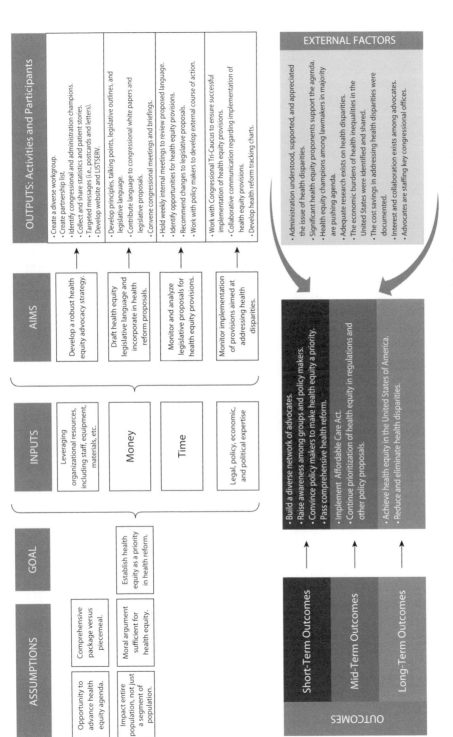

Figure 3.7. Health equity advocacy model. Daniel E. Dawes, JD, and Shanell L. McCoy, PhD, MPH.

July 14, 2009

The Honorable George Miller
Chair
Committee on Education and Labor
U.S. House of Representatives
Washington, DC 20515

The Honorable Charles Rangel
Chair
Committee on Ways and Means
U.S. House of Representatives
Washington, DC 20515

The Honorable Henry A. Waxman
Chair
Committee on Energy and Commerce
U.S. House of Representatives
Washington, DC 20515

Dear Representatives Miller, Rangel, and Waxman

We are writing in support of the *Health Equity and* ...
sion in the final health reform legislation. As you ...
health reform legislation, the undersigned coalitio ...
strengthen the commitment to addressing health i ...
health care disparities reduction and elimination is ...

Health disparities, which exist along the lines not ...
gender, gender identity, disability, geography, sexu ...
socioeconomics, have a direct and detrimental imp ...
and thus, well-being of millions of people in our c ...
legislation that ensures equity and accountability. ...
of 2009 provides the best opportunity for individu ...
comprehensive as well as culturally and linguistic ...
health services, and to achieve positive health out ...

Comprehensive health reform is essential to impr ...
populations and communities that suffer from hea ...
care and public health services. Therefore, we urg ...
Accountability Act of 2009 in health reform legisl ...

We would like to take this opportunity to thank yo ...
to eliminating health disparities. We look forward ...
of health reform legislation that includes the *Heal* ...
to ensure that all populations affected by health an ...
quality health care and experience optimal health. ...

July 14, 2009

The White House
1600 Pennsylvania Avenue, NW
Washington, DC 20500

Dear President Obama:

We are writing in support of the *Health Equity and Accountability Act of 2009* and its inclusion in the final health reform legislation. As you and your colleagues continue to work on health reform legislation, the undersigned coalitions), groups, and organizations urge you to strengthen the commitment to addressing health inequities and make certain that health and health care disparities reduction and elimination is prioritized.

Health disparities, which exist along the lines not only of race and ethnicity, but also gender, gender identity, disability, geography, sexual orientation, national origin, and socioeconomics, have a direct and detrimental impact on the health care, health outcomes, and thus, well-being of millions of people in our country. We envision health reform legislation that ensures equity and accountability. The *Health Equity and Accountability Act of 2009* provides the best opportunity for individuals affected by health disparities to access comprehensive as well as culturally and linguistically appropriate health care and public health services, and to achieve positive health outcomes.

Comprehensive health reform is essential to improving health across the lifespan of populations and communities that suffer from health disparities and barriers to health care and public health services. Therefore, we urge you to include the *Health Equity and Accountability Act of 2009* in health reform legislation.

We would like to take this opportunity to thank you for your leadership and commitment to eliminating health disparities. We look forward to working with you to secure passage of health reform legislation that includes the *Health Equity and Accountability Act of 2009* to ensure that all populations affected by health and health care disparities have access to quality health care and experience optimal health.

We would also like to thank you for your thoughtful consideration of this request and offer our assistance in addressing this critical issue. Please contact Daniel E. Dawes, J.D., at ***-**** or ***@***, if you would like any additional information.

Sincerely,

Figure 3.8. Third National Working Group health reform letter, sent in support of including the Tri-Caucus health equity legislation in health reform

In July 2009, the National Working Group conducted a comprehensive strategic advocacy campaign, which entailed holding meetings with key officials over several weeks to underscore the impact of health disparities on the population. We argued that including health equity provisions in health reform legislation would result in greatly improved health and thousands of lives saved. The National Working Group at this time also sent a third letter to Congress urging support for the inclusion of the comprehensive Health Equity and Accountability Act of 2009, in health reform proposals. It had been introduced in every Congress since 2003 by the Tri-Caucus.

Tea Parties and Death Panels

At this time, as health reform bills in the House were taking shape and negative ads against health reform efforts in Congress were sweeping the country, several congressional members and staff who were supportive of health equity and passing comprehensive health reform legislation contacted advocates, urging us to more publicly demonstrate our support for health reform. They expressed concern that they were hearing only from individuals who oppose the legislation, so a strong show of support for health reform legislation would be needed to secure enough votes for passage. Emotions were high, Democrats were on edge, and many were politically fatigued because of the ambitious legislative undertaking they had endured since the beginning of the year—from tackling the financial bailout of major banking institutions to stimulating the economy out of the Great Recession to climate change as well as other major bills.

The concern about the show of support from health reform champions arose in part from the increasing complexity of the health reform bills and the emergence earlier in the year of the Tea Party, a conservative populist movement characterized by ire against the federal government and what they perceived as excessive taxation. Many Democratic lawmakers were concerned about how comprehensive the bill had become, and "few in the caucus of 256 House Democrats [understood] the emerging 1,000-page bill."[30] To rectify this internal problem, House Democratic leaders organized several briefings during various stages of the bills to keep members informed about what was taking place in the committees that were working on the bills.

While congressional leaders addressed concerns internally in their caucus, they relied on external groups to help them more broadly inform the public about the health reform proposals and stave off rampant misinformation that was engulfing districts across the United States. Tea Party members were virulently opposed to health reform and expended much effort in protesting it. Their protests were spurred on by one-time vice presidential nominee Sarah Palin, who claimed that the health reform legislation would create "death panels" of government employees who would decide who could receive care. Palin was at the time referring to a provision in the early bill that would allow Medicare to cover end-of-life counseling.

The furor from Palin's claim led to this provision's removal from the legislation. Palin later claimed that she was referring to the Independent Payment Advisory Board, a committee tasked with controlling the rate of Medicare spending.[31] Though inaccurate, Palin's notion of "death panels" took hold among the public, adding fuel to the fires of Tea Party resistance.

The leaders of the National Working Group therefore reached out to our members, mobilizing our grassroots to send a clear message to Congress that we supported this vital legislation. With the rise of the Tea Party movement, health reform champions were faced with a new, bold, and uncooperative force opposing the passage of any health reform bill. Members of the Tea Party fanned the flames of resentment, amplified the opposition's voice, and retaliated with the fiercest measures. Nonetheless, during this time of increased opposition, congressional health reformers demonstrated indefatigable courage and resolve, continuing to push for comprehensive health reform despite the tide of external pressures and the unrelenting campaign to dismantle any health reform package that had advanced in the House and Senate. Like previous Congresses, the 111th Congress found itself at a critical juncture in our nation's history, one that presented both an opportunity and a challenge: whether to stand up for what is right even though it may not be popular at the time.

In a surprising turnaround, the American Medical Association on July 16, 2009, boldly announced its support for the House's health reform bill. The AMA in a press release spoke favorably of the bill's provisions that were "key to effective, comprehensive health reform," including providing choice of plans through health insurance exchanges, ending coverage denials based on preexisting conditions, and providing additional funding for primary care services. In an interview on the subject the following week, AMA president Dr. James Rohack explained the organization's decision to support health care reform: "The AMA is clearly committed to health reform this year. We believe the status quo is unacceptable. We want to make sure patients have access to a healthcare system that has affordable health insurance coverage for everybody. As we took a look at those principles and the bill that was being proposed, we knew that our endorsement would be helpful to keep the legislative process moving forward."[32]

Given the history of the advocacy around health reform and the fact that the American Medical Association had in the past been its fiercest opponent, this reversal from one of the most powerful associations in health care was a major boon for the prospects of enacting health reform.

Reform for All, Not Reform for Some!

Despite making strides with the White House and lawmakers, the secondary treatment of the issue of health disparities was still evident during negotiations. Nevertheless, our group, finding strength in numbers and harnessing the power of collaboration, pushed forward, arguing that it was imperative for policy makers to acknowledge the severity of the problems and enact health reforms to curb them. Health equity advocates frequently and consistently argued that eliminating disparities should be a key component of health reform since it will improve health status, save lives, and increase longevity and quality of life for the nation's most vulnerable populations. The National Working Group's tag line became *Health Reform should be reform for all, not reform for some!*

The National Working Group on Health Disparities and Health Reform, which by August 2009 had grown to include well over three hundred national organizations, associations, and coalitions, tirelessly advocated for health equity provisions, which endured multiple attacks from those opposed to health equity or those simply ignorant about these issues. For several months, we made the argument that including health equity provisions in health reform would result in greatly improved health and thousands of lives saved. We thought this moral argument would be sufficient to ensure the inclusion of health equity provisions, and it seemed to resonate with many members of Congress and their staff. But then the focus shifted to costs and cost savings. The Congressional Budget Office, after conducting an analysis of the provisions of the health reform bills, stated that they would cost more than a $1 trillion, so House and Senate health reformers felt tremendous pressure to reduce the estimated costs of their bills.[33] The White House was also feeling pressure to counter arguments that health reform was unaffordable, that the country could not afford to pass a health reform package with that price tag that would increase the national deficit.

Obviously, it was important for the group to react and reframe our message to accommodate this new focus and demonstrate the cost burden that health and health care disparities have on our country. That was easier said than done. Up to this point, group members had tried our best to engage in proactive advocacy, but the shift in focus by policy makers forced us to employ a more reactive advocacy strategy to accommodate this new shift and ensure the continued relevance of health equity provisions in the larger debate on health reform. When congressional staff requested information on the costs of health disparities and the cost savings that would be realized by reducing these disparities, the National Working Group was able to share only two very small studies focusing on Colorado and California.

Fortunately, the Joint Center for Political and Economic Studies released a groundbreaking report by Johns Hopkins University and George Washington University scholars Drs. Thomas A. LaVeist, Darrell J. Gaskin, and Patrick Richard on the costs of health disparities in our country, which put things into perspective.[34] The numbers were more frightening than many thought. But at least now, health equity advocates were able to convince congressional staff that they could not afford to ignore health disparities in health reform. Our group ardently voiced support for the notion that cost savings would be realized not only by improving the health of populations and communities that experience health disparities and barriers to health care and public health services but by reducing the costs resulting from the disproportionate burden of disease faced by these populations. Unfortunately, demonstrating the cost savings that would accrue to the United States if it reduced and eliminated health disparities was not enough to convince policy makers for long, because the focus for health reform shifted once again. At this time, policy makers moved away from calling health reform "comprehensive health reform" to "health insurance reform" once opposition to the bill started to intensify. On August 8, 2009, in his weekly address, President Obama for the first time referred to health reform as "health insurance reform."[35]

At first, many members of the National Working Group thought this was a smart shift—vilifying the insurance companies. But then we became very concerned when many government officials started taking a very narrow approach to health reform, primarily discussing health insurance coverage provisions and barely mentioning the other provisions around quality, prevention, and workforce. As a result, health equity advocates argued that health insurance coverage is crucial, but addressing it alone would not necessarily equate to access and access would not necessarily equate to quality services, treatment, and better outcomes. The group further argued that we envisioned health reform legislation that ensured equity and accountability, provided individuals with the ability to access comprehensive and culturally and linguistically appropriate health care and public health services, and achieve health outcomes consistent with the rest of the population.

From "Comprehensive Health Reform" to "Health Insurance Reform"

■ On March 5, 2009, during a special forum on health reform, President Obama declared, "Our goal will be to enact *comprehensive health reform* by the end of this year."[1]

■ On April 20, 2009, Senator Kennedy (chair of Senate HELP Committee) and Senator Baucus (chair of Senate Finance Committee) sent a letter to President Obama affirming their mutual commitment to passing *"comprehensive health reform"* and marking up legislation in early June.[2]

■ On May 13, 2009, the president wrote in his first e-mail newsletter, "The Vice President and I just met with leaders from the House of Representatives and received their commitment to pass a *"comprehensive health care reform"* bill by July 31."[3]

■ On June 2, 2009, President Obama sent a lengthy letter to both Senators Edward Kennedy and Max Baucus, where it was clear the administration had nixed "comprehensive" when describing health care reform. He commended them for "the hard work your Committees are doing on *health care reform"* and stated *"health care reform* is not a luxury." He went on to say, "We simply cannot afford to postpone *health care reform* any longer" and *"health care reform* must not add to our deficits over the next 10 years." He then concluded by mentioning "health care reform" three more times, including that he was "committed to working with the Congress to fully offset the cost of *health*

care reform," that there was "a valuable tool to help achieve *health care reform*," and that he "look[ed] forward to working with [them] so that the Congress can complete *health care reform* by October."[4] In all, the president mentioned health care reform seven times in his letter. This was a noticeable change in strategy— moving from "comprehensive health reform" to "health care reform," which occurred at the height of the Tea Party's emergence, when congressional staffers were asking health reform proponents to make their voices heard more.

■ On June 15, 2009, President Obama during his speech at the annual conference of the AMA, continued referencing "health care reform" and moved away from using "comprehensive health reform," except one time when he referred to "comprehensive reform." He said, "After all, Presidents have called for *health care reform* for nearly a century." Later on he mentioned, "We know the moment is right for *health care reform*" and *"health care reform* should be guided by a simple principle: Fix what's broken and build on what works." He also emphasized, *"Health care reform* must be, and will be, deficit-neutral in the next decade," and "the best thing for our charities is the stronger economy that we will build with *health care reform*." And he stated, "We've put $950 billion on the table, taking us almost all the way to covering the full cost of *health care reform*," and "I look forward to working with Congress to make up the difference so that *health care reform* is fully paid for."[5]

■ On July 17, 2009, President Obama made remarks pledging to get *health care reform* done that year. Remarks did not include the term "comprehensive."[6]

■ On August 8, 2009, President Obama in his weekly address stated, "We must lay a new foundation for future growth and prosperity, and a key pillar of a new foundation is *health insurance reform*—reform that we are now closer to achieving than ever before."[7]

■ On October 29, 2009, Speaker Nancy Pelosi and the House Democratic Caucus held an event at the Capitol on *health insurance reform*.

■ On November 21, 2009, Senator Patrick Leahy, speaking on the floor of the senate stated, "Decision time is near on *health insurance reform*."[8]

■ On December 24, 2009, President Obama, after the vote in the Senate, made remarks that included reference to health insurance reform three times. First he remarked, "In a historic vote that took place this morning members of the Senate joined their colleagues in the House of Representatives to pass a landmark *health insurance reform package*." Second he asserted, "We are now finally poised to deliver on the promise of real, meaningful *health insurance reform*." Third he stated, "We are now incredibly close to making *health insurance reform* a reality in this country."[9]

■ On March 21, 2010, Speaker Pelosi spoke on the House floor before the vote on the Patient Protection and Affordable Care Act: "today, we have the opportunity to complete the great unfinished business of our society and pass *health insurance reform* for all Americans that is a right and not a privilege."[10]

Notes

1. Obama, "Remarks by the President at the Opening of the White House Forum on Health Reform" (emphasis added).
2. Newton-Small, "And. Here. We. Go" (emphasis added).
3. Lee, "Health Reform" (emphasis added).
4. Lee, "The President Spells Out His Vision on Health Care Reform" (emphasis added).
5. Obama, "Remarks by the President to the Annual Conference of the American Medical Association" (emphasis added).
6. Brandon, "President on Health Care" (emphasis added).
7. Obama, "President Obama Calls Health Insurance Reform Key to Stronger Economy and Improvement on Status Quo" (emphasis added).
8. Cong. Rec. S11907–S11967 (November 21, 2009, emphasis added).
9. Obama, "Remarks by the President on Senate Passage of Health Insurance Reform" (emphasis added).
10. Pelosi, "Today, We Have the Opportunity to Complete the Great Unfinished Business of Our Society and Pass Health Insurance Reform for All Americans" (emphasis added).

NOTES

1. Moffit, "McCain Health Care Plan."

2. *Seizing the New Opportunity for Health Reform* (opening statement of Senator Chuck Grassley).

3. Ibid.

4. *Seizing the New Opportunity for Health Reform* (testimony of Tommy Thompson, emphasis mine).

5. "Ted Kennedy and Health Care Reform."

6. Dwyer, "After a Death Seen on Tape, Change Is Promised"; Snow and Fantz, "Woman Who Died on Hospital Floor Called 'Beautiful Person.'"

7. Kaiser Family Foundation, "Eliminating Racial/Ethnic Disparities in Health Care." Senators Barack Obama and John McCain were the candidates in this election cycle.

8. Obama, Plan for a Healthy America.

9. Baucus, "Finance Chairman Baucus Unveils Blueprint for Comprehensive Health Care Reform."

10. Hilda Solis was nominated by President Obama for the Secretary of Labor cabinet post during December 2008 and was confirmed by the United States Senate on February 24, 2009. She became the first Latina cabinet member.

11. Seabrook, "Healthcare Overhaul Boosts Pelosi's Clout."

12. Martin, "Obama Calls for Health-Care Reform in 2009."

13. Obama recognized that the American Recovery and Reinvestment Act laid the foundation for health reform and appointed Sebelius and DeParle to his team. Obama, "Remarks by President Obama, HHS Secretary-designate Kathleen Sebelius, and White House Office of Health Reform Director Nancy-Ann DeParle."

14. See chapter 6 for details about comparative effectiveness research.

15. Obama, "Remarks by the President at the Opening of the White House Forum on Health Reform."

16. Cooper et al., *Unclaimed Children Revisited*.

17. Executive Order 13507, Establishment of the White House Office of Health Reform.

18. Newton-Small, "And. Here. We. Go."

19. US Senate Committee on Finance, "Finance Leaders Release Health Care Reform Policy Options."

20. Darrel Thompson, the senior advisor to the Senate majority leader, Harry Reid; Mayra Alvarez, who served as a health policy advisor to Senator Richard Durbin, the assistant majority leader—the second-highest ranking position in the Senate; Mona Shah, the senior health policy advisor to Senator Barbara Mikulski; and Priscilla Ross, the policy director for Senator Benjamin Cardin, worked closely with their colleagues to ensure that the health reform package included robust provisions to advance health equity and elevate the health of all communities.

21. Burris, the only African American senator at the time, had filled President Obama's Senate seat.

22. US Senate Committee on Finance, "Health Care Reform from Conception to Final Passage"; US Senate Committee on Finance, "Baucus, Grassley Release Policy Options for Expanding Health Care Coverage."

23. Obama, "Text of a Letter from the President to Senator Edward M. Kennedy and Senator Max Baucus."

24. Congressional Black Caucus to Barak Obama, June 5, 2009, in the author's possession.

25. *Addressing Disparities in Health and Healthcare.*

26. Invited speakers included Garth Graham, MD, MPH, deputy assistant secretary for minority health, US Department of Health and Human Services; Louis W. Sullivan, MD, chair of the Sullivan Alliance to Transform the Health Professions, former secretary, US Department of Health and Human Services, and president emeritus, Morehouse School of Medicine; Sally Satel, MD, resident scholar, American Enterprise Institute; Rubens J. Pamies, MD, vice chancellor for academic affairs at the University of Nebraska Medical Center; Peter B. Bach, MD, Memorial Sloan-Kettering Cancer Center, pulmonary and critical care physician, former senior advisor to the administrator of the Centers for Medicare and Medicaid Services; Amitabh Chandra, PhD, professor of public policy, Harvard University Kennedy School of Government; Herman A. Taylor Jr., MD, principal investigator/director, Shirley Professor for the Study of Health Disparities, Jackson Heart Study; Barbara Howard, PhD, principal investigator, Strong Heart Study, Medstar Research Institute; William Lewis, MD, for the American Heart Association's Get with the Guidelines; and Bruce Siegel, MD, codirector, Expecting Success: Excellence in Cardiac Care, of the Robert Wood Johnson Foundation Quality Improvement Collaborative, George Washington University School of Public Health and Health Services.

27. *Health Care Disparities* (testimony of Sally Satel).

28. *Health Care Disparities.*

29. Roybal-Allard, "Congresswoman Lucille Roybal-Allard, Healthcare Equality Advocates 'Light the Night.'"

30. Murray and Kane, "Pelosi Vows Passage of Health-Care Overhaul."

31. Kessler, "Sarah Palin, 'Death Panels' and 'Obamacare.'"

32. American Medical Association, "AMA Supports H.R. 3200, 'America's Affordable Health Choices Act of 2009'"; Garber, "AMA: Healthcare Reform Bill a 'Starting Point.'"

33. The Senate proposal was estimated to cost the federal government $1.6 trillion.

34. From 2003 to 2006 the combined cost of health disparities totaled $1.24 trillion in our country. This report also found that in the same time period, eliminating certain health disparities would have reduced direct health care

expenditures by $229.4 billion. LaVeist, Gaskin, and Richard, *Economic Burden of Health Inequalities in the United States*.

35. Obama, "President Obama Calls Health Insurance Reform Key to Stronger Economy and Improvement on Status Quo."

BIBLIOGRAPHY

Addressing Disparities in Health and Healthcare: Issues of Reform; Hearing Before the Subcommittee on Health of the Committee on Ways and Means US House of Representatives, 110th Cong. Second session, June 10, 2008. http://www.gpo .gov/fdsys/pkg/CHRG-110hhrg47453/pdf/CHRG-110hhrg47453.pdf.

Agency for Healthcare Research and Quality. *Clinician Summary: Attention Deficit Hyperactivity Disorder in Children and Adolescents*. Rockville, MD, 2011. Retrieved September 10, 2012, from http://effectivehealthcare.ahrq.gov/ehc /products/191/1149/adhd_clin_fin_to_post.pdf.

———. *National Healthcare Disparities Report: Summary*. Rockville, MD, 2004. Retrieved August 22, 2011, from http://www.ahrq.gov/qual/nhdr03/nhdrsum03.htm.

———. *National Healthcare Disparities Report*. Rockville, MD, 2006. Retrieved August 22, 2011, from http://www.ahrq.gov/qual/nhdr06/nhdr06.htm.

———. *National Healthcare Disparities Report*. Rockville, MD, 2011. Retrieved August 22, 2012, from http://www.ahrq.gov/qual/qrdr11.htm.

———. *National Healthcare Quality Report*. Rockville, MD, 2011. Retrieved August 22, 2012, from http://www.ahrq.gov/qual/qrdr11.htm.

American Medical Association. "AMA Supports H.R. 3200, 'America's Affordable Health Choices Act of 2009.'" Press release, July 16, 2009. http://www.ama -assn.org/ama/pub/news/news/ama-supports-hr-3200.page.

American Psychological Association. "Psychological and Behavioral Perspectives on Health Disparities." Communique, March 2009. Washington, DC. http://www.apa.org/pi/oema/resources/communique/2009/03/march.pdf.

Baucus, Max. "Finance Chairman Baucus Unveils Blueprint for Comprehensive Health Care Reform." US Senate Committee on Finance. Press release, November 12, 2008. http://www.finance.senate.gov/newsroom/chairman /release/?id=a36a2265-d3ea-41c3-904c-d02620103acb.

Brandon, Katherine. "The President on Health Care: 'We are Going to Get this Done.'" *White House Blog*, July 17, 2009. http://www.whitehouse.gov/blog /The-President-on-Health-Care-We-are-Going-to-Get-this-Done.

Breakey, W. R., P. J. Fischer, M. Kramer, G. Nestadt, A. J. Romanoski, A. Ross, R. M. Royall, and O. Stine. "Health and Mental Health Problems of Homeless Men and Women in Baltimore." *Journal of the American Medical Association* 262 (1989): 1352-1357.

Breslau, J., S. Aguilar-Gaxiola, K. Kendler, S. Maxwell, D. Williams, and R. Kessler. "Specifying Race-Ethnic Differences in Risk for Psychiatric Disorder in a USA National Sample." *Psychological Medicine* 36, no. 1 (2006): 57-68.

Centers for Disease Control and Prevention. *Childhood Obesity Facts*. Hyattsville, MD: 2012. Retrieved May 29, 2012, from http://www.cdc.gov/obesity/data /childhood.html.

———. Table 61. In *Health, United States, 2007 with Chartbook on Trends in the Health of Americans*. Hyattsville, MD: 2007, 262-263.

———. National Center for Health Statistics. *Health, United States, 2011: With Special Feature on Socioeconomic Status and Health*. Hyattsville, MD, 2012. Retrieved May 29, 2012, from http://www.cdc.gov/nchs/data/hus/hus11 .pdf#listfigures.

Cochran, S., J. Sullivan, and V. Mays. "Prevalence of Mental Disorders, Psychological Distress, and Mental Health Services Use among Lesbian, Gay, and Bisexual Adults in the United States." *Journal of Consulting and Clinical Psychology* 71 (2003): 53-61.

Congressional Record. "Service Members Home Ownership Tax Act of 2009—Motion to Proceed." S11907-S11967 (November 21, 2009). http://www .gpo.gov/fdsys/pkg/CREC-2009-11-21/html/CREC-2009-11-21-pt1-PgS11907-2 .htm.

Cooper, J., Y. Aratani, J. Knitzer, A. Douglas-Hall, R. Masi, P. Banghart, and S. Dababnah. *Unclaimed Children Revisited: The Status of Children's Mental Health Policy in the United States*. New York: National Center for Children in Poverty, 2008.

Dawes, Daniel. "Health Reform: A Bridge to Health Equity." In *Child and Family Advocacy: Bridging the Gaps between Research, Practice, and Policy,* edited by Anne McDonald Culp, 35-49. New York: Springer, 2013.

Dwyer, Jim. "After a Death Seen on Tape, Change Is Promised." *New York Times,* July 12, 2008. http://www.nytimes.com/2008/07/12/nyregion/12about.html? _r=0.

Evans, Jennifer, and Jaclyn Schiff. "A Timeline of Kennedy's Health Care Achievements and Disappointments." *Kaiser Health News,* August 26, 2009. http://www.kaiserhealthnews.org/stories/2009/august/26/kennedy-health -care-timeline.aspx.

Executive Order 13507. Establishment of the White House Office of Health Reform. April 8, 2009. https://www.whitehouse.gov/the-press-office /executive-order-establishing-white-house-office-health-reform.

Garber, Kent. "AMA: Healthcare Reform Bill a 'Starting Point.'" *US News,* July 29, 2009. http://www.usnews.com/news/national/articles/2009/07/29/ama -healthcare-reform-bill-a-starting-point.

Health Care Disparities: A Briefing before the United States Commission on Civil Rights. US CCR briefing report, December 2010. Washington, DC. http://www.usccr .gov/pubs/Healthcare-Disparities.pdf.

Institute of Medicine. *The Health of Lesbian, Gay, Bisexual and Transgender People: Building a Foundation to Better Health.* Washington, DC: National Academies Press, 2011.

———. *How Far Have We Come in Reducing Health Disparities? Progress since 2000; Workshop Summary.* Washington, DC: National Academies Press, 2012.

———. *Unequal Treatment: Confronting Racial and Ethnic Disparities in Healthcare.* Washington, DC: National Academies Press, 2002.

Janssen, I., W. Craig, W. Boyce, and W. Pickett. "Associations between Overweight and Obesity with Bullying Behaviors in School-Aged Children." *Pediatrics*, 113 (2004): 1187-1194.

Kaiser Family Foundation. "Eliminating Racial/Ethnic Disparities in Health Care: What Are the Options?" Issue brief, October 2008. http://kaiserfamilyfoundation.files.wordpress.com/2013/01/7830.pdf.

———. "President Obama's Campaign Position on Health Reform and Other Health Care Issues." November 01, 2008. http://kff.org/disparities-policy/issue-brief/president-obamas-campaign-position-on-health-reform/.

Kennedy, Edward. *Fighting for Quality, Affordable Health Care.* http://tedkennedy.org/service/item/health_care.

Kessler, Glenn. "Sarah Palin, 'Death Panels' and 'Obamacare.'" *Washington Post*, June 27, 2012. http://www.washingtonpost.com/blogs/fact-checker/post/sarah-palin-death-panels-and-obamacare/2012/06/27/gJQAysUP7V_blog.html.

Koegel, P. M., A. Burnam, and R. K. Farr. "The Prevalence of Specific Psychiatric Disorders among Homeless Individuals in the Inner City of Los Angeles." *Archives of General Psychiatry* 45 (1988): 1085-1093.

LaVeist, T., D. Gaskin, and P. Richard. *The Economic Burden of Health Inequalities in the United States.* Washington, DC: Joint Center for Political and Economic Studies Report, September 2009.

Lee, Jesse. "Health Reform: 'Urgency and Determination.'" *White House Blog*, May 3, 2009. http://www.whitehouse.gov/blog/Health-Reform-Urgency-and-Determination.

———. "The President Spells Out His Vision on Health Care Reform." *White House Blog*, June 3, 2009. https://www.whitehouse.gov/blog/2009/06/03/president-spells-out-his-vision-health-care-reform.

Low, N., and J. Hardy. "Psychiatric Disorder Criteria and Their Application to Research in Different Racial Groups." *BMC Psychiatry* 7, no. 1 (2007). doi: 10.1186/1471-244X-7-1.

Martin, David. "Obama Calls for Health-Care Reform in 2009." *CNN*, February 24, 2009. http://www.cnn.com/2009/POLITICS/02/24/obama.health.care/index.html?_s=PM:POLITICS.

Minority Health and Health Disparities Research and Education Act of 2000. P.L. 106-525, 114 Stat. 2495.

Moffit, Robert E. "The McCain Health Care Plan: More Power to Families." *Heritage Foundation.* Backgrounder, October 15, 2008. http://www.heritage.org/research/reports/2008/10/the-mccain-health-care-plan-more-power-to-families.

Murray, Shailagh, and Paul Kane. "Pelosi Vows Passage of Health-Care Over-
haul." Politics. *Washington Post*, July 27, 2009. http://www.washingtonpost
.com/wp-dyn/content/article/2009/07/26/AR2009072602856.html.
National Alliance on Mental Illness. "Mental Illness: Facts and Numbers."
Arlington, VA, 2013. Retrieved August 26, 2015, from http://www2.nami.org
/factsheets/mentalillness_factsheet.pdf.
National Association of State Mental Health Program Directors. *Measurement of
Health Status for People with Serious Mental Illnesses*. Alexandria, VA, 2008.
Retrieved September 7, 2012, from http://www.nasmhpd.org/content
/measurement-health-status-people-serious-mental-illnesses.
National Federation of Independent Business v. Sebelius, 132 U.S. 2566.
Newton-Small, Jay. "And. Here. We. Go." *Time*, April 20, 2009. http://swampland
.time.com/2009/04/20/and-here-we-go/.
Obama, Barak. Plan for a Healthy America. http://www.nytimes.com/packages
/pdf/politics/factsheet_healthcare.pdf.
———. "President Obama Calls Health Insurance Reform Key to Stronger
Economy and Improvement on Status Quo." Weekly address, August 8, 2009.
http://www.whitehouse.gov/the-press-office/weekly-address-president
-obama-calls-health-insurance-reform-key-stronger-economy-a.
———. "Remarks by President Obama, HHS Secretary-designate Kathleen
Sebelius, and White House Office of Health Reform Director Nancy-Ann
DeParle." Press release, March 2, 2009. https://www.whitehouse.gov/the
-press-office/remarks-president-obama-hhs-secretary-designate-kathleen
-sebelius-and-white-house-o.
———. "Remarks by the President at the Opening of the White House Forum on
Health Reform." Press release, March 5, 2009. http://www.whitehouse.gov
/the-press-office/remarks-president-opening-white-house-forum-health
-reform.
———. "Remarks by the President on Senate Passage of Health Insurance
Reform." Press release, December 24, 2009. http://www.whitehouse.gov/the
-press-office/remarks-president-senate-passage-health-insurance-reform.
———. "Remarks by the President to the Annual Conference of the American
Medical Association." Press release, June 15, 2009. https://www.whitehouse
.gov/the-press-office/remarks-president-annual-conference-american
-medical-association.
———. "Text of a Letter from the President to Senator Edward M. Kennedy and
Senator Max Baucus." The White House. June 2, 2009. http://www
.whitehouse.gov/the_press_office/Letter-from-President-Obama-to
-Chairmen-Edward-M-Kennedy-and-Max-Baucus.
Obama, Barak, and Joe Biden. "The Obama-Biden Plan." Office of the President-
Elect. http://change.gov/agenda/health_care_agenda/.
Patient Protection and Affordable Care Act. P.L. 111-148.

Pelosi, Nancy. "Today, We Have the Opportunity to Complete the Great Unfinished Business of Our Society and Pass Health Insurance Reform for All Americans." Press release, March 21, 2010. http://pelosi.house.gov/news /press-releases/pelosi-today-we-have-the-opportunity-to-complete-the-great -unfinished-business.

Roybal-Allard, Lucille. "Congresswoman Lucille Roybal-Allard, Healthcare Equality Advocates 'Light the Night' for Reform, Demand Congressional Action on Disparities." Press release, June 24, 2009. http://roybal-allard .house.gov/news/documentsingle.aspx?DocumentID=134906.

Sack, Kevin, Shan Carter, Jonathan Ellis, Farhana Hossain, and Alan Mclean. "Election 2008—On the Issues: Health Care." *New York Times*, May 23, 2012. http://elections.nytimes.com/2008/president/issues/health.html.

Seabrook, Andrea. "Health Care Overhaul Boosts Pelosi's Clout." *NPR*, March 29, 2010. http://www.npr.org/templates/story/story.php?storyId =125294497.

Seizing the New Opportunity for Health Reform: Hearing of the Committee on Finance. 110th Congress, Second session, Tuesday, May 6, 2008.

Smith, Emily. "Timeline of the Health Care Law." *CNN.com*, June 17, 2012. http://www.cnn.com/2012/06/17/politics/health-care-timeline/.

Snow, Mary, and Ashley Fantz. "Woman Who Died on Hospital Floor Called 'Beautiful Person.'" *CNN*, July 3, 2008. http://www.cnn.com/2008/US/07/03 /hospital.woman.death/.

Stagman, S., and J. Cooper. *Children's Mental Health: What Every Policymaker Should Know.* New York: National Center for Children in Poverty, 2010.

Substance Abuse and Mental Health Services Administration. *Risk of Suicide among Hispanic Females Aged 12 to 17.* National Household Survey on Drug Abuse Report. Rockville, MD: SAMHSA, 2003. Retrieved September 1, 2011, from http://www.oas.samhsa.gov/2k3/LatinaSuicide/LatinaSuicide.htm.

Swartz, M., R. Wagner, J. Swanson, B. Burns, L. George, and D. Padgett. "Administrative Update: Utilization of Services." *Community Mental Health Journal* 34, no. 2 (1998): 133–144.

"Ted Kennedy and Health Care Reform." *Newsweek*, July 17, 2009. http://www .newsweek.com/ted-kennedy-and-health-care-reform-82011.

Teplin, L. A. "The Prevalence of Severe Mental Disorder among Male Urban Jail Detainees: Comparison with the Epidemiologic Catchment Area Program." *American Journal of Public Health* 80 (1990): 663–669.

Thomas, Peter. "White House Summit on Health Care Reform." External memorandum to CCD Health and Long Term Services Task Forces and interested parties, March 10, 2009, in the author's possession.

Thrush, Glenn. "Black Caucus Pushes Obama on Health Equity." *Politico*, June 8, 2009. http://www.politico.com/blogs/glennthrush/0609/Black_Caucus _pushes_Obama_on_health_equity.html.

US Department of Health and Human Services. *Mental Health: Culture, Race, and Ethnicity—A Supplement to Mental Health: A Report of the Surgeon General*. Rockville, MD: US Department of Health and Human Services, 2001.

US Department of Health and Human Services, Advisory Committee on Minority Health, Office of Minority Health. *Ensuring That Health Care Reform Will Meet the Health Care Needs of Minority Communities and Eliminate Health Disparities: A Statement of Principles and Recommendations*. Rockville, MD, 2009. Retrieved September 10, 2011, from http://minorityhealth.hhs.gov /Assets/pdf/Checked/1/ACMH_HealthCareAccessReport.pdf.

US Department of Health and Human Services, New Freedom Commission on Mental Health. *Achieving the Promise: Transforming Mental Health Care in America—Final Report*. Rockville, MD, 2003.

US Department of Health and Human Services, Office of Minority Health. *Native Hawaiian/Other Pacific Islander Profile*. Rockville, MD, 2012. Retrieved May 29, 2012, from http://minorityhealth.hhs.gov/templates/content.aspx ?lvl=3&lvlID=4&ID=8593.

US Senate Committee on Finance. "Baucus, Grassley Release Policy Options for Expanding Health Care Coverage." Press release, May 11, 2009. http://www .finance.senate.gov/newsroom/chairman/release/?id=e135f9d6-6140-4d57 -87ab-4b80647283ff.

———. "Finance Leaders Release Health Care Reform Policy Option." Press release, April 28, 2009. http://www.finance.senate.gov/newsroom/chairman /release/?id=f8ea4f72-b3af-4c93-8bf1-922f61714dfd.

———. "Health Care Reform from Conception to Final Passage: Timeline of the Finance Committee's Work to Reform America's Health Care System." http://www.finance.senate.gov/issue/?id=32be19bd-491e-4192-812f -f65215c1ba65.

Vernez, G. M., M. A. Burnam, E. A. McGlynn, S. Trude, and B. Mittman. *Review of California's Program for the Homeless Mentally Ill Disabled*. Report No. R3631-CDMH. Santa Monica, CA: RAND, 1988.

Wells, K., R. Klap, A. Koike, and C. Sherbourne. "Ethnic Disparities in Unmet Need for Alcoholism, Drug Abuse, and Mental Health Care." *American Journal of Psychiatry* 158 (2001): 2027-2032.

"White House Forum on Health Reform Attendees and Breakout Session Participants." Press release, March 5, 2009. https://www.whitehouse.gov/the -press-office/white-house-forum-health-reform-attendees-and-breakout -session-participants.

Williams, D., H. Gonzalez, H. Neighbors, R. Nesse, J. Abelson, J. Sweetman, and J. Jackson. "Prevalence and Distribution of Major Depressive Disorder in African Americans, Caribbean Blacks, and Non-Hispanic Whites: Results from the National Survey of American Life." *Archives of General Psychiatry* 64 (2007): 305-315.

The Fight Is On
Final Efforts to Pass ObamaCare

The leadership belongs not to the loudest, not to those who beat the drums or blow the trumpets, but to those who day in and day out, in all seasons, work for the practical realization of a better world—those who have the stamina to persist and remain dedicated.—*Congressman Gus Hawkins*

Disappointed but Not Defeated

During August 2009, the period that Congress typically takes off to visit constituents, the Tea Party movement executed a strategy to target town halls that were convened by Democrats. These town halls resulted in heated exchanges between the member of Congress and the audience. House Speaker Nancy Pelosi, echoing the sentiments of many in her caucus, declared, "The town hall meetings were really an orchestration. What is out there's where people who want to stop a progress, exploit and hijack the good intentions of people who have legitimate concerns. So you have to be able to differentiate among those who are obstructionists and those who have real concerns."[1] Health reform supporters did their best to mobilize their base and ensure that the dialogue was balanced, but they were no match for the opposition groups who heckled lawmakers and effectively spread their ringing propaganda.

Toward the end of the month, on August 25, 2009, the great champion for health reform, Senator Kennedy, passed away; just one month after his Senate Health, Education, Labor and Pensions Committee passed the Affordable Health Choices Act. So strong was Senator Kennedy's passion for health reform that, in 2008, he ignored his doctors' advice and gave a speech at the Democratic National Convention in Denver about health care reform. In May 2009 he repeated his feelings in a letter to President Obama, which his wife Vicki delivered after his passing. "You will be the president who at long last signs into law the health care reform that is the great unfinished business of our society," Kennedy wrote. "For me, this cause stretched across decades; it has been disappointed, but never finally defeated. It was the cause of my life."[2] A few weeks later President Obama gave remarks to a Joint Session of Congress on health care, supporting the ongoing negotiations in Congress, and reemphasizing his commitment to reform. President Obama spoke about Senator Kennedy during his remarks.

Now, I have no interest in putting insurance companies out of business. They provide a legitimate service, and employ a lot of our friends and neighbors. I just want to hold them accountable. (Applause.) And the insurance reforms that I've already mentioned would do just that. But an additional step we can take to keep insurance companies honest is by making a not-for-profit public option available in the insurance exchange. (Applause.) Now, let me be clear. Let me be clear. It would only be an option for those who don't have insurance. No one would be forced to choose it, and it would not impact those of you who already have insurance. In fact, based on Congressional Budget Office estimates, we believe that less than 5 percent of Americans would sign up.

Despite all this, the insurance companies and their allies don't like this idea. They argue that these private companies can't fairly compete with the government. And they'd be right if taxpayers were subsidizing this public insurance option. But they won't be. I've insisted that like any private insurance company, the public insurance option would have to be self-sufficient and rely on the premiums it collects. But by avoiding some of the overhead that gets eaten up at private companies by profits and excessive administrative costs and executive salaries, it could provide a good deal for consumers, and would also keep pressure on private insurers to keep their policies affordable and treat their customers better, the same way public colleges and universities provide additional choice and competition to students without in any way inhibiting a vibrant system of private colleges and universities. (Applause.)

Now, it is—it's worth noting that a strong majority of Americans still favor a public insurance option of the sort I've proposed tonight. But its impact shouldn't be exaggerated—by the left or the right or the media. It is only one part of my plan, and shouldn't be used as a handy excuse for the usual Washington ideological battles. To my progressive friends, I would remind you that for decades, the driving idea behind reform has been to end insurance company abuses and make coverage available for those without it. (Applause.) The public option—the public option is only a means to that end—and we should remain open to other ideas that accomplish our ultimate goal. And to my Republican friends, I say that rather than making wild claims about a government takeover of health care, we should work together to address any legitimate concerns you may have. (Applause.)

I received one of those letters a few days ago. It was from our beloved friend and colleague, Ted Kennedy. He had written it back in May, shortly after he was told that his illness was terminal. He asked that it be delivered upon his death.

In it, he spoke about what a happy time his last months were, thanks to the love and support of family and friends, his wife, Vicki, his amazing children, who are all here tonight. And he expressed confidence that this would be the year that health care reform—"that great unfinished business of our society," he called it—would finally pass. He repeated the truth that health care is decisive for our future prosperity, but he also reminded me that "it concerns more than material things." "What we face," he wrote, "is above all a moral issue; at stake are not just the details of policy, but fundamental principles of social justice and the character of our country."

I've thought about that phrase quite a bit in recent days—the character of our country. One of the unique and wonderful things about America has always been our self-reliance, our rugged individualism, our fierce defense of freedom and our healthy skepticism of government. And figuring out the appropriate size and role of government has always been a source of rigorous and, yes, sometimes angry debate. That's our history.[3]

After fighting to make sure that other health equity provisions remained a priority during this shift to "health insurance reform," advocates endured additional battles and had to make sure that we remained diligent in our advocacy in order to keep these provisions intact. On September 2, 2009, we were contacted by officials at the White House warning us that several of our health equity provisions were slated for the chopping block. We were surprised to hear this and conveyed to White House officials our concerns. Then, the following morning, the *New York Times* published an article titled "Obama Aides Aim to Scale Back Health Bills," which detailed plans by some officials to eliminate provisions in health reform proposals around data collection and school-based health clinics.[4] We were disappointed but determined to keep pushing back against any attempts to repeal our critical provisions.

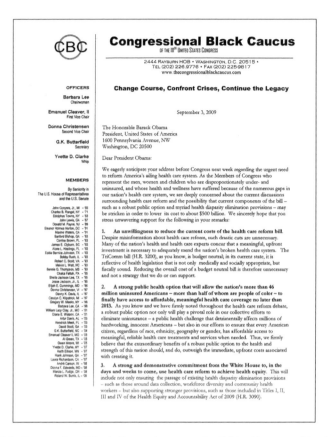

Figure 4.1. Congressional Black Caucus Letter to the White House pushing back on attempts to eliminate health equity-focused provisions

The Congressional Black Caucus was also deeply concerned about the possibility that the public option and key health equity provisions could be stricken. The next day, on September 3, 2009, the CBC struck back by declaring its strong opposition to any attempts to cut the myriad of health disparity elimination provisions. Anticipating the president's address before a Joint Session of Congress in one week, the CBC used its letter to highlight its key priorities as health reform continued to move forward: (1) shifting the focus away from the substance of the bill to the cost of the bill would be ineffective, (2) the need for a strong public option, (3) commitment from the White House to use health reform to achieve health equity, (4) inclusion of provisions to ensure equity and parity for individuals in the US territories, and (5) using the savings from the prevention and public health provisions to pay for or offset the costs of the legislation.

In response to the CBC's letter, the White House convened a conference call with leaders of the Quad-Caucus, which included the CBC, CHC, CAPAC, and the Progressive Caucus. During the call with President Obama, these congressional leaders stressed the importance of expanding prevention and wellness services and the need for health equity provisions—such as data collection, workforce diversity, and community health workers. They emphasized that these provisions were necessary to address the root causes of the health inequities that disproportionately and detrimentally affect racial and ethnic minorities, women, rural Americans, and Americans in the US territories. According to Representative Barbara Lee, the "discussion with President Obama was a useful and productive conversation." The consensus was that the president appreciated their input and was taking their views seriously. The congressional Tri-Caucus iterated its commitment to working diligently on health reform to the president.

The National Working Group responded to the *New York Times* article by sending a letter to the White House urging the Obama administration to keep the data-collection provisions in the health reform legislation. Fortunately, four days prior, the Institute of Medicine had released a report on August 31, 2009, titled *Race, Ethnicity, and Language Data: Standardization for Health Care Quality Improvement,* that demonstrated the importance of collecting and reporting demographic data. This report helped to bolster our arguments for more accurate and robust data collection and reporting. Later on, it all made sense to us why the White House was pressed to find provisions to cut that would reduce the costs of the bills.

One week after the White House had contacted us, on September 9, 2009, President Obama spoke before a Joint Session of Congress and promised that his health reform proposal would not add to the deficit and would not cost more than $900 billion. This meant that the White House had to find ways to fulfill this promise, as did the congressional architects of the legislation who were also worried about public perception. Lawmakers were determined to meet the president's ceiling on the cost of the bill, while we were determined to continue arguing the fact that our provisions would not only significantly reduce costs but also help to elevate the health of all Americans once implemented.

Having pushed back on attempts to undermine the health equity agenda that had been achieved in various reform bills, advocates faced another

September 8, 2009

The White House
1600 Pennsylvania Avenue, NW
Washington, DC 20500

Dear President Obama:

The undersigned coalitions, groups, and organizations wish to express our concern with recent information indicating the possibility of eliminating data collection provisions in health reform legislation. As noted in an article published in the New York Times on September 3, 2009 titled, *Obama Aides Aim to Simplify and Scale Back Health Bills*, it was stated, "White House officials said Congress could also drop proposals requiring the government to create school-based health clinics and collect nationwide data on health and health care by race, sex, sexual orientation and 'gender identity.'"

As you know, data collection is essential to track use and quality of care, document disparities and tailor interventions. Without data, it will not be possible to identify and properly address disparities in health and health care in a culturally and linguistically appropriate way.

Your Administration has continued to be supportive of data collection, including provisions in the *American Recovery and Reinvestment Act* (ARRA). This statute requires the Department of Health and Human Services (HHS) to develop standards for collecting race, ethnicity and language data for electronic health records. The inclusion of this important provision was made with the support of your Administration and without any objection by the public or Congress.

Earlier this week, the Institute of Medicine released its report, *Race, Ethnicity, and Language Data: Standardization for Health Care Quality Improvement*. The report, commissioned by the Agency for Healthcare Research and Quality (AHRQ), notes the need for standardizing collection of race, ethnicity and language data for quality improvement and provides a number of recommendations. The report notes, "there is strong evidence that the quality of health care varies as a function of race, ethnicity, and language. Having quality metrics stratified by race, Hispanic ethnicity, granular ethnicity, and language need can assist in improving overall quality and promoting equity."

We strongly urge you to continue your ongoing support of data collection and respectfully request the inclusion of specific data collection provisions in health reform legislation. Critical provisions impacting data collection have been included in health reform legislation including those for race, ethnicity, gender, gender identity, language, sexual orientation, and disability status. A final bill should include the data collection provisions outlined in the Senate Finance Committee's *Description of Policy Options Expanding Health Care Coverage: Proposals to Provide Affordable Coverage to All Americans*, Sec. 3301 from the *Affordable Health Choices Act, and Title III from the Health Equity and Accountability Act of 2009*.

Thank you for your ongoing leadership and support of issues impacting populations and communities that continue to suffer grave health and health care disparities. We would also like to thank you for your thoughtful consideration of this request and offer our assistance in addressing this critical issue. Please contact Daniel E. Dawes, J.D., at ***-**** or ***@***, if you would like any additional information.

Sincerely

Figure 4.2. National Working Group letter to White House in response to *New York Times* article

serious issue that needed to be addressed immediately. The US Commission on Civil Rights had submitted to President Obama and congressional leaders a letter criticizing inclusion of the workforce provisions in the House health reform bill (H.R. 3200) that prioritized giving grants to health professional schools to increase outreach to and training of underrepresented and disadvantaged groups. Health equity advocates were quite surprised because, as they had remembered, the commission in 1999 had released a report on health care disparities that underscored the importance of addressing this specific issue in public policy.[5] The Energy and Commerce staff asked us to meet with them immediately to discuss our reactions to the letter and what steps they should take to address this issue. Some staff thought that perhaps they should just negate these provisions, but that was not an option we would entertain. We pushed back and underscored the fact that, just ten years ago, this same commission had been pushing for just such a provision and now all of a sudden they were backpedaling. We argued that the provision was not advocating affirmative action policies but instead was urging schools to recognize that the increased diversity in patients warranted more culturally and linguistically appropriate care. How else could one deliver effective care without understanding the cultural and linguistic issues impacting it? we argued. Congressional staff then raised these arguments with the White House, and it was decided that they would be left in.

Making a Mark: The Bipartisan Health Reform Bill

In late September, the Senate Finance Committee continued debating its health reform proposal, the America's Healthy Future Act. During the fiery negotiations, the Senate Finance Committee convened a bipartisan group of senators, the "Gang of Six," which included three Republicans and three Democrats. The senators met thirty-one times to try to reach consensus. Senator Baucus, describing this process, stated, "We held exhaustive meetings. We met for more than 61 hours. We went the extra mile. And now, we've held an open and exhaustive markup. I put out the mark[up] and posted it on the Web on September 16. That was nearly a week before we started the markup. In a first for this Committee, we posted every amendment—all 564 of them—on the Web." The seven days of meetings leading up to the committee vote were long and stressful; no other bill under consideration by the Senate Finance Committee in the previous twenty-two years had demanded that amount of time for consideration.[6] At the end of the markup, the Senate Finance Committee approved the America's Healthy Future Act with a bipartisan vote of 14-9. The lone Republican voting in favor of the bill was Senator Olympia Snowe of Maine. In all, the committee had conducted seventy-nine roll call votes and adopted forty-one amendments. Meanwhile, on the House side, Speaker Pelosi promised that congressional members would have seventy-two hours—three days—to read their health reform bill before voting on it. Although some House members were upset by the time constraint, like

Congresswoman Michele Bachmann (R-MN), who thought they should be given three months instead, most members did not argue that this was insufficient time to read a bill of that size.[7]

As advocates, our heads were swirling trying to keep up with the lightning speed at which negotiations were taking place and learning whether our priorities would be considered and included. We saw this time as one of the last opportunities to have our public policy priorities included in the omnibus health reform legislation. We worked diligently to ensure that amendments that were proffered to advance health equity were adopted, including Senator Ben Cardin's amendment to transfer the Office of Minority Health at the US Department of Health and Human Services from the Office of the Assistant Secretary to the Office of the Secretary, establish six additional offices of minority health at various federal agencies, and elevate the National Center on Minority Health and Health Disparities to an institute at the National Institutes of Health.

One stalwart health equity champion in Maryland, Senator Shirley Nathan-Pulliam, demonstrated how lessons learned at the state level could help strengthen federal policies, and she worked with Senator Cardin's office to develop this amendment. Through her work in the state legislature, she recognized an opportunity to elevate these entities at the federal level and, with Dr. Britt Weinstock, director of the CBC Health Braintrust; and Priscilla Ross, senior policy advisor to Senator Cardin, pushed this amendment internally in Congress. Weinstock and Ross worked tirelessly into the early morning hours to educate and advocate for this amendment to ensure that it was considered and adopted. Even though Democrats led the House, the Senate, and the White House, surprisingly these two congressional staff had to fight to get their colleagues on the Democratic side to agree to include it in the health reform bill.

We also urged support for Senator Roland Burris's proposed amendment, the Health Entities Community Reinvestment Assistance Act, which would enable hospitals and other health care entities to appropriately respond to their local community health care needs and provide the technical assistance and training required to address critical disparities in health care. The amendment would strengthen the Senate Finance health reform bill's section on hospitals conducting community health needs assessments. It was significantly reduced to a couple sentences but was finally adopted by the committee along with Senator Cardin's amendments and ultimately included in the final bill.

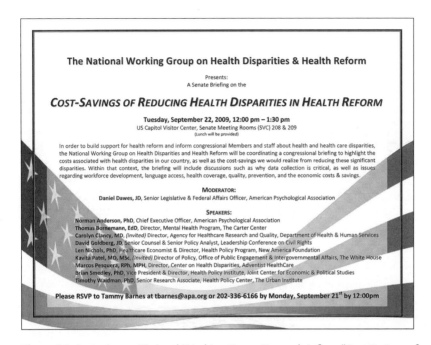

The National Working Group on Health Disparities & Health Reform

Presents:
A Senate Briefing on the

COST-SAVINGS OF REDUCING HEALTH DISPARITIES IN HEALTH REFORM

Tuesday, September 22, 2009, 12:00 pm – 1:30 pm
US Capitol Visitor Center, Senate Meeting Rooms (SVC) 208 & 209
(Lunch will be provided)

In order to build support for health reform and inform congressional Members and staff about health and health care disparities, the National Working Group on Health Disparities and Health Reform will be coordinating a congressional briefing to highlight the costs associated with health disparities in our country, as well as the cost-savings we would realize from reducing these significant disparities. Within that context, the briefing will include discussions such as why data collection is critical, as well as issues regarding workforce development, language access, health coverage, quality, prevention, and the economic costs & savings.

MODERATOR:
Daniel Dawes, JD, Senior Legislative & Federal Affairs Officer, American Psychological Association

SPEAKERS:
Norman Anderson, PhD, Chief Executive Officer, American Psychological Association
Thomas Bornemann, EdD, Director, Mental Health Program, The Carter Center
Carolyn Clancy, MD, *(invited)* Director, Agency for Healthcare Research and Quality, Department of Health & Human Services
David Goldberg, JD, Senior Counsel & Senior Policy Analyst, Leadership Conference on Civil Rights
Len Nichols, PhD, Healthcare Economist & Director, Health Policy Program, New America Foundation
Kavita Patel, MD, MSc, *(invited)* Director of Policy, Office of Public Engagement & Intergovernmental Affairs, The White House
Marcos Pesquera, RPh, MPH, Director, Center on Health Disparities, Adventist HealthCare
Brian Smedley, PhD, Vice President & Director, Health Policy Institute, Joint Center for Economic & Political Studies
Timothy Waidman, PhD, Senior Research Associate, Health Policy Center, The Urban Institute

Please RSVP to Tammy Barnes at tbarnes@apa.org or 202-336-6166 by Monday, September 21st by 12:00pm

Figure 4.3. Invitation to National Working Group Senate briefing: "Cost-Savings of Reducing Health Disparities in Health Reform"

During September, the National Working Group coordinated our largest event, a congressional briefing titled "Cost-Savings of Reducing Health Disparities in Health Reform." The lead-up to the event was stressful and time consuming, but because of a great deal of hard work and the outstanding help and support we received, we put together an exceptional briefing. Our partners included the National Dental Association, WomenHeart: The National Coalition for Women with Heart Disease, the National Health Equity Coalition, Community Catalyst, National League for Nursing, National Korean-American Service and Education Consortium, and the Asian & Pacific Islander American Health Forum. Many different groups provided support either financially or by lending us staff to develop signage, create fact sheets for distribution, or direct traffic flow. Members of the group committed to sending out invitations to their contacts and following up with congressional offices. It was an excellent example of effective collaboration. The briefing would highlight the costs associated with health care inequalities among certain populations in the United States and include discussions of issues such as workforce development, language access, health coverage, quality, and prevention.

One of our biggest challenges was deciding which speakers to invite, but we agreed they should be as diverse as possible. We needed an expert on health disparities to give an overview, so we invited Dr. Norman Anderson, CEO of the American Psychological Association. We wanted to keep the White House closely linked to the event and hear how it was prioritizing health equity, so we invited Dr. Kavita Patel, director of policy in the White House Office of Public Engagement and Intergovernmental Affairs, who had championed our health equity priorities at the White House. We also invited Dr. Carolyn Clancy, director of the Agency for Healthcare Research and Quality at HHS, whose agency had been instrumental in illustrating the disparities in the system with their *National Healthcare Disparities Reports*.

We needed experts who understood the economic burden health inequities were to our country, so we invited Dr. Brian Smedley, Dr. Len Nichols, and Dr. Timothy Waidmann to highlight these issues and unveil two seminal reports. We also needed an expert from a group representing the civil rights organizations to highlight legal and policy issues impacting vulnerable groups, and so we invited David Goldberg, Esq., senior counsel of the Leadership Conference on Civil Rights. In addition to these policy experts, we wanted the briefing to include not only health policy experts with expertise on the national level but also experts on the state and local level, so we invited speakers such as Dr. Thomas Bornemann of the Carter Center and Marcos Pesquera of Adventist Healthcare's Center on Health Disparities, who were actually working within underresourced communities.

At the briefing, which we dedicated to the late Senator Kennedy, we unveiled two landmark reports on the costs of health disparities—one by the Urban Institute and one by the Joint Center for Political and Economic Studies.[8] The standing-room-only audience of more than 150 people included congressional staff from Democratic and Republican offices, representatives from the American Hospital Association, advocates from numerous health coalitions, and academic experts in health policy. The panelists addressed the issue of health equity from a national to a regional to a local level. During the event, it was challenging to keep presenters on message. Some of the talking points we wanted speakers to focus on were not adhered to, with some addressing their individual priorities instead of the broader ones of the National Working Group. But, despite those challenges, in the end our message rang loud and clear, and the briefing was a great success.

Remembering the Forgotten Faces

Just a few days after our major congressional briefing, members attended the Congressional Black Caucus's fall 2009 Health Braintrust on September 25. The event was themed "Addressing the Forgotten Faces and Voices of Health Reform" and focused on health care reform, its impact on individuals, communities, providers, and businesses and its role in health equity. Panelists included Nancy-Ann DeParle, director of the White House Office of Health Reform. I was a panelist in the session "Opportunities in Health Care Reform: Filling in the Gaps Around Scoring, Prevention and Health Equity" and delivered remarks about the role that health reform would play in reducing health disparities and improving the health of all communities affected by them. I laid out the case for addressing the less popular disparities issues, like mental/behavioral and dental health. Previously, we focused on physical health disparities, and I was becoming frustrated that in the larger debate these lesser-addressed issues were being neglected.

At this conference, we told the story of a woman in her thirties with uncontrolled diabetes who lived with her two children and a relative in South Carolina. She did not qualify for Medicaid under South Carolina's guidelines because she had not yet been found disabled by the Social Security Administration. Since she had no treating physician, every time her blood sugar went too high or too low, she went to the local emergency room for treatment. She continually complained to the ER staff that she had a sore on her right foot that would not heal. No one evaluated her for this because they were concerned about getting her blood sugar under control. Every ER visit had notations of her unhealing sores but provided no treatment. Eventually, she insisted that the doctor look at the worsening sores on her foot. Once the doctor saw her foot, she was immediately admitted and the next day her leg was amputated below the knee. The surgeon could not remove all of the leg that needed to be removed and wanted to wait a few days because it would be too much of a shock to her system. The sores were so bad that, even with the amputation, osteomyelitis had set in, and before the next surgery could be performed she died. Access to affordable health care would have enabled her to better manage her diabetes and could have saved her life.[9]

From: Dawes, Daniel ***@***
Date: Fri, Oct 16, 2009 at 2:52 PM
Subject: For your records - Congressional Letters with List of Signatories
To: "Dawes, Daniel" ***@***

Good afternoon—

Please find attached, for your records, a copy of the final sign-on letter with the list of signatories urging Congress and the Administration to leave intact the health equity provisions in health reform legislation, including (Data Collection, Health Care Quality Improvements, Prevention and Wellness, Language Access, and Health Workforce and Infrastructure).

This letter was delivered to Congress and the White House yesterday. Thanks to all who signed-on and continue to support the inclusion of health disparities reduction and elimination efforts in health reform. **Over 250 organizations and coalitions signed-on in support of these provisions and more continue to sign-on!!!**

If you wanted to sign-on, but was late in getting back to me, please send a letter directly to the Members addressed and cc'd on this letter.

Thanks so much for your cooperation and diligence with these matters.

Respectfully,

Daniel

Daniel E. Dawes, J.D. | Senior Legislative & Federal Affairs Officer,
Public Interest Directorate
American Psychological Association
750 First Street NE, Washington, DC 20002-4242
Tel: ***-**** | Fax: ***-****
email: ***@*** | www.apa.org

Figure 4.4. Grassroots e-mail to health equity advocates sharing the final National Working Group letter and highlighting the continued strong support for health equity priorities

As health reform legislation continued moving forward, we forged ahead with our agenda to ensure that health equity was a major factor in the final bill. We drafted and sent another letter to Congress and the White House urging them to leave intact the health equity provisions secured in the health reform bills. These critical provisions addressed data collection, health care quality improvements, prevention and wellness, language access, and health workforce and infrastructure.

Within Reach

On October 29, 2009, Representative John Dingell Jr. introduced the Affordable Health Care for America Act (H.R. 3962), the House's version of the health reform legislation. The bill was a revised version of an earlier, unsuccessful measure, the America's Affordable Health Choices Act (H.R. 3200), which had been introduced on July 14, 2009. The bill was revised to meet certain goals outlined in the president's September address

October 15, 2009

The Honorable Harry Reid
Majority Leader
U.S. Senate
Washington, DC 20510

The Honorable Max Baucus
Chair
Finance
U.S. Senate
Washington, DC 20510

The Honorable Tom Harkin
Chair
Health, Education, Labor & Pensions
U.S. Senate
Washington, DC 20510

Dear Senators Reid, Baucus, Harkin, and Dodd:

As you and your colleagues continue to work on h
undersigned coalitions and organizations urge you
includes provisions to address health inequities an
health care disparities.

A recent report from the Joint Center for Political
2003 to 2006 the combined cost of health dispariti
This report also found that in the same time period
would have reduced direct health care expenditure
ings would be realized not only by improving the
that suffer from health disparities and barriers to h
by reducing the costs resulting from the dispropor
populations. As a result, the final health reform leg

- **Data Collection, Analyses, and Quality**
  on race, ethnicity, gender, disability status
  status, primary language, sexual orientatic
  subpopulation groups, as well as the deve
  factors to improve health status and qualit
- **Health Care Quality Improvements**, inc
  Improvements in Health Care, Quality Me
  Needs Assessment, and Cultural and Ling
  public health services by providing grants
  research and community-based programs
  barriers to health services through educati
  disease prevention activities, and health li

October 15, 2009

The Honorable Nancy Pelosi
Speaker
U.S. House of Representatives
Washington, DC 20515

The Honorable Steny Hoyer
Majority Leader
U.S. House of Representatives
Washington, DC 20515

The Honorable James Clyburn
Majority Whip
U.S. House of Representatives
Washington, DC 20515

Dear Representatives Pelosi, Hoyer, and Clyburn:

As you and your colleagues continue to work on health reform legislation, the over 250 undersigned coalitions and organizations urge you to ensure that the final legislation includes provisions to address health inequities and to reduce and eliminate health and health care disparities.

A recent report from the Joint Center for Political and Economic Studies found that from 2003 to 2006 the combined cost of health disparities totaled $1.24 trillion in our country. This report also found that in the same time period, eliminating certain health disparities would have reduced direct health care expenditures by $229.4 billion. These potential savings would be realized not only by improving the health of populations and communities that suffer from health disparities and barriers to health care and public health services, but by reducing the costs resulting from the disproportionate burden of disease faced by these populations. As a result, the final health reform legislation must, at a minimum, include:

- **Data Collection, Analyses, and Quality** to ensure collection and reporting of data on race, ethnicity, gender, disability status, geographic location, socioeconomic status, primary language, sexual orientation, gender identity, and, especially for subpopulation groups, as well as the development of standards for measuring these factors to improve health status and quality in health care.
- **Health Care Quality Improvements**, including the National Strategy for Quality Improvements in Health Care, Quality Measure Development, Community Health Needs Assessment, and Cultural and Linguistic Competence in health care and public health services by providing grants and demonstration projects to support research and community-based programs designed to reduce health disparities and barriers to health services through education and outreach, health promotion and disease prevention activities, and health literacy and services.
- **Health Workforce and Infrastructure Investment** to strengthen the recruitment, retention, training, and continuing education of health professionals, and increase their diversity, distribution, cultural competence, and knowledge of treating the

Figure 4.5. Final National Working Group letter making the economic impact of health disparities argument

to the Joint Session of Congress. Before House Democrats unveiled their health reform bill, they convened a meeting in the Capitol building's basement for a final briefing with Speaker Pelosi and other leaders. All agreed at that time that the moment of compromise had finally arrived. No longer could the conservative and liberal factions of the caucus afford to continue fighting. The consensus at the meeting was that they had to pass the bill. The House of Representatives passed the Affordable Health Care for

America Act on November 7, 2009, in a 220-215 vote.[10] One Republican, Congressman Joseph Cao of Louisiana, voted in favor of the bill. If the Senate would go on to pass its own bill, the House and Senate bills would have to be reconciled into one document and voted on again.

Over in the Senate, Majority Leader Harry Reid and Senators Max Baucus, Tom Harkin, and Chris Dodd worked together to merge the Finance Committee's health reform bill, the America's Healthy Future Act, with the bill passed by the Health Education Labor and Pensions Committee, the Affordable Health Choices Act. Since the Constitution requires all revenue-related bills to originate in the House, the Senate adopted H.R. 3590, a bill regarding housing tax breaks for service members, because it was first passed by the House as a revenue-related modification to the Internal Revenue Code.[11] The Senate then revised the content of the bill, using it as their vehicle for health reform legislation. The result was the Patient Protection and Affordable Care Act, which on November 19, 2009, was sent to the Senate floor for debate. Republicans were eager to drag out this debate for weeks, if not longer, while Democrats were eager to have the health reform bill passed and enacted into law by the end of the following month.

Republicans used their time to question whether the bill would actually reduce health care costs to Americans. They questioned the legitimacy of the cost of the health reform bill itself, which the nonpartisan Congressional Budget Office now concluded would equate to approximately $850 billion. Republicans also questioned the methodology for arriving at that figure, as well as policy decisions or tactics used by Democrats to ensure the bill would not exceed $1 trillion in costs. Democrats, by contrast, discussed key provisions that were included in the bill and argued for additional policies they believed strongly should be included. They also argued for the continued inclusion of a public health insurance option that Americans could choose when purchasing health insurance coverage in the proposed health insurance exchange or marketplace. Democrats argued that reforming health care would improve the economy and emphasized that the health reform bill included provisions that would reduce the deficit and reduce costs to both state and federal governments while increasing access to health care and improving health outcomes. On December 24, 2009, the Senate passed the Patient Protection and Affordable Care Act, 60-39. Every Democratic Senator voted in favor of the bill, while every Republican opposed it.

As 2010 dawned, the enactment of health reform legislation was just within reach. Then, in a potentially devastating development for health reform, Republican Scott Brown won Senator Kennedy's Massachusetts Senate seat in a special election. This meant that the Democrats no longer held a supermajority in the Senate, so the Republicans could sustain a filibuster and block health reform. At this point, with the Senate already having passed the Patient Protection and Affordable Care Act in December, the most viable option for passing health reform was for the House to abandon its own bill, the Affordable Health Care for America Act, and pass the Senate's bill instead. However, House Democrats were not satisfied with the content of the Senate bill and had expected to be able to negotiate changes in a House-Senate conference before passing a final bill. They compromised and instead drafted the Health Care and Education Reconciliation Act, a bill that would be used to amend the Senate bill to House Democrats' satisfaction and that could be passed via budget reconciliation.

There was a great deal of tension and concern among health equity advocates regarding what Scott Brown's election would mean for health reform and our work to advance health equity. One year after the presidential election, we were finally seeing the light at the end of the tunnel, and now all that progress was in jeopardy. We were getting calls and e-mails from advocates concerned about the health equity provisions in the House and Senate health reform legislation. We responded that we could not remain quiet about our support for the health disparities provisions that we worked so hard to secure and that it was crucial not to give up at this point. The momentum that we had seen from congressional health reformers seemed to be slowing now. For some, it felt as though the wind had been taken out of their sails. This alarmed us. Health equity advocates were frustrated by the hesitation or second guessing of congressional champions on whether to continue pushing health reform. We all had worked too hard up to that point to ensure that health disparities reduction and elimination remained a priority in health reform to give up now!

We urged advocates to contact their members of Congress, especially leadership in the House and Senate, voicing their strong support for moving the Senate-passed bill, which included provisions aimed at reducing health disparities and improving the health status of all population groups. We contacted lawmakers, urging them to pass health reform quickly before the window of opportunity closed. We wanted to remind these leaders that these provisions would potentially save more than $60 billion a year in direct health care expenditures and countless lives saved. While our advocacy campaign continued in high gear, Families USA, the Raising Women's Voices coalition, and the National Partnership for Women and Families, which were members of our working group, including approximately fifty academics from across the country, sent out action alerts or circulated their own letters to Congress urging them to not delay passing health reform. Instead, we argued, they should focus their energies on moving health reform forward to its needed enactment. We stressed the belief that now was the time to speak up before it became too late.

Health reformers in Congress and the White House had been proposing several strategies to move forward with health reform. One major strategy that was being debated by the White House and congressional champions involved moving away from comprehensive health care reform legislation to piecemeal legislation. Another major strategy that was increasingly gaining support involved using the "more popular and less controversial" components of the two health care reform bills. This ambiguous strategy was concerning to health equity advocates, because we were not sure whether health equity provisions would fall into that category and thus be included in the final bill.

In the weeks leading up to the final vote on the combined health reform proposal, we continued to urge congressional champions of health reform and health equity to stay the course and keep the package intact. We then started seeing senior officials in the administration and Congress becoming more vocal and agreeing that approach was the best alternative in light of the circumstances. More Democratic lawmakers soon argued that they believed it was crucial to pass a bill and show some success after negotiating for more than a year. And in March 2010, on the weekend prior to the vote on the Patient Protection and Affordable Care Act, the National Working Group organized massive final grassroots efforts to urge lawmakers to vote in support of health reform.

A Promise Fulfilled

The American Medical Association announced on the Friday before the final vote that it endorsed the revised health reform legislation. According to the president of the AMA, "This is certainly not the bill we would have written, but we cannot let the perfect be the enemy of the good."[12] The AMA had earlier announced support for the House version of the bill that passed in November and the Senate version that passed in December.

From: Dawes, Daniel
Date: Fri, Mar 19, 2010 at 9:29 PM
Subject: Urgent - Action Needed: Health Disparities in Health Reform!
To: "Dawes, Daniel"

Greetings—

This is it! There is a major health reform vote scheduled for Sunday afternoon and Members of Congress need to continue hearing from supporters. It is critical that you and your networkscall Congress to seize this historic opportunity and pass meaningful health reform legislation as soon as possible.

I've been getting lots of calls and e-mails concerning the health equity provisions in the reconciliation bill - H.R. 4872, The Health Care & Education Affordability Reconciliation Act of 2010. As it currently stands:

1. The health disparities provisions in the Senate health reform bill are left intact.
2. The reconciliation bill adds language to strengthen those provisions in the Senate health reform bill, including funding for the territories for Medicaid and health insurance exchanges, increased funding for disproportionate share hospitals (DSH) and community health centers, and increased funding to minority universities and colleges to train more scientists, etc. To review the text and summaries of the reconciliation bill, please click on the following link.

http://energycommerce.house.gov/index.php?option=com_content&view=article&id=1931:health-care-reform&catid=169:legislation&Itemid=55

Opponents of health reform have been casting it in a false light and have been advising their listeners to kill health reform. According to Roll Call, "House administrators estimate that Capitol switchboard operators are fielding roughly 40,000 calls per hour from constituents and that perhaps twice as many callers are experiencing busy signals a full day after radio host Rush Limbaugh gave his listening audience the Capitol switchboard phone number and encouraged them to call it."

Before this email gets buried in your inbox I urge you to take the following action immediately – before it's too late. We need to make sure that our Representatives know the truth about health reform and vote in support of the health reform bill so that we can ensure that people suffering from health and health care disparities will be given the necessary services, programs, and supports they need. You can find the number for your Representative's district office by clicking here.

This is the time that health equity advocates have been waiting for! I know many of you have been sending in your letters and e-mails and making numerous calls to encourage your Representative to vote in support, but we must continue to advocate and keep our voices loud and clear. As a nation, we have come too far and have reached too many areas of consensus to accept inaction. Now is the time to move beyond discussions of process, partisanship, or political philosophy to enact health reforms that will create system-wide sustainability and equity, increase access, improve quality of care, and improve health outcomes for vulnerable populations.

Respectfully,
Daniel

Daniel E. Dawes, J.D.

Figure 4.6. Grassroots e-mail to health equity advocates urging final push for health reform

On Sunday, March 21, 2010, arguably the most emotionally riveting and the most pivotal day in the health reform debate, the US House of Representatives was scheduled to vote at 1 p.m. on the health reform package that had previously been voted on by the Senate a few months earlier on Christmas Eve. The actual vote would not take place until much later that evening. On that day, the pressure from opponents of health reform intensified, with protesters active outside the Capitol. While congressional proponents were walking to the Capitol to cast their historic votes, many were taunted, vilified, and even spat on. Congressman John Lewis (D-GA), a strong proponent of health reform even during the Clinton negotiations, when recalling his most memorable time during the health reform negotiations, stated that it was during the march to the Capitol to cast his historic vote that he remembers most fondly.[13] It is a day neither he nor other congressional champions will soon forget. Among the ranks of advocates were many supporters of the health reform bill urging the lawmakers not to stand down but to be courageous and vote in support of this bill even though it may not be popular at this time. No matter what either side was advocating for, the final votes were sure to be extremely close. Finally, at 10:49 p.m., the House passed the bill in a 219-212 vote. All 178 Republicans opposed it, along with 34 Democrats.[14]

On March 23, 2010, President Obama signed into law the Patient Protection and Affordable Care Act.

> After a century of striving, after a year of debate, after a historic vote, health care reform is no longer an unmet promise. It is the law of the land. It is the law of the land.
>
> And although it may be my signature that's affixed to the bottom of this bill, it was your work, your commitment, your unyielding hope that made this victory possible. When the special interests deployed an army of lobbyists, an onslaught of negative ads, to preserve the status quo, you didn't give up. You hit the phones and you took to the streets. You mobilized and you organized. You turned up the pressure and you kept up the fight.[15]

It was a groundbreaking piece of legislation, which advocates hoped would bring coverage to more than thirty-two million uninsured Americans. The law contained many provisions concerning health equity and the elimination of health disparities, and it was the most significant federal effort directly addressing health disparities in the country's history.[16] However, though the Affordable Care Act had finally been enacted and all this promise had been achieved, its proponents had to temper our celebrations. We would soon be forced to tackle many obstacles in the path of the ACA's implementation. As advocates and lawmakers would soon realize, getting the law enacted was the shockingly easy part. The hardest part was yet to come.

NOTES

1. Weir, "Nancy Pelosi Fights for Health Care Reform."

2. Saslow and Rucker, "Ted Kennedy Is Celebrated for His Longtime Support of Health-Care Reform."

3. Obama, "Remarks by the President to a Joint Session of Congress on Health Care."

4. Pear and Calmes, "Obama Aides Aim to Simplify and Scale Back Health Bills."

5. US Commission on Civil Rights, *Health Care Challenge.*

6. US Senate Committee on Finance, "Baucus Opening Statement at Mark-up of the America's Healthy Future Act"; US Senate Committee on Finance, "Health Care Reform from Conception to Final Passage."

7. Stewart, "Bachmann."

8. Waidmann, *Estimating the Cost of Racial and Ethnic Health Disparities;* LaVeist, Gaskin, and Richard, *Economic Burden of Health Inequalities in the United States.*

9. *Joint Hearing on Eliminating the Social Security Disability Backlog* (testimony of Peggy Hathaway).

10. Final Vote Results for Roll Call 887, Affordable Health Care for America Act.

11. US Const. art. I, § 7, cl. 1.

12. Johnson, "AARP, AMA Announce Support for Health Care Bill: Largest Doctors and Retiree Groups Backing Legislation."

13. Personal interview, September 15, 2014.

14. Final Vote Results for Roll Call 165, Patient Protection and Affordable Care Act.

15. Obama and Biden, "Remarks by the President and Vice President on Health Insurance Reform at the Department of the Interior."

16. US Department of Health and Human Services, *HHS Action Plan to Reduce Racial and Ethnic Health Disparities.*

BIBLIOGRAPHY

Agency for Healthcare Research and Quality. *Clinician Summary: Attention Deficit Hyperactivity Disorder in Children and Adolescents.* Rockville, MD, 2011. Retrieved September 10, 2012, from http://effectivehealthcare.ahrq.gov/ehc /products/191/1149/adhd_clin_fin_to_post.pdf.

———. *National Healthcare Disparities Report: Summary.* Rockville, MD, 2004. Retrieved August 22, 2011, from http://www.ahrq.gov/qual/nhdr03 /nhdrsum03.htm.

———. *National Healthcare Disparities Report.* Rockville, MD, 2006. Retrieved August 22, 2011, from http://www.ahrq.gov/qual/nhdr06/nhdr06.htm.

———. *National Healthcare Disparities Report.* Rockville, MD, 2011. Retrieved August 22, 2012, from http://www.ahrq.gov/qual/qrdr11.htm.

———. *National Healthcare Quality Report.* Rockville, MD, 2011. Retrieved August 22, 2012, from http://www.ahrq.gov/qual/qrdr11.htm.

American Psychological Association. "Psychological and Behavioral Perspectives on Health Disparities." Communique, March 2009. Washington, DC. http://www.apa.org/pi/oema/resources/communique/2009/03/march.pdf.

Brandon, Katherine. "The President on Health Care: 'We Are Going to Get This Done.'" *White House Blog,* July 17, 2009. http://www.whitehouse.gov/blog /The-President-on-Health-Care-We-are-Going-to-Get-this-Done.

Breakey, W. R., P. J. Fischer, M. Kramer, G. Nestadt, A. J. Romanoski, A. Ross, R. M. Royall, and O. Stine. "Health and Mental Health Problems of Homeless Men and Women in Baltimore." *Journal of the American Medical Association* 262 (1989): 1352-1357.

Breslau, J., S. Aguilar-Gaxiola, K. Kendler, S. Maxwell, D. Williams, and R. Kessler. "Specifying Race-Ethnic Differences in Risk for Psychiatric Disorder in a USA National Sample." *Psychological Medicine* 36, no. 1 (2006): 57-68.

Centers for Disease Control and Prevention. *Childhood Obesity Facts.* Hyattsville, MD: 2012. Retrieved May 29, 2012, from http://www.cdc.gov/obesity/data /childhood.html.

———. Table 61. In *Health, United States, 2007 with Chartbook on Trends in the Health of Americans.* Hyattsville, MD: 2007, 262-263.

———. National Center for Health Statistics. *Health, United States, 2011: With Special Feature on Socioeconomic Status and Health.* Hyattsville, MD: 2012. Retrieved May 29, 2012, from http://www.cdc.gov/nchs/data/hus/hus11 .pdf#listfigures.

Cochran, S., J. Sullivan, and V. Mays. "Prevalence of Mental Disorders, Psychological Distress, and Mental Health Services Use among Lesbian, Gay, and Bisexual Adults in the United States." *Journal of Consulting and Clinical Psychology* 71 (2003): 53-61.

Congressional Record. "Service Members Home Ownership Tax Act of 2009—Motion to Proceed." S11907-S11967 (November 21, 2009). http://www .gpo.gov/fdsys/pkg/CREC-2009-11-21/html/CREC-2009-11-21-pt1-PgS11907-2 .htm.

Evans, Jennifer, and Jaclyn Schiff. "A Timeline of Kennedy's Health Care Achievements and Disappointments." *Kaiser Health News,* August 26, 2009. http://www.kaiserhealthnews.org/stories/2009/august/26/kennedy-health -care-timeline.aspx.

Final Vote Results for Roll Call 165, Patient Protection and Affordable Care Act. http://clerk.house.gov/evs/2010/roll165.xml.

Final Vote Results for Roll Call 887, Affordable Health Care for America Act. http://clerk.house.gov/evs/2009/roll887.xml.

Health Care and Education Reconciliation Act of 2010. P.L. 111-152.

Institute of Medicine. *The Health of Lesbian, Gay, Bisexual and Transgender People: Building a Foundation to Better Health.* Washington, DC: National Academies Press, 2011.

——. *How Far Have We Come in Reducing Health Disparities? Progress since 2000; Workshop Summary.* Washington, DC: National Academies Press, 2012.

——. *Race, Ethnicity, and Language Data: Standardization for Health Care Quality Improvement.* Washington, DC: National Academies Press, 2009.

Janssen, I., W. Craig, W. Boyce, and W. Pickett. "Associations between Overweight and Obesity with Bullying Behaviors in School-Aged Children." *Pediatrics*, 113 (2004): 1187-1194.

Johnson, Carla K. "AARP, AMA Announce Support for Health Care Bill: Largest Doctors and Retiree Groups Backing Legislation." *Huffington Post*, March 19, 2010. http://www.huffingtonpost.com/2010/03/19/aarp-ama-announce -support_n_506060.html.

Joint Hearing on Eliminating the Social Security Disability Backlog, before the Subcommittee on Social Security and Subcommittee on Income Security and Family Support of the House Committee on Ways & Means. Testimony of Peggy Hathaway, representing the Consortium for Citizens with Disabilities, March 24, 2009; http://www.c-c-d.org/fichiers/CCD-W&M-Jt-Subomm -testimony3-24-09.doc. Story retold by Day Al-Mohamed, Why Do We Need Health Reform Anyway? *Day in Washington Blog*, September 2009. http:// dayinwashington.com/?p=350.

Kaiser Family Foundation. "President Obama's Campaign Position on Health Reform and Other Health Care Issues." November 01, 2008. http://kff.org /disparities-policy/issue-brief/president-obamas-campaign-position-on-health -reform/.

Kennedy, Edward. *Fighting for Quality, Affordable Health Care.* http://tedkennedy .org/service/item/health_care.

Koegel, P. M., A. Burnam, and R. K. Farr. "The Prevalence of Specific Psychiatric Disorders among Homeless Individuals in the Inner City of Los Angeles." *Archives of General Psychiatry* 45 (1988): 1085-1093.

LaVeist, T., D. Gaskin, and P. Richard. *The Economic Burden of Health Inequalities in the United States.* Washington, DC: Joint Center for Political and Economic Studies Report, September 2009.

Lee, Jesse. "Health Reform: 'Urgency and Determination.'" *White House Blog*, May 3, 2009. http://www.whitehouse.gov/blog/Health-Reform-Urgency-and -Determination.

Low, N., and J. Hardy. "Psychiatric Disorder Criteria and Their Application to Research in Different Racial Groups." *BMC Psychiatry* 7, no. 1 (2007). doi: 10.1186/1471-244X-7-1.

National Alliance on Mental Illness. "Mental Illness: Facts and Numbers."
Arlington, VA, 2013. Retrieved August 26, 2015, from http://www2.nami.org
/factsheets/mentalillness_factsheet.pdf.

National Association of State Mental Health Program Directors. *Measurement of Health Status for People with Serious Mental Illnesses.* Alexandria, VA, 2008. Retrieved September 7, 2012, from http://www.nasmhpd.org/content /measurement-health-status-people-serious-mental-illnesses.

National Federation of Independent Business v. Sebelius, 132 U.S. 2566.

Obama, Barack. "Remarks by the President to a Joint Session of Congress on Health Care." Press release, September 9, 2009. http://www.whitehouse.gov /the_press_office/Remarks-by-the-President-to-a-Joint-Session-of-Congress -on-Health-Care/.

———. "Remarks by the President on Senate Passage of Health Insurance Reform." Press release, December 24, 2009. http://www.whitehouse.gov/the -press-office/remarks-president-senate-passage-health-insurance-reform.

Obama, Barack, and Joe Biden. "The Obama-Biden Plan." Office of the President-Elect. http://change.gov/agenda/health_care_agenda/.

———. "Remarks by the President and Vice President on Health Insurance Reform at the Department of the Interior." Press release, March 23, 2010. http://www.whitehouse.gov/the-press-office/remarks-president-and-vice -president-health-insurance-reform-bill-department-interi.

Patient Protection and Affordable Care Act. P.L. 111-148.

Pear, Robert, and Jackie Calmes. "Obama Aides Aim to Simplify and Scale Back Health Bills." *New York Times,* September 2, 2009.

Pelosi, Nancy. "Today, We Have the Opportunity to Complete the Great Unfinished Business of Our Society and Pass Health Insurance Reform for All Americans." Press release, March 21, 2010. http://pelosi.house.gov/news /press-releases/pelosi-today-we-have-the-opportunity-to-complete-the-great -unfinished-business.

Sack, Kevin, Shan Carter, Jonathan Ellis, Farhana Hossain, and Alan Mclean. "Election 2008—On the Issues: Health Care." *New York Times,* May 23, 2012. http://elections.nytimes.com/2008/president/issues/health.html.

Saslow, Eli, and Philip Rucker. "Ted Kennedy Is Celebrated for His Longtime Support of Health-Care Reform." *Washington Post,* March 24, 2010. http:// www.washingtonpost.com/wp-dyn/content/article/2010/03/23 /AR2010032303883.html.

Stagman, S., and J. Cooper. *Children's Mental Health: What Every Policymaker Should Know.* National Center for Children in Poverty. New York, 2010.

Stewart, Martina. "Bachmann: House Dems 'Embarrassed' by Their Health Care Bill." CNN, October 6, 2009. http://politicalticker.blogs.cnn.com/2009/10/06 /bachmann-house-dems-embarrassed-by-their-health-care-bill/comment -page-7/.

Substance Abuse and Mental Health Services Administration (SAMHSA). *Risk of Suicide among Hispanic Females Aged 12 to 17.* National Household Survey on Drug Abuse Report. Rockville, MD: SAMSHA, 2003. Retrieved September 1, 2011, from http://www.oas.samhsa.gov/2k3/LatinaSuicide/LatinaSuicide .htm.

Swartz, M., R. Wagner, J. Swanson, B. Burns, L. George, and D. Padgett. "Administrative Update: Utilization of Services." *Community Mental Health Journal* 34, no. 2 (1998): 133-144.

Teplin, L. A. "The Prevalence of Severe Mental Disorder among Male Urban Jail Detainees: Comparison with the Epidemiologic Catchment Area Program." *American Journal of Public Health* 80 (1990): 663-669.

Thomas, Peter. "White House Summit on Health Care Reform." External memorandum to CCD Health and Long Term Services Task Forces and interested parties, March 10, 2009, in the author's possession.

Thrush, Glenn. "Black Caucus Pushes Obama on Health Equity." *Politico,* June 8, 2009. http://www.politico.com/blogs/glennthrush/0609/Black_Caucus _pushes_Obama_on_health_equity.html.

US Commission on Civil Rights. *The Health Care Challenge: Acknowledging Disparity, Confronting Discrimination, and Ensuring Equality.* September 1999.

US Constitution. Article I, § 7, clause 1.

US Department of Health and Human Services. *HHS Action Plan to Reduce Racial and Ethnic Health Disparities: A Nation Free of Disparities in Health and Health Care.* Rockville, MD: US Department of Health and Human Services, 2011.

———. *Mental Health: Culture, Race, and Ethnicity—A Supplement to Mental Health: A Report of the Surgeon General.* Rockville, MD: US Department of Health and Human Services, 2001.

US Department of Health and Human Services, Advisory Committee on Minority Health, Office of Minority Health. *Ensuring That Health Care Reform Will Meet the Health Care Needs of Minority Communities and Eliminate Health Disparities: A Statement of Principles and Recommendations.* Rockville, MD, 2009. Retrieved September 10, 2011, from http://minorityhealth.hhs.gov /Assets/pdf/Checked/1/ACMH_HealthCareAccessReport.pdf.

US Department of Health and Human Services, New Freedom Commission on Mental Health. *Achieving the Promise: Transforming Mental Health Care in America—Final Report.* Rockville, MD, 2003.

US Department of Health and Human Services, Office of Minority Health. *Native Hawaiian/Other Pacific Islander Profile.* Rockville, MD, 2012. Retrieved May 29, 2012, from http://minorityhealth.hhs.gov/templates/content.aspx ?lvl=3&lvlID=4&ID=8593.

US Senate Committee on Finance. "Baucus Opening Statement at Mark-Up of the America's Healthy Future Act." Press release, October 13, 2009.

http://www.finance.senate.gov/newsroom/chairman/release/?id=a2728d6d
-ecf6-45fa-903f-d2a430147156.

———. "Health Care Reform from Conception to Final Passage: Timeline of the Finance Committee's Work to Reform America's Health Care System." http://www.finance.senate.gov/issue/?id=32be19bd-491e-4192-812f -f65215c1ba65.

Vernez, G. M., M. A. Burnam, E. A. McGlynn, S. Trude, and B. Mittman. *Review of California's Program for the Homeless Mentally Ill Disabled*. Report No. R3631-CDMH. Santa Monica, CA: RAND, 1988.

Waidmann, T. *Estimating the Cost of Racial and Ethnic Health Disparities*. Washington, DC: Urban Institute, September 2009.

Weir, Bill. "Nancy Pelosi Fights for Health Care Reform." *ABC News*, October 31, 2009. http://abcnews.go.com/GMA/Weekend/nancy-pelosi-works-hard -health-care-reform/story?id=8961771&page=2.

Wells, K., R. Klap, A. Koike, and C. Sherbourne. "Ethnic Disparities in Unmet Need for Alcoholism, Drug Abuse, and Mental Health Care." *American Journal of Psychiatry* 158 (2001): 2027-2032.

"White House Forum on Health Reform Attendees and Breakout Session Participants." Press release, March 5, 2009. https://www.whitehouse.gov/the -press-office/white-house-forum-health-reform-attendees-and-breakout -session-participants.

Williams, D., H. Gonzalez, H. Neighbors, R. Nesse, J. Abelson, J. Sweetman, and J. Jackson. "Prevalence and Distribution of Major Depressive Disorder in African Americans, Caribbean Blacks, and Non-Hispanic Whites: Results from the National Survey of American Life." *Archives of General Psychiatry* 64 (2007): 305-315.

Brushes with Death
How Many Lives Does ObamaCare Have?

Members of this Court are vested with the authority to interpret the law; we possess neither the expertise nor the prerogative to make policy judgments. Those decisions are entrusted to our Nation's elected leaders, who can be thrown out of office if the people disagree with them. It is not our job to protect the people from the consequences of their political choices.—*Chief Justice John Roberts, Supreme Court of the United States*

Before the ink could even dry on the Patient Protection and Affordable Care Act, opponents of health reform began filing lawsuits challenging the law's validity. They primarily challenged two issues: the individual mandate, which would require individuals to purchase health insurance or pay a penalty, and the Medicaid expansion provision, which would expand Medicaid to all individuals under the age of sixty-five making less than 138 percent of the federal poverty level. Within the first six months, opponents initiated at least twenty-six lawsuits across the nation. As these cases moved through the courts, the appellate courts diverged on the constitutionality of the individual mandate, giving both supporters and opponents of the health law hope. The Sixth Circuit Court of Appeals found the mandate constitutional, while the Eleventh Circuit Court of Appeals held that it was not. The Department of Justice filed an appeal with the Supreme Court after the Eleventh Circuit's ruling, and in November 2011 the Court agreed to review the case. The Supreme Court's holding could have dismantled the Affordable Care Act, and the nation waited with bated breath to learn if this was going to be the case.

On Thursday, June 28, 2012, the morning the Supreme Court was due to release its decision regarding these two provisions, I was at the airport heading to Washington, DC. Before getting on the plane that morning, I had experienced confusion, outrage, and bitter disappointment after receiving word of the news media's erroneous reports that the Court had held the health reform law unconstitutional. Perhaps this is one of the reasons for Justice Sonia Sotomayor's observation, "I realized that in this fast-paced internet world, reporters are no longer reading about cases before they comment on them."[1] Once airborne, I immediately accessed the Supreme Court website and was overwhelmed with relief when I realized that the law had in fact been upheld. I settled in to carefully read the Court's decision and determine its impact on the Affordable Care Act as well as the implications moving forward. This decision could have been the end of the ACA; however, it was not the first time that the law narrowly escaped a brush with death. This chapter will describe the many instances that could have been the end of health reform.

The Vice President's Hesitation

After the presidential election in 2008 and after the transition of administrations, the first brush with death for health reform occurred when Vice President Joe Biden suggested that the president should reconsider tackling health reform so early on in his administration. He was afraid that attempting to enact sweeping health reform might jeopardize the president's reelection. The nation was then in the midst of a major recession and crippling job losses, and Biden thought that the Obama administration should focus on creating jobs instead. He suggested this approach despite the fact that congressional leaders had already been holding meetings and hearings exploring this issue. President Obama disagreed with the vice president, however, and decided to move forward. He believed that comprehensive health reform would have a positive impact and would help to create new jobs and stimulate the economy. Later on at the American Medical Association's annual conference on June 15, 2009, the president stated, "Make no mistake: The cost of our health care is a threat to our economy. It's an escalating burden on our families and businesses. It's a ticking time bomb for the federal budget. And it is unsustainable for the United States of America."[2] The president decided to risk losing his own reelection and the Democratic majorities in both chambers of Congress.

Senator Ted Kennedy's Passing

The second brush with death for the Affordable Care Act occurred when Senator Edward M. Kennedy lost his battle with cancer on August 25, 2009. An ardent champion for the most vulnerable and marginalized and a champion for universal health coverage, Senator Kennedy had been instrumental in the passage of major health-related legislation. When he died, there was a sense that we had lost a great leader, one who through experience had the wherewithal to finally help usher in the successful passage of health reform. Perhaps realizing the impact his death could have on passing the health reform legislation if Democrats lost their 60-vote majority in the Senate, Kennedy had earlier requested that the Massachusetts legislature enact a law allowing the governor to appoint a temporary replacement until a special election could be held. The legislature did so, and Massachusetts governor Deval Patrick appointed Paul G. Kirk Jr. (D-MA), a former aide of the late senator, to fill his seat until a special election on January 19, 2010.

However, under the Massachusetts Constitution, unless a law is an emergency or declared so by the governor, it cannot take effect earlier than ninety days after it is passed. Governor Patrick declared that Kirk's appointment was indeed an emergency. However, while Kirk enjoyed tremendous support from President Obama and other Democratic leaders, Republicans were not especially pleased with his selection. They argued that it was unconstitutional for the governor to make an emergency declaration in this case and set out to get an injunction to prevent the appointment from taking effect. Their efforts were not successful, and Senator Kirk's appointment would soon prove crucial during the December 24, 2009, vote in the Senate on the health reform legislation.

The Christmas Eve Senate Vote

The third brush with death for health reform occurred when the Senate convened a vote for the Patient Protection and Affordable Care Act on Christmas Eve morning. The vote was the culmination of twenty-five consecutive days of intense debate, the second-longest run in Senate history and the first Christmas Eve Senate session since 1985. Before the vote, Senate majority leader Harry Reid asserted, "Opponents of this bill have used every trick in the book to delay this day. And yet, here we are, minutes away from doing what many have tried, but none has ever achieved. We are here because facts will always defeat fear. And though one might slow the speed of progress, its force cannot be stopped."[3]

With Senator Kirk seated, Democrats once again had the sixty votes needed to pass their health reform bill, but there was no guarantee that all the Democratic senators would vote in its favor. Just as they did years earlier with the Clinton health reform proposal, the National Federation of Independent Business and other probusiness lobbying groups worked determinedly to prevent the Obama health reform proposal from gaining any further momentum. Certain senators had leveraged their votes to gain concessions for their states and key stakeholders. Senator Lieberman of Connecticut, a former Democrat turned Independent, refused to vote in favor of any bill that included a public option that would compete with the private insurers in his state. Senator Ben Nelson (D-NE) agreed to vote in favor of the law only if Nebraska's Medicaid expansion was fully paid for by the federal government and language was included restricting federal funding from paying for abortion coverage. Senator Bill Nelson (D-FL) demanded protections for Medicare Advantage plans in Florida, and Senator Mary Landrieu (D-LA) was promised $300 million for Louisiana's Medicaid program, which came to be referred to as the "Louisiana Purchase."[4]

In the end, Majority Leader Harry Reid was able to cut enough deals to gain the support of every member of the Democratic caucus. On Christmas Eve morning, the Patient Protection and Affordable Care Act passed on a 60-39 party-line vote. Shortly after the vote, President Obama declared, "We are now finally poised to deliver on the promise of real, meaningful health insurance reform that will bring additional security and stability to the American people." As tough as it was to pass this bill with the fierce winds of opposition continually blowing, Senate minority leader Mitch McConnell vowed after the vote to continue fighting against health reform: "The public is on our side. This fight is not over."[5] Four years later one-third of the Democrats who voted in favor of the bill would no longer be in the Senate. Some passed away, including Robert Byrd of West Virginia, Daniel Inouye of Hawaii, Arlen Specter of Pennsylvania, and Frank Lautenberg of New Jersey.[6] Others retired or were defeated in their reelection campaigns. During the fifth anniversary of the passage of the ACA, more Democrats found themselves defeated in their bid for reelection or decided to retire at the end of the 113th Congress. As for Republicans, four years after passage of the ACA, 40 percent of their senators who voted against the bill were no longer in the Senate. Some lost in primary challenges by more conservative Tea Party candidates, which actually helped Democrats fare better than expected in the 2012 elections.

Scott Brown's Election Win

The fourth brush with death for health reform occurred when Scott Brown won Senator Kennedy's senate seat in the Massachusetts special election. When Brown, a Tea Party-backed Republican who ran on a platform of opposing health reform, won the election, many feared the opportunity to pass comprehensive health reform had been lost to history. The January 19, 2010, special election was between Brown and Martha Coakley, the state's attorney general, who had been widely expected to win. Instead, Scott Brown won, with 52 percent of the vote. The election result stunned the nation, especially proponents of health reform. Massachusetts had always voted reliably Democratic, so this was supposed to have been a relatively safe seat. The political ramifications of such a liberal-leaning state electing a candidate who strongly opposed health reform were major, in particular because Massachusetts had earlier enacted its own health insurance reforms.

Scott Brown's victory left Democrats just short of the sixty votes needed for a filibuster-proof majority in the Senate, which meant that Republicans would now be able to obstruct the progress and passage of any bill. His victory thus left Democrats scrambling to determine how to proceed. Soon after the election results, Senator Jim Webb of Virginia, a moderate Democrat, called on his Senate colleagues to hold off on voting on the health reform legislation until Senator-elect Scott Brown was sworn into office. He firmly believed that the election was a referendum on health reform. Majority Leader Reid decided to hold off on the vote until Brown was sworn in, stating, "We're going to wait until the new senator arrives until we do anything more on health care."[7]

The strategy all along had been to pass two health reform bills—one in the Senate and one in the House—that could be merged together in conference. The combined bill would then be voted on again; however, with Brown's victory, it was now unlikely that a health reform bill could make it through the Senate. Democrats therefore decided to avoid a second Senate vote by having the House pass the bill that the Senate had passed on Christmas Eve a month prior. However, some House Democrats had concerns about passing the Senate bill. Although both bills contained many similar priorities, there were some major provisions that differentiated the two. The House bill, for example, had a public option and imposed taxes on wealthy individuals, while the Senate bill did not have a public option and taxed only expensive health insurance plans. House members were also wary of passing the Senate bill, especially during an election year, because of the inclusion of certain provisions that were deemed kickbacks for various states, including Florida, Louisiana, and Nebraska. Whether House members' expressed discontent with the Senate-passed bill was a political strategy to gain some concessions and include priorities from their own bill, it was clear that these lawmakers would not accept the Senate-passed plan without some changes.

Speaker Pelosi, understanding the incredible and rare opportunity before the House, seized the moment and went about implementing a strategy that would prove successful in regaining her caucus's faith and their acceptance of the Senate version of the health care bill. She decided to utilize a reconciliation bill, which would require only a majority vote by both chambers, to address her colleagues' concerns with the Senate-approved bill. The result of Speaker Pelosi's work was the Health Care and Education Reconciliation Act, which would make several changes to the Patient Protection and Affordable Care Act. It would get rid of many of the concessions given to certain states, such as Nebraska's Medicaid expansion kickback. It would also increase tax credits for purchasing insurance, reduce the penalty for not purchasing insurance, provide full reimbursement for doctors who care for Medicaid patients, among many other amendments. Although opponents of the law tried in vain to argue their point to the parliamentarian why certain provisions of the ACA were not germane to the reconciliation procedure, with the strategy executed and House Democrats on board, the stage was now set for the House to vote on the Patient Protection and Affordable Care Act.

The March 21 Congressional Vote for ObamaCare

The fifth brush with death for the health reform legislation took place during the historic vote on March 21, 2010, after a brutal congressional battle. Despite the Democrats having control of the House, the votes to pass the bill were never guaranteed. The intense congressional negotiations over health reform had led to increased partisanship and gridlock, limiting Congress's ability to introduce and pass other major bills. House members were particularly worried about casting a "dangerous" vote and of potential backlash from their constituents. The White House expended considerable time and energy hosting meetings with wavering Democrats in the House and all but begged them to vote in favor of the Patient Protection and Affordable Care Act. Leading unions were not happy with the final package but decided to lend their support to the administration and congressional lawmakers. Pro-life advocates urged conservative antiabortion Democrats to vote against the package. The White House was eager to allay any concerns these "Blue Dog Democrats" may have had, and President Obama promised them that no abortions would be funded under the act.

That Sunday at 2 p.m., the House of Representatives convened to vote on the health reform bill. The vote carried with it major political ramifications for the future. All day long, the Representatives argued over H.R. 3590 and H.R. 4872, the health reform package. Congressman John Lewis, a civil rights icon who had helped spearhead the historic civil rights march from Selma to Montgomery, urged his colleagues not to be fearful and to "answer the call of history." In a passionate and stern manner, House minority leader John Boehner (R-OH) warned his colleagues that voting in favor of the act would be "denying the will of the American people."[8] A little after 10:45 that night the announcement came that the bill had finally passed the House by the incredibly slim margin of 219-212—just seven votes—with no Republicans voting in favor of the bill. The vote had been agonizingly close, right up to the last minute, but the results were now clear. Health reform champions inside and outside of Congress that night erupted in cheers. Opponents of health reform were more subdued and promised to use every resource and tactic they could to ensure that the bill would never be implemented.

The 2010 Midterm Elections and an Effective Strategy for Undermining the Law

The next brush with death for the Patient Protection and Affordable Care Act took place eight months after its enactment, with the 2010 midterm elections. The health reform law was a major issue in midterm election campaigns, with many Republican candidates vowing to repeal the law. Poll after poll showed public confusion and dissatisfaction with the ACA, and it seemed that the Republican strategy of vilifying the law was resonating with voters. Proponents feared that the election would lead to the repeal of the health law or at least undermine it in such a way that it would never achieve its purpose.

The elections took place on Tuesday, November 2, 2010, and the results were discouraging for Democrats and for proponents of health reform. Democrats suffered major defeats both nationally and at the state level and lost their majority in the House of Representatives. Emboldened after the election, Republicans sought to fulfill their promise of dismantling the Affordable Care Act, and one of the first votes held by the new 112th Congress was on H.R. 2, the Repealing the Job-Killing Health Care Law Act, which passed the House by a 245-189 vote.[9] However, though Republicans had gained control of the House, Democrats had retained their Senate majority.

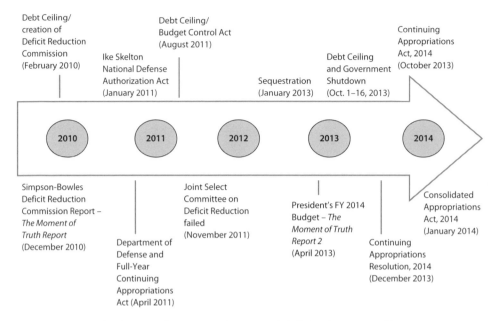

Figure 5.1. Budget, appropriations, and deficit reduction timeline

With President Obama in the White House, successful repeal of the Affordable Care Act was thus highly unlikely for the next two years.

Since opponents lacked enough votes to repeal the Affordable Care Act, they instead focused on crippling its implementation by conducting intense oversight of the law via hearings and appropriations and budget negotiations. While proponents of the law in the Senate used their hearing power to shed a positive light on the law, opponents in the House used their hearing power to shed a negative light.[10] This again had the effect of causing much confusion in the public arena, but it was not this strategy that had the biggest impact on chipping away at the law. Rather, after winning the House in 2010, Republicans cleverly used the must-pass bills—primarily appropriations, budget, debt ceiling, and deficit reduction bills—to modify or repeal certain provisions of the Affordable Care Act.

In almost every negotiation between 2010 and 2014, when Congress and the Obama administration got into a heated exchange over the federal budget, raising the debt ceiling, reducing the deficit, or appropriations, the result was that at least one provision of the Affordable Care Act was chipped away either by modification or outright repeal. In the first four years of the law's existence, opponents successfully amended the law at least twenty times.

While Republicans were pressuring President Obama to address the nation's fiscal challenges, it was not until two Democratic senators who were up for reelection in 2012 voiced concern about raising the debt ceiling in early 2010 that action took place. On February 18, 2010, the Obama administration by executive order formally established a bipartisan commission to identify and make policy recommendations that would thoughtfully tackle the federal deficit problem. Members of the National Commission on Fiscal Responsibility and Reform or the Simpson-Bowles Deficit Reduction Commission were appointed by the president and bipartisan, bicameral congressional leaders and were charged with meeting once a month while Congress was in session. The commission was expected to develop a report highlighting meaningful policies to address the fiscal challenges by December 1, 2010, but after eight months of meeting, the commission could not muster the votes needed to approve the final report.[11] This report, however, later served as a template for subsequent deficit reduction proposals over the next several years by the Obama administration and members of Congress from both sides of the aisle. Because of these various deficit reduction proposals from the White House and Congress, several key health equity programs that had been established right after the civil rights movement, including the Area Health Education Centers, Health Careers Opportunity Program, and the Racial and Ethnic Approaches to Community Health program were slated for termination.

Many of the recommendations promulgated by the report and subsequent proposals by the White House and Congress would have detrimentally impacted many health equity programs if they were actually acted upon. Recommendations in this report called for both reductions in discretionary and mandatory programs as well as tax increases. Three years after convening the commission, however, both cochairs of the commission, Alan Simpson and Erskine Bowles, released another report, *A Bipartisan Path Forward to Securing America's Future,* which went even further than the first report by recommending stringent cuts to discretionary and mandatory federal programs.

The Supreme Court's Decision: Anything but Final

The seventh brush with death for the Affordable Care Act occurred with the Supreme Court decision in June 2012. After its enactment, opponents of the Patient Protection and Affordable Care Act had taken

Timeline of ACA Repeal and Modification Efforts

Effective	Bill	Description
		111th CONGRESS
04/26/2010	H.R. 4887	**TRICARE Affirmation Act** Reclassifies the coverage provided by the TRICARE program and the Non-appropriated Fund Health Benefits Program of the Department of Defense as minimum essential coverage under the PPACA.
05/27/2010	H.R. 5014	**To clarify the health care provided by the Secretary of Veterans Affairs that constitutes minimum essential coverage.** Care and services received through the Department of Veterans Affairs (VA) constitutes minimum essential coverage.
09/27/2010	H.R. 5297	**Small Business Jobs Act of 2010** Amends PPACA Sec. 9006 concerning Treatment of Rental Property Expense Payments: a person receiving rental income from real estate shall be considered to be engaged in a trade or business of renting property.
12/15/2010	H.R. 4994	**Medicare and Medicaid Extenders Act of 2010** Amends the PPACA 12-month special Medicare Part B enrollment period to apply to elections made on and after enactment of PPACA for military retirees, their spouses, and dependent children.
12/17/2010	H.R. 4853	**Tax Relief, Unemployment Insurance Reauthorization, and Job Creation Act of 2010** Separate Sunset for Expansion of Adoption Benefits under the Patient Protection and Affordable Care Act
01/07/2011	H.R. 6523	**Ike Skelton National Defense Authorization Act for Fiscal Year 2011** Directs the comptroller general (CG) to report on costs associated with compliance with the PPACA and the Health Care and Education Reconciliation Act of 2010.
		112th CONGRESS
04/14/2011	H.R. 4	**Comprehensive 1099 Taxpayer Protection and Repayment of Exchange Subsidy Overpayments Act of 2011** Expansion of IRS reporting requirements (1099)
04/15/2011	H.R. 1473	**Department of Defense and Full-Year Continuing Appropriations Act, 2011** Free choice vouchers
02/22/2012	H.R. 3630	**Middle Class Tax Relief and Job Creation Act of 2012** 1) Special adjustment to federal medical assistance percentage (FMAP) determination for certain states recovering from a major disaster—technical correction 2) Medicaid disproportionate share hospitals (DSH) payments—rebases state DSH allotments for FY 2021 3) Prevention and Public Health Fund—i) no funds may be used for propaganda purposes, ii) $6.25 billion cut
01/02/2013	H.R. 8	**American Taxpayer Relief Act of 2012** 1) Federal program to assist establishment and operation of nonprofit, member-run health insurance issuers (co-ops) 2) Repealed Community Living Assistance Services and Supports Act

Timeline of ACA Repeal and Modification Efforts

Effective	Bill	Description
		113th CONGRESS
10/17/2013	H.R. 2775	**Continuing Appropriations Act, 2014** Eligibility verifications for premium tax credits and cost-sharing for health exchanges
12/26/2013	H.R. 59	**Continuing Appropriations Resolution, 2014** Provides additional short-term funding for state health insurance programs, area agencies on aging, Aging and Disability Resource Centers, and the contract with the national center for benefits and outreach enrollment.
01/07/2014	H.R. 3547	**Consolidated Appropriations Act, 2014** 1) Discontinues the Obama administration's flexible use of the Prevention and Public Health Fund, instead reallocating funds for specific programs. 2) Requires establishment of a publicly accessible website regarding use of the Prevention and Public Health Fund. 3) Requires the identification of federal full-time employees and contractors who are implementing the PPACA. 4) Publish the uses of all funds used by CMS specifically for health insurance marketplaces.
10/07/2015	H.R. 1624	**Protecting Affordable Coverage for Employees Act, 2015** Amends the ACA to include employers with 51 to 100 employees as large employers for purposes of health insurance markets. States have the option to treat these employers as small employers.
11/02/2015	H.R. 1314	**Bipartisan Budget Act of 2015** Repeals the requirement for employers who have more than 200 full-time employees and offers health benefit plans to automatically enroll their employees in such a plan.

to the courts in droves to attempt to get the law declared invalid. The largest suit was filed jointly by the attorneys general of Florida, South Carolina, Nebraska, Texas, Utah, Louisiana, Alabama, Michigan, Colorado, Pennsylvania, Washington, Idaho, and South Dakota. Other states soon began joining the suit, and eventually the plaintiffs consisted of twenty-six states, two individuals, and the National Federation of Independent Business.[12] The multistate lawsuit challenged the individual mandate as unconstitutional under the Commerce Clause and under Congress's taxing powers, and it alleged that the law violated the Tenth Amendment by infringing on state sovereignty. The district court ruled the individual mandate unconstitutional and found that it could not be severed from the rest of the Affordable Care Act and so struck down the entire law. The Eleventh Circuit Court of Appeals then reversed that decision in part, agreeing with the district court that the individual mandate was unconstitutional but finding that it could be severed from the rest of the act, the remainder of which was thus upheld. The Supreme Court granted certiorari to review the case and scheduled oral arguments for the spring of 2012.

The questions that the Supreme Court had to consider included whether the individual mandate and the expansion of the Medicaid program were within Congress's constitutional power. Specifically the Court was charged with first determining whether the suit was barred by the Anti-Injunction Act, which would prevent them from considering the substantive arguments raised by appellants. If the suit was not barred, then the Court had to consider whether the mandate could be upheld under the Commerce Clause, the Necessary and Proper Clause, or the Taxing Clause. The second issue the Court was charged with determining was whether the Medicaid expansion provision was constitutional.

Although it seemed that most people dismissed these legal challenges, a few health equity advocates were extremely concerned that the Supreme Court agreed to review the Medicaid expansion provision. No appellate court had reviewed that provision prior to the Eleventh Circuit Court of Appeals, which found it constitutional. Supporters of the law started worrying once oral arguments began in the *National Federation of Independent Business v. Sebelius* Supreme Court case in March 2012. They criticized Solicitor General Donald B. Verrilli Jr., who took over from Acting Solicitor General Neal Katyal, for his vacillating performance during the oral arguments.[13]

They also criticized the Obama administration for not developing legal arguments tailored to the Court's conservative wing. Legal scholars won-

March 2010 – Sept. 2010	District Courts 2010–2011	Appeals Courts 2011	U.S. Supreme Court 2012

26 cases filed against ACA	• 3 cases overturned ACA in whole or in part
	
	• 7 cases ruled ACA ➡ constitutional and dismissed case
	
	• 15 cases dismissed for lack of standing or procedural reasons
		• 6th Circuit Ct (6/1/11) oral arguments
		  • 6/29/11 held const. *(2-1)*
		  • District Ct held const.
		• 11th Circuit Ct (6/8/11) oral arguments
		  • 8/12/11 held unconst. *(2-1)*
		  • District Ct held unconst.
		• 4th Circuit Ct (5/10/11) oral arguments
		  • 9/8/11 dismissed – lack of ➡ jurisdiction
		  • District Ct disagreed:
		  1 court const.
		  1 court unconst.
		• D.C. Circuit Ct (9/23/11) oral arguments
		  • 11/8/11 held const. *(2-1)*
		  • District Ct held const.
		• 8th Circuit Ct (4/26/11) oral arguments
		  • 10/4/12 dismissed – lack of standing
		  • District Ct dismissed for failure to state a claim upon which relief may be granted.
			January 6
			• Federal government and other amici curiae filed briefs
			February 6
			• Respondents filed briefs
			March 7
			• Federal government ➡ filed reply brief
			March 26–28
			• Supreme Court heard 11th Circuit ACA case in 5½ hours of oral argument
			June
			• Supreme Court decided case and published its opinion on June 28

Figure 5.2. ACA progress through the courts

dered why the administration had not argued that the Militia Act of 1792 signed by the nation's first president, George Washington, obligating every free adult man eighteen or older to purchase a firearm and ammunition, supported their case. Or that a 1798 statute signed by President John Adams, An Act for the Relief of Sick and Disabled Seamen, strengthened their case. They could have argued that the Seamen's Act was indeed the first federal health insurance mandate, since it expressly mandated that ship owners purchase medical insurance for their crew and that sailors purchase hospital insurance for themselves.

The administration chose instead to primarily argue that health care was a unique marketplace that Congress, under the Constitution's interstate commerce clause, could regulate by imposing the requirement that consumers buy insurance before receiving treatment or pay a penalty. Solicitor General Verrilli pushed the argument that Congress's taxing powers justified the mandate because the penalty for those who do not buy insurance, written into the internal revenue code, can be viewed as a tax. Though it was politically risky to argue during an election year that the president supported a tax, it was a strong legal argument.

As time got closer to the date when the decision was expected by the Court, tensions continued to increase over the prospect of the five conservative justices dismantling the Affordable Care Act. Proponents worried that after the *Citizens United* case, the five conservative justices would strike not only the heart and guts of the ACA but the entire law. A few weeks before the decision was expected, proponents started to play the blame game and questioning Obama's strategies and tactics. However, the administration pushed back, stating that its "arguments were thoroughly analyzed, vetted and discussed."[14]

Arguably, no proponent was more concerned than President Obama, who was confronting the real possibility that his signature legislative accomplishment could be struck down. Proponents thought the administration should have used delay tactics such as filing motions, seeking full review of the case by certain appellate courts instead of just a select panel of judges on the court, or even making arguments that might have delayed the case past the 2012 elections into 2014. With the stakes high and the chips stacked against him, the president, despite criticisms that he was trying to intimidate the justices, made remarks at a press conference relating to his health reform law while the Supreme Court was in session:

> I am confident the Supreme Court will not take what would be an unprecedented, extraordinary step of overturning a law that was passed by a strong majority of a democratically-elected Congress . . .
>
> I just remind conservative commentators that for years we have heard the biggest problem on the bench was judicial activism or a lack of judicial restraint. That an unelected group of people would somehow overturn a duly constituted and passed law. Well, this is a good example and I am pretty confident that this Court will recognize that and not take that step . . .
>
> As I said, . . . I am confident this will be upheld because it should be upheld. And again, that is not just my opinion. That is the opinion of a whole lot of constitutional law professors and academics and judges and lawyers who have examined this law, even if they're not particularly sympathetic to this piece of legislation or my presidency.[15]

The next day, the president expounded on what he meant, saying his point was simply that, as the Supreme Court is the arbiter of the Constitution and has a great deal of power in that regard, the Court has traditionally deferred to Congress and was thus unlikely to strike down the Affordable Care Act. Obama's remarks and the way they were perceived by the media and opponents of health reform caused the law's proponents additional heartburn. Proponents were concerned that the Supreme Court justices would deem the president's comments inappropriate and that any justice who was on the fence would thus end up voting against the Affordable Care Act. It was certainly understandable that a health care overhaul law that affects virtually every American—from cradle to grave—would test the boundaries of constitutional permissibility. So it was not surprising that lawsuits contested the most contentious provisions included in the statute, including the individual mandate, Medicaid expansion, women's preventive services, the employer mandate, and the Independent Payment Advisory Board.

The Court's Revelation

On the day the decision came out, Thursday, June 28, 2012, there was a lot of nail biting and prayers ascending. Thankfully, the law narrowly escaped death, once again, when the Supreme Court decided to uphold the constitutionality of the health reform law and its provisions aimed at addressing health disparities.

Under the ACA, individuals who do not receive insurance from an employer or government program must purchase private insurance. Those who did not comply and enroll in a health plan by 2014 would be subject to the penalty or "shared responsibility payment," which would be assessed and collected in the same manner as tax penalties. The Court ruled that the Anti-Injunction Act did not bar them from considering this suit. The Court reasoned that although the act stipulates, "No suit for the purpose of restraining the assessment or collection of any tax shall be maintained in any court by any person," and the case before the Court sought to restrain collection of the shared responsibility payment, it was not applicable because a statute must contain the word "tax" for purposes of triggering the applicability of the act. The Affordable Care Act did not use the word "tax" when referring to the penalty, so the Court decided it could consider the merits of this case.

Once the justices determined that the Anti-Injunction Act did not bar the suit, they thoughtfully analyzed the constitutionality of the individual mandate under the Commerce Clause of the US Constitution. The Court ruled that the mandate was not a valid exercise of Congress's power under the Commerce Clause because the framers gave Congress the power to regulate commerce, not compel it. Essentially, the Court argued that the individual mandate to purchase health insurance did not regulate existing activity. Instead, it compelled individuals to become active in commerce by purchasing a product.

The Court then went on to determine whether the individual mandate could be upheld under the Necessary and Proper Clause. Again the Court ruled that it could not be sustained under the Necessary and Proper Clause as an integral part of the Affordable Care Act. The justices reasoned that the mandate vested Congress with extraordinary ability to create the necessary predicate to the exercise of an enumerated power and draw within its regulatory scope those who would not otherwise be outside it. In other words, the Court argued that even if the individual mandate were necessary to the rest of the law, such expansion of federal power is not a proper means for making those reforms effective.

Finally, the Court examined whether the individual mandate was within Congress's power to "lay and collect taxes." In a remarkable twist, the Court held that the mandate was within Congress's power under the Taxing Clause even though the ACA described the shared responsibility payment as a "penalty," not a "tax." Chief Justice Roberts stated that the Court must "[disregard] the designation of the exaction, and [view] its substance and application." As a result, the Court argued that the "shared responsibility payment" could be considered a tax. In expounding further, the Court reasoned that the payment is not so high that there is no choice but to buy health insurance; the payment is not limited to willful violations, as penalties for unlawful acts often are; and the payment is collected solely by the Internal Revenue Service (IRS) through the normal means of taxation. Therefore, the mandate need not be read to declare that failing to purchase health insurance is unlawful.

The Court, in effect, agreed with the solicitor general's argument that the mandate could be upheld as a proper exercise of Congress's taxing power. This was similar to the ruling that the Court had made when it voted 5-4 upholding the Social Security Act as a valid exercise of the federal government's taxing power. However, the Court also held that the Medicaid expansion was not a proper exercise of Congress's spending power because the legitimacy of Spending Clause legislation depends on whether a state voluntarily and knowingly accepts the terms of such programs.[16] The Court explained, when Congress threatens to terminate other grants as a means of pressuring a state to accept a Spending Clause program, the legislation runs counter to this nation's system of federalism. Therefore, the Court prohibited the federal government from refusing

Medicaid funding to states that refused to expand Medicaid. This was due in part to the notion that the threatened loss of more than 10 percent of a state's overall budget is economic "dragooning" that leaves the states with no real option but to acquiesce in Medicaid expansion.

Furthermore, the Court argued that the expansion of Medicaid to everyone under age sixty-five with incomes below 138 percent of the federal poverty level transformed the Medicaid program so drastically that it was a shift in kind, not degree. Since this provision was found unconstitutional, the Court was then tasked with determining whether the Medicaid expansion provision could be severed from the rest of the statute or whether the whole law must be struck. In another nail-biting analysis, the Court reasoned that the violation is fully remedied by precluding the secretary of health and human services from enforcing the penalty of withdrawing existing Medicaid funds for failure to comply. Consequently, the remaining Affordable Care Act provisions could be left intact. This ruling essentially left Medicaid expansion under the health reform law optional for states, which was likely to lead to fewer uninsured or underinsured individuals having access to affordable health insurance coverage. The Medicaid expansion provision was a key aspect of the statute's efforts to expand coverage to vulnerable populations, so while proponents were rejoicing they were also grieving that the Court had weakened this provision. One of their greatest fears had come to pass.

Unfortunately, the decision from the Supreme Court did not settle the issue once and for all. Instead, it led to a resurgence of opposition. Opponents were determined to use the political process to undermine the law, and they saw the opportunity to do so in the upcoming 2012 presidential elections. In a strongly worded section from his majority opinion in *NFIB v. Sebelius*, Chief Justice John Roberts asserted, "Members of this Court are vested with the authority to interpret the law; we possess neither the expertise nor the prerogative to make policy judgments. Those decisions are entrusted to our Nation's elected leaders, who can be thrown out of office if the people disagree with them. It is not our job to protect the people from the consequences of their political choices."[17] This statement essentially punted the issue of dismantling the law back in the political arena.

The 2012 Presidential Election

The eighth brush with death occurred during the 2012 presidential election. So long as President Obama remained in the White House, any attempts at repeal from Congress were doomed to fail, as the president would almost certainly exercise his veto power on any repeal bill that made it to his desk. However, were he to lose the election to a Republican president, the Affordable Care Act would be in danger of repeal or dismantling. Obama's opponent this time was former Massachusetts governor Mitt Romney, who by May had clinched the Republican Party's nomination. President Obama's health reform law was a major issue in the election campaign, along with the usual campaign issues such as immigration and foreign policy. The Republican Party was of course firmly opposed to "ObamaCare," and former governor Romney campaigned on the promise that he would "repeal and replace" the law if he won the election.[18]

However, Mitt Romney found himself in the awkward position of advocating against the Affordable Care Act while having enacted health reform while he was governor of Massachusetts. The Massachusetts law, which Romney enacted with the help of Senator Ted Kennedy, has been described as a model for the Affordable Care Act: it mandates that all individuals purchase health insurance, requires businesses to offer health insurance plans to employees, and created an online health insurance exchange called the Health Connector.[19] At the time of its enactment, Romney said the law would provide "every citizen with affordable, comprehensive health insurance."[20] Critics pounced on Romney for his arguably contradictory position opposing the Affordable Care Act while defending his own health insurance reform achievement. Romney fired back, declaring that the Massachusetts law was tailored to that state's needs, whereas the ACA places the mandate on all Americans. The voters finally had their say on Tuesday, November 6, 2012, and President Obama won the election decisively, winning both the popular vote and the electoral college vote. Whether opponents of health reform were correct in their assessment that the election was a referendum on the health reform law, President Obama would be staying in the White House, and the Affordable Care Act would continue to be implemented for the next four years.

In Congress, there were also difficult battles. All seats in the House of Representatives were up for election. Six incumbent Democrats lost their seats to Republicans, while sixteen incumbent Republicans lost their seats to Democratic challengers. Republicans maintained their House majority, 234–201. In the Senate, thirty-three seats were contested, and some of the campaigns involved major controversies. Missouri incumbent Senator Claire McCaskill ran against Republican Todd Akin. Akin found himself at the center of a nationwide controversy after making the claim in an interview that women rarely become pregnant as a result of "legitimate rape," as "the female body has ways to try and shut that whole thing down."[21] The comments were met with a huge uproar and likely contributed to Akin only gaining 39.2 percent of the vote to McCaskill's 54.7 percent.

Then, in Indiana, during a debate two weeks before the election, Republican Senate nominee Richard Mourdock, in speaking about abortion, said, "I just struggled with it myself for a long time but I came to realize: Life is that gift from God that I think even if life begins in that horrible situation of rape, that it is something that God intended to happen."[22] His comments were also hugely controversial and may have resulted in his losing to Democratic nominee Joe Donnelly. In the end, the Democrats gained two seats in the 2012 election, increasing their majority in the Senate. With the House remaining in Republican control and the Senate in Democratic hands, the bitter struggles between the two chambers would continue for another two years.

The 2013 Government Shutdown

The ninth brush with death occurred in 2013, during the historic federal government shutdown when Congress failed to enact appropriations legislation for fiscal year 2014. House Republicans had continued with their efforts to undermine the Affordable Care Act and in late 2013 insisted that any spending bill should include provisions to defund or delay the law. Several key provisions of the ACA were set to take effect in 2014, most notably the individual mandate, so opponents had intensified their efforts. The Republican-led House on September 20 thus passed an appropriations bill containing a provision that would defund the Affordable Care Act. The Democratic-led Senate, however, refused to pass a bill that would negatively affect the ACA. Republican Senator Ted Cruz gave a twenty-one-hour speech against the law, charging his colleagues to pass the appropriations bill and advocating government shutdown unless the Democrats made compromises. Nevertheless, the Senate removed the defunding provision and sent the bill back to the House. House Republicans then switched tactics and presented a proposal that would delay implementation of the law for a year. The Senate rejected this proposal on September 30 and rejected the subsequent proposals that would also delay the implementation of the law. The two chambers failed to reach a compromise by midnight on September 30, 2013, the end of the 2013 fiscal year.

On the start of the 2014 fiscal year, October 1, 2013, the federal government shut down, and eight hundred thousand federal employees were furloughed. President Obama gave a speech that day, lambasting Republicans for their actions.

> No, this shutdown is not about deficits, it's not about budgets. This shutdown is about rolling back our efforts to provide health insurance to folks who don't have it. It's all about rolling back the Affordable Care Act. This, more than anything else, seems to be what the Republican Party stands for these days. I know it's strange that one party would make keeping people uninsured the centerpiece of their agenda, but that apparently is what it is.
>
> And of course, what's stranger still is that shutting down our government doesn't accomplish their stated goal. The Affordable Care Act is a law that passed the House; it passed the Senate. The Supreme Court ruled it constitutional. It was a central issue in last year's election. It is settled, and it is here to stay.[23]

The House immediately began approving bills to restart certain popular government programs, such as the national parks and museums, the Food and Drug Administration, and National Institutes of Health medical research. The Senate rejected these piecemeal bills as a tactic by Republicans to allow the shutdown to drag on longer. House Republican leaders met with President Obama but failed to reach an agreement, and bills proposed by Speaker John Boehner failed to receive full support. In the Senate, however, a bipartisan group worked together on a bill to end the shutdown. On October 16, 2013, the Reid-McConnell bill was put to a vote and passed the Senate 81-18. The bill would fund the government through January 15 and included no provisions to defund or delay the Affordable Care Act. The only modification to the law was a tightening of the income verification rules for Americans applying for tax credits on the health insurance exchanges. The House passed the bill a few hours later, on a 285-144 vote. President Obama signed it into law at about 12:30 a.m. Thursday, and the federal government reopened. Speaker Boehner admitted defeat in an interview after the House vote: "We fought the good fight. We just didn't win."[24]

SCOTUScare, Pure Applesauce, and Jiggery-Pokery—*King v. Burwell*

The tenth brush with death occurred during 2015 when the Affordable Care Act faced its second major challenge in the Supreme Court of the United States.[25] This case could have seriously undermined the health care law and totally disrupt the gains that had been achieved in increasing health insurance coverage for millions of Americans. Despite ObamaCare's positive impact on communities across the country, opponents of the ACA continued to wage their battles. Though proponents may have hoped that the Supreme Court's June 2012 *NFIB v. Sebelius* decision would decisively settle the issue of the Affordable Care Act's constitutionality, opponents continued trying to chip away at the law in the courts.

Since the 2012 Supreme Court ruling, lawsuits have challenged other aspects of the Affordable Care Act. In June 2014, the Supreme Court ruled in *Burwell v. Hobby Lobby* that the contraceptive mandate violates the Religious Freedom Restoration Act by requiring employers to provide coverage for female employees' contraceptives. The Court ruled that closely held corporations may be exempt from a law its owners religiously object to if there is a less restrictive means of furthering the law's interest. While a huge blow for increasing women's preventive services, especially for women who work in these corporations, this case did not have the potential to unravel the Affordable Care Act like the *King v. Burwell* and *Halbig v. Burwell* cases, which challenged the premium subsidies offered to beneficiaries on the federal health insurance exchange.

Together the petitioners in these cases argued that the federally established exchanges are not legally an "exchange established by the State under section 1311" as was interpreted by the IRS in regulation and should thus be exempt from receiving federal subsidies. The DC Circuit Court of Appeals, which heard the *Halbig v. Burwell case*, was the first appeals court to decide the issue. In a 2-1 decision, the court ruled against the Obama administration, holding that the statutory language was not ambiguous and that the IRS had overstepped its authority. This came as quite a shock to proponents of the ACA, but that disappointment would not last long since the Fourth Circuit Court of Appeals, which heard a parallel case, *King v. Burwell*, just a few hours later unanimously upheld the IRS's regulation providing for premium subsidies in states with a federally run or federally facilitated exchange. In its ruling, the court held that the ACA's provision on this point is ambiguous, which means the IRS has the authority to reasonably interpret the ACA. As a result, there was now a split between the appellate courts, which increased the likelihood of the Supreme Court intervening to decide the issue.

Before the Supreme Court intervened, however, the Obama administration petitioned the DC Court of Appeals to set aside its ruling and rehear the case en banc, meaning before the entire court. The court agreed, but the rehearing was put on hold after the Supreme Court announced it would hear the *King v. Burwell* case. Although there is no requirement that there has to be a split for such a review by the high Court, this caused many proponents unease. They questioned the Court's intentions for breaking from its normal practice, since the case no longer met the usual criteria for Supreme Court review. Nevertheless, once the Supreme Court granted certiorari in the *King v. Burwell* case on November 7, 2014, one thing was certain: the ACA was about to face its tenth brush with death. The Court now put itself in the position of being the final determiner of whether the Affordable Care Act's tax credits or premium subsidies to purchase insurance are available to states that have a federal exchange rather than a state-based exchange.

The Obama administration interpreted the provision to authorize subsidies both in states that operate their own exchanges and the thirty-four states that rely on the federal government to run their exchanges. Opponents of the ACA challenged the administration's ruling, arguing that a plain text reading does not permit subsidies in states with exchanges operated by the federal government. Interestingly, a significant majority of states who joined on amicus briefs to the Court, both Republican controlled and Democrat controlled, sided with the Obama administration and urged the Court to uphold the final IRS regulation implementing the premium tax credit provision of the Affordable Care Act.[26] Even Republicans came out in support of the federal government's position, including former senator Olympia Snowe of Maine. Although she had voted against the final bill, she argued, "I don't ever recall any distinction between federal and state exchanges in terms of the availability of subsidies. It was never part of our conversations at any point. Why would we have wanted to deny people subsidies? It was not their fault if their state did not set up an exchange."[27] The Supreme Court heard oral arguments in the *King v. Burwell* case on March 4, 2015, and a decision regarding the permissibility of these subsidies for federal health insurance exchange beneficiaries was promulgated on Thursday, June 25, 2015.

Chief Justice John Roberts authored the opinion of the Court, just like he had with the first major case challenging the Affordable Care Act three years earlier. Unlike the case in 2012, however, he was joined by another conservative justice, Anthony Kennedy, making it a 6–3 decision. He wrote that when analyzing an agency's interpretation of a statute, the Court often applies a two-step framework that involves whether the statute is ambiguous and whether the agency's interpretation is reasonable. This approach, he wrote, was premised on the theory that a statute's ambiguity constitutes an implicit delegation from Congress to the agency to fill in the statutory gaps. However, he went on to state that, in extraordinary cases, there may be reason to hesitate before concluding that Congress has intended such an implicit delegation, and *King v. Burwell* represented such a case. He argued that because of the billions of dollars spent on these tax credits or subsidies and the effect they have on the price of health insurance for millions of people, this presented a question of deep economic and political significance. So if Congress had intended to assign that question to an agency, it surely would have done so expressly. Therefore, it was the Court, not the IRS, who was tasked with determining the correct reading of the ACA's provision regarding the application of tax credits to enrollees in the federally facilitated exchange.

In his reasoning, the chief justice added that, to determine the meaning or ambiguity of certain words or phrases, they must be read in their context and with a view to their place in the overall statutory scheme. For it was the Court's duty to construe statutes, not isolated provisions. After analyzing the statute to determine the meaning of the phrase that was at the center of the debate, Chief Justice Roberts went on to criticize the inartful drafting of the Affordable Care Act as well as the process for crafting the statute. He argued that, because of these issues, "the Act does not reflect the type of care and deliberation that one might expect of such significant legislation."[28] Nonetheless, the Court held that a fair reading of the statute demanded a fair understanding of the legislative plan, which was to improve health insurance markets, not destroy them. Therefore, the subsidies did apply to enrollees not only in state-based health insurance exchanges but also the federally facilitated health insurance exchanges in thirty-four states.

Justice Antonin Scalia, in a passionate and scathing dissent, repeatedly argued that the Court's "interpretation [in the 2012 and now 2015 ACA cases] seem always to yield to the overriding principle of the present Court: The Affordable Care Act must be saved." He argued that the Court was rewriting the law, instead of interpreting it, thus making it futile to challenge the Affordable Care Act in the future under the Roberts Court. Scalia concluded that we might as well start calling ObamaCare SCO-TUScare and described the Court's reasoning as "pure applesauce" and "jiggery-pokery."[29]

In what appears to be a direct rebuttal to the chief justice's statement in *NFIB v. Sebelius* regarding the Court's exact role, Justice Scalia stated, "This Court holds only the judicial power—the power to pronounce the law as Congress has enacted it. We lack the prerogative to repair laws that do not work out in practice, just as the people lack the ability to throw us out of office if they dislike the solutions we concoct. We must always remember, therefore, that '[o]ur task is to apply the text, not improve upon it.'" Despite his belief that the decision that day by the majority was erroneous, one thing both proponents and opponents of ObamaCare can agree with Scalia on is that the "Court's two decisions on the Act will surely be remembered through the years."[30]

One More Brush with Death?

Interestingly, just like in *NFIB v. Sebelius*, Chief Justice Roberts in *King v. Burwell* included a caveat that, in a democracy, the power to make laws rests with those chosen by the people and so the Court could only interpret the law or say what it is. This, once again, effectually punted the Affordable Care Act into the political process whereby opponents would have to legislatively work to undermine the law or repeal and replace it with another policy. To successfully do that, it was clear that the 2016 presidential election would be the next best opportunity to knock down the ACA, since Republicans gained control of both Houses of Congress after the 2014 midterm elections. This result was widely expected and did not cause the same level of angst that the 2010 and 2012 elections did because there was no indication that this would result in the supermajority needed to override a presidential veto.

The Affordable Care Act has survived many brushes with death, proving that it has more lives than a cat, and it is most likely to experience more brushes as time passes. As elections come and go and new policy makers take office, proponents of the law will rightly be concerned about the act's future. There is always a chance that the political winds could shift and support for the law could diminish as a result. However, the Affordable Care Act can be compared in many ways to two other sweeping laws impacting many citizens' access to health care: the Social Security Act and Medicare and Medicaid.

Both Social Security and Medicare and Medicaid were strongly opposed by many Republicans at first and for quite a while after their enactment, but they then gained acceptance through the ensuing years. In fact, according to Wilbur Cohen, one of the architects of Medicare and Medicaid, "For 9 years (1957-65), Medicare and Medicaid were highly controversial issues."[31] This is the best-case scenario for the Affordable Care Act, a fate that even Justice Scalia acknowledged in *King v. Burwell* was a real possibility: "perhaps the Patient Protection and Affordable Care Act will attain the enduring status of the Social Security Act or the Taft-Hartley Act." A major difference, however, is that Medicare and Medicaid as well as Social Security were established when Republicans and Democrats were not as sharply divided as they are now.

In remarks after the Supreme Court released its decision on the *King v. Burwell* case, President Obama stated that the ACA had moved away from being an abstract thing to something that people can now see is working, and "working better than we expected it would." While acknowledging that ObamaCare is now woven into the fabric of America, he recognized that, unlike "Social Security or Medicare, a lot of Americans still don't know what Obamacare is beyond all the political noise in Washington. Across the country, there remain people who are directly benefitting from the law but don't even know it. . . . There's no card that says 'Obamacare' when you enroll. But that's by design, for this has never been a government takeover of health care, despite cries to the contrary."[32] For now, in any case, the Affordable Care Act is still in limbo, so its proponents must remain vigilant to ensure that its next brush with death is not fatal.

NOTES

1. Justice Sotomayor in an interview with George Stephanopoulos on *This Week, Sunday,* June 22, 2014, when discussing why she read her dissent on Affirmative Action from the bench.

2. Obama, "Remarks by the President at the Annual Conference of the American Medical Association."

3. Shaw, "Senate Passes Historic Bill to Reform the U.S. Health Care System"; Reid, "Historic Health Reform Vote Marks a New Beginning to Deal with Old Challenges."

4. Cohn, "How They Did It"; *Miami Herald,* "Nelson for the Senate."

5. US Senate roll call votes, 111th Cong., 1st sess.; Obama, "Remarks by the President on Senate Passage of Health Insurance Reform"; Pear, "Senate Passes Health Care Overhaul on Party-Line Vote."

6. In April 2009, Senator Specter had switched from Republican to Democrat, stating that his views no longer aligned with the Republican philosophy. In addition, Al Franken won his seat in Minnesota, giving Democrats the 60 seats needed for a filibuster-proof majority. When Senator Specter ran for his seat in the November 2010 elections as a Democrat, he lost, before passing away in 2012.

7. Lovley, "Harry Reid: We'll Wait on Scott Brown for Health Care Vote."

8. Winerman, "House Votes Cap Day of Debate on Health Reform."

9. Bill summary and status, H.R. 2.

10. The party in control of the chamber decides which hearings to convene, exploring various issues.

11. The commission was named after Alan Simpson, a former Republican senator from Wyoming and Erskine Bowles, a former chief of staff to President Clinton. Only eleven of the eighteen members voted to approve the report. www.fiscalcommission.gov; White House, *Moment of Truth*.

12. The National Federation of Independent Business had led the campaign to block Clinton's health reform efforts, and was instrumental in the efforts to bring down Obama's health reform legislation.

13. Neal Katyal filled in when Elena Kagan, who served as solicitor general from March 2009 to August 2010, was appointed as a justice to the US Supreme Court. Though some claimed Justice Kagan had helped the Department of Justice develop a defense strategy for Affordable Care Act cases, she refused to recuse herself from the case, saying that she had not played a significant role in those decisions.

14. Wallsten, "Obama's Legal Tactics Seen as Possibly Hurting Chances to Save Health-Care Law."

15. Aigner-Treworgy, "President Obama: Overturning Individual Mandate Would Be 'Unprecedented, Extraordinary Step.'"

16. The Spending Clause grants power to "pay the Debts and provide for the . . . general Welfare of the United States." US Const. art. I, §8, cl. 1.

17. *National Federation of Independent Business v. Sebelius.*

18. Hancock, "Election Will Decide Health Law's Future."

19. While the Romney proposal served as a blueprint for the Obama proposal, there is a clear distinction between the two. The Romney proposal focused specifically on health insurance reforms, whereas the Obama proposal focused also on delivery system and payment reforms, bolstering research and workforce development, prevention, and more.

20. CNN Election Center.

21. Jaco, "Full Interview with Todd Akin."

22. Groer, "Indiana GOP Senate Hopeful Richard Mourdock Says God 'Intended' Rape Pregnancies."

23. Obama, "Remarks by the President on the Affordable Care Act and the Government Shutdown."

24. US Senate roll call votes, 113th Cong., 1st sess., H.R. 2775; Final vote results for Roll Call 550, H.R. 2775; Weisman and Parker, "Republicans Back Down, Ending Crisis over Shutdown and Debt Limit."

25. Sometimes abbreviated SCOTUS or the Court.

26. The following states filed an amicus brief with the Supreme Court in support of the Obama administration: California, Connecticut, Delaware, the District of Columbia, Hawaii, Illinois, Iowa, Kentucky, Maine, Maryland, Massachusetts, Mississippi, New Hampshire, New Mexico, New York, North

Carolina, North Dakota, Oregon, Pennsylvania, Rhode Island, Vermont, Virginia, and Washington. Seven states sided with the challengers and filed an amicus brief with the Court: Alabama, Georgia, Indiana, Nebraska, Oklahoma, South Carolina, and West Virginia.

27. Pear, "Four Words That Imperil Health Care Law Were All a Mistake, Writers Now Say."

28. *King v. Burwell.*

29. Ibid.

30. Ibid.

31. Cohen, "Reflections on the Enactment of Medicare and Medicaid."

32. Obama, "Remarks by the President on the Supreme Court's Ruling of the Affordable Care Act."

BIBLIOGRAPHY

Aigner-Treworgy, Adam. "President Obama: Overturning Individual Mandate Would Be 'Unprecedented, Extraordinary Step.'" *The 1600 Report* (blog). CNN. April 2, 2012. http://whitehouse.blogs.cnn.com/2012/04/02/president -obama-overturning-individual-mandate-would-be-unprecedented -extraordinary-step/.

Bill summary and status. 112th Congress (2011–2012). H.R. 2. Library of Congress. http://thomas.loc.gov/cgi-bin/bdquery/z?d112:HR00002:@@@R.

Burwell v. Hobby Lobby Stores, Inc., 134 U.S. 2751 (2014).

CNN Election Center. http://www.cnn.com/election/2012/campaign-issues .html#healthcare.

Cohen, Wilbur. "Reflections on the Enactment of Medicare and Medicaid." Supplement, *Health Care Financing Review* (December 1985): 3–11. http:// www.ncbi.nlm.nih.gov/pmc/articles/PMC4195078/.

Cohn, Jonathan. "How They Did It." *New Republic*, May 21, 2010. http://www .newrepublic.com/article/75077/how-they-did-it.

Final vote results for Roll Call 550, H.R. 2775. http://clerk.house.gov/evs/2013 /roll550.xml.

Groer, Annie. "Indiana GOP Senate Hopeful Richard Mourdock Says God 'Intended' Rape Pregnancies." *Washington Post*, October 24, 2012. http://www .washingtonpost.com/blogs/she-the-people/wp/2012/10/24/indiana-gop -senate-hopeful-richard-mourdock-says-god-intended-rape-pregnancies/.

Halbig v. Burwell, 758 F. 3d 390 (2014).

Hancock, Jay. "Election Will Decide Health Law's Future. *Kaiser Health News*, November 5, 2012. http://www.kaiserhealthnews.org/Stories/2012 /November/06/election-future-of-health-law.aspx.

Jaco, Charles. "Jaco Report: Full Interview with Todd Akin." *Fox2now*, August 19, 2012. http://fox2now.com/2012/08/19/the-jaco-report-august-19 -2012/.

King v. Burwell. 576 U.S. (14-114) (2015).

Lovley, Erika. "Harry Reid: We'll Wait on Scott Brown for Health Care Vote," *Politico*, January 20, 2010. http://www.politico.com/news/stories/0110/31734 .html.

Miami Herald. "Nelson for the Senate." Nelson for Senate website. http:// nelsonforsenate.com/nelson-for-the-senate.

National Federation of Independent Business v. Sebelius. 567 U.S. 648 F.3d 1235 (2012).

Pear, Robert. "Four Words That Imperil Health Care Law Were All a Mistake, Writers Now Say." *New York Times*, March 25, 2015.

———. "Senate Passes Health Care Overhaul on Party-Line Vote." *New York Times*, December 24, 2009. http://www.nytimes.com/2009/12/25/health /policy/25health.html.

Obama, Barack. "Remarks by the President at the Annual Conference of the American Medical Association." Press release, June 15, 2009. http://www .whitehouse.gov/the-press-office/remarks-president-annual-conference -american-medical-association.

———. "Remarks by the President on Senate Passage of Health Insurance Reform." Press Release, December 24, 2009. http://www.whitehouse.gov /the-press-office/remarks-president-senate-passage-health-insurance -reform.

———. "Remarks by the President on the Affordable Care Act and the Government Shutdown." Press release, October 1, 2013. http://www.whitehouse .gov/the-press-office/2013/10/01/remarks-president-affordable-care-act-and -government-shutdown.

———. "Remarks by the President on the Supreme Court's Ruling of the Affordable Care Act." Press release, June 25, 2015. https://www.whitehouse.gov /the-press-office/2015/06/25/remarks-president-supreme-courts-ruling -affordable-care-act.

Reid, Harry. "Historic Health Reform Vote Marks a New Beginning to Deal with Old Challenges." US Senate Democrats. Press release, December 24, 2009. http://democrats.senate.gov/2009/12/24/reid-historic-health-reform-vote -marks-a-new-beginning-to-deal-with-old-challenges/#.U9qOhrHGujo.

Shaw, Donny. "Senate Passes Historic Bill to Reform the U.S. Health Care System." *OpenCongress* (blog), December 24, 2009. http://www.opencongress .org/articles/view/1421-Senate-Passes-Historic-Bill-to-Reform-the-U-S-Health -Care-System.

Sotomayor, Sonia. Interview by George Stephanopoulos. *This Week, Sunday.* June 22, 2014,

US Senate roll call votes. 111th Congress, first Session. H.R. 359. http://www .senate.gov/legislative/LIS/roll_call_lists/roll_call_vote_cfm.cfm?congress =111&session=1&vote=00396.

US Senate roll call votes. 113th Congress, first Session. H.R. 2775. http://www
.senate.gov/legislative/LIS/roll_call_lists/roll_call_vote_cfm.cfm?congress
=113&session=1&vote=00219.

Wallsten, Peter. "Obama's Legal Tactics Seen as Possibly Hurting Chances to
Save Health-Care Law." *Washington Post*, June 23, 2012. http://www
.washingtonpost.com/politics/obamas-legal-tactics-seen-as-possibly-hurting
-chances-to-save-health-care-law/2012/06/23/gJQA4VqsxV_story.html.

Weisman, Jonathan, and Ashley Parker. "Republicans Back Down, Ending Crisis
over Shutdown and Debt Limit." *New York Times*, October 16, 2013. http://
www.nytimes.com/2013/10/17/us/congress-budget-debate.html.

White House. *The Moment of Truth: Report of the National Commission on Fiscal
Responsibility and Reform.* Washington, DC, December 2010.

Winerman, Lea. "House Votes Cap Day of Debate on Health Reform." *PBS
NewsHour.* March 21, 2010. http://www.pbs.org/newshour/rundown/as-floor
-debate-begins-democrats-predict-health-reform-will-pass/.

Breaking Down the Law
Understanding the Policy and the Politics

It will be of little avail to the people that the laws are made by men of their own choice if the laws be so voluminous that they cannot be read, or so incoherent that they cannot be understood.
—*President James Madison*

Early in our nation's history, President Madison recognized that it was not enough for lawmakers who were elected by the people to make and pass laws on their behalf. These laws also had to be easily understood and manageable. Some of the biggest criticisms from opponents of the health reform law are that it is too complicated, too overreaching, and too voluminous. Opponents of the Affordable Care Act railed not only against the process for passing this law but also the breadth, scope, and complexity of the bill. Some of these criticisms may be justified, but, when looking back at the process, proponents of the Affordable Care Act provided ample opportunities to all lawmakers to review and provide feedback. In fact, some even argue that from the time the Senate Finance Committee held the first health reform hearing in May 2008 to the time the law was enacted—almost two years—every lawmaker had a reasonable amount of time to engage in the process and work collaboratively to develop the legislation. At each step of the process, committee chairs and House and Senate leaders allowed more time than usual for review of the bill before voting on it.

Although this health care law included comprehensive reforms, it could have been even more voluminous. Many amendments had been introduced and considered during committee meetings that were never included in the final package because Democrats believed they were intended to slow the passage of the health reform law or water down certain requirements. Some of those proposed amendments included limiting Medicaid expansion until the current Medicaid program reached an enrollment of 90 percent of eligible beneficiaries or until Medicaid fraud was reduced or requiring the Office of Management and Budget to certify the elimination of the federal deficit before the provisions could go into effect. Other proposed amendments required members of Congress to have Medicaid insurance instead of continuing to participate in the Federal Employees Health Benefits Program or required all members to read the bill before casting a vote.

Contrary to statements made by opponents of the ACA, the majority of its provisions have long enjoyed bipartisan support. In fact, bills that were negotiated, introduced, and approved by both Republicans and Democrats decades before in previous Congresses provided much of the framework for the current law. During negotiations many amendments that were offered by Republican lawmakers or in conjunction with Republican lawmakers were incorporated in the final bill and had the effect of strengthening provisions or adding value, including the physician payment sunshine disclosure requirement, the community health needs assessment requirement for nonprofit hospitals, school-based health centers, and comparative effectiveness research.[1] So it should come as no surprise that both Democrats and Republicans have their fingerprints all over the ACA.

With the process argument aside, the next issue is whether the Affordable Care Act is so voluminous that it is impossible to read or so incoherent that people cannot understand it. One of the chief complaints I often get from ordinary citizens is that the law is confusing. I then follow up and ask is it confusing because of what you read or because of what you have heard. Most individuals admit it is what they have heard that has been the source of their confusion. While some may argue that a nearly two-thousand-page bill is lengthy, and I would concede that point, I disagree that it cannot be read. Yes, it would take several hours, but it is not incomprehensible, as some opponents of the law would like people to believe. This chapter will serve to help clarify any misinformation or misunderstandings.

This chapter aims to break down the provisions of the ACA and provide concrete examples of how they will work—highlighting the provisions that have generated the most controversy, those that have received widespread support, and those that have gotten less attention. Since the main focus of the opposition has been on the provisions expanding health insurance coverage, those provisions will be considered first.

The Mandate and Exceptions

Not surprisingly, the majority of opposition early on to the ACA centered on the health insurance reforms. This has also been the case during its implementation phase. Perhaps the most controversial provision of the law was the individual mandate to purchase health insurance, even after being upheld by the US Supreme Court.[2] The Affordable Care Act requires virtually every citizen, legal permanent resident, refugee, and other documented immigrant in the United States to obtain minimum essential coverage by January 1, 2014, and thereafter or else pay a tax penalty of $95 per year or 1 percent of income—whichever is greater. That penalty will increase to $325 per year, or 2 percent of income, by 2015 and to $695 per year, or 2.5 percent of income, by 2016. After 2016, the penalty will increase annually as indicated by cost-of-living adjustments. For purposes of the law, those who have employer-sponsored coverage, Medicare, Medicaid, CHIP, most TRICARE plans (for active duty military personnel), Veterans Health Administration, and certain other coverage, meet the requirement of having minimum essential coverage and do not have to purchase health insurance coverage through the health insurance marketplace or elsewhere.[3]

Those who do not have minimum essential coverage are required to pay the penalty unless they fall into one of the following exceptions: they are undocumented immigrants, they experience financial hardship, they have a bona fide religious objection, they are incarcerated, they have incomes below the tax filing threshold, they are members of an American Indian tribe, they have been without coverage for less than three months, or their lowest-cost plan option exceeds 8 percent of their household income. Interestingly, in addition to being exempt from the individual mandate, undocumented immigrants are prohibited from obtaining benefits under the ACA, including purchasing health insurance coverage through the health insurance exchanges even if they purchase it with their own funds.

While undocumented immigrants are prohibited from accruing benefits under the ACA, legal permanent residents and refugees are eligible for the same benefits and protections as US citizens under the health care law, since they are considered lawfully present immigrants. Prior to the enactment of the ACA, in 2009, Obama signed into law the Children's Health Insurance Program Reauthorization Act of 2009, which eliminated the five-year waiting period required of immigrant children and youth before they are allowed to enroll in the Children's Health Insurance Program.

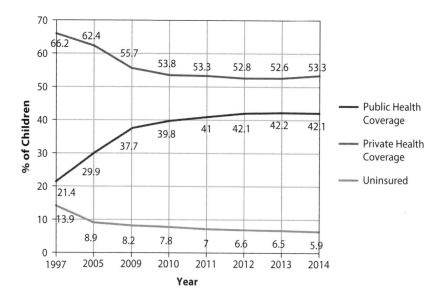

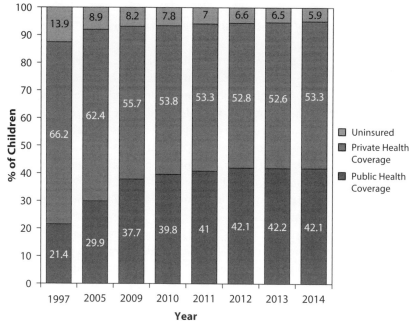

Figures 6.1 and 6.2. Health coverage status for children aged 0-17. Centers for Disease Control and Prevention, National Health Interview Survey, 2014.

This statute included a new option for states to provide Medicaid and CHIP coverage to children, youth, and pregnant women who are lawfully residing in the United States, including those within their first five years of having certain legal status. According to the Centers for Medicare and Medicaid Services (CMS), twenty-nine states, including the District of Columbia and the Northern Mariana Islands, have elected to provide Medicaid coverage to lawfully present children or pregnant women without a five-year waiting period, with twenty-one of these states also covering lawfully present children or pregnant women in CHIP. The impact of this policy has, undoubtedly, been to increase the number of children who have health insurance coverage nationally. However, for nonpregnant adults seeking Medicaid eligibility, a five-year waiting period still is required. Legal permanent residents who fall below 100 percent of the federal poverty level are actually able to receive subsidies to purchase health insurance in the exchanges. US citizens at that income level do not have that option, but they are eligible to get covered under Medicaid, which is why there is a push to expand Medicaid.

Expanding Health Insurance Protections and Coverage

Prior to the enactment of the Affordable Care Act, reports documented the difficult and sometimes insurmountable barriers to gaining health insurance coverage or to accessing health services once insured. The health reform law sought to provide individuals and families with more comprehensive coverage and protections than was typically provided in the marketplace prior to its passage. The goal was to ensure that all people have access to health care not only by prohibiting certain exclusions, rescissions, limitations, and restrictions that previously left people without coverage or care but also by requiring all "qualified health plans" to meet minimum standards.

Prior to the passage of the ACA, health insurance plans frequently charged patients more for, limited, or even denied coverage to people who had a preexisting illness or disability. Those who managed to acquire health insurance found their policies rescinded or cancelled when they got too sick and the cost of treatment got too high. The ACA directly addresses these issues, prohibiting health plans from excluding an individual from coverage due to preexisting conditions such as diabetes, cancer, or mental illness. It also prohibits health plans from canceling or rescinding a person's coverage solely because the person's treatment becomes expensive or because of an unintentional mistake on an application form. In cases where clear fraud was committed, health insurers may still rescind that individual's coverage. This prohibition ensures that vulnerable populations who suffer from high rates of chronic conditions, such as diabetes, HIV/AIDS, serious mental illnesses, substance use, cancer, and heart disease, are able to obtain coverage and remain insured once they have satisfied their obligations such as payment of premiums and copays.

Health insurance plans commonly had annual and lifetime limits on the dollar amount of care that people could receive, which left many individuals faced with a health crisis financially vulnerable. Such limits caused great financial hardship to people fighting serious or chronic illnesses and conditions. Although the ACA initially restricted all health plans from imposing unreasonable annual limits, the ACA now completely bans health plans from imposing lifetime and annual coverage limits on essential health benefits. The ACA does, however, allow the US Department of Health and Human Services to waive restrictions on annual limits in cases where a health plan or employer shows they would result in a significant increase in premiums or a significant decrease in access to benefits for covered members. Moreover, it should be noted that lifetime and annual coverage limits on what are deemed nonessential health benefits are still allowed.

Prohibiting Discrimination in Health Insurance Coverage Eligibility

The ACA recognizes and strengthens existing protections against discrimination based on race, ethnicity, age, sex, color, religion, and disability, as provided in the Civil Rights Act of 1964, the Americans with Disabilities Act, and the Genetic Information Nondiscrimination Act. It also goes further by incorporating the Health Insurance Portability and Accountability Act nondiscrimination provisions for group health plans and extending them to consumers seeking individual health insurance coverage (coverage not provided by an employer). As a result, it prohibits most health plans from using any of the following overlapping health factors to determine eligibility for coverage, providing different benefits, or charging different premiums or copays to consumers:

- Health status
- Medical condition (including both physical and mental illnesses)
- Claims experience (frequency and history of claims)

- Receipt of health care
- Medical history
- Genetic information
- Evidence of insurability or proof of good health (plans are prohibited from considering conditions arising out of acts of domestic violence as well as participation in risky activities such as motorcycling, snowmobiling, all-terrain vehicle riding, horseback riding, skiing, and other similar activities)
- Disability
- Any other health status factor determined appropriate by the secretary of health and human services

There is, however, one exception to this rule prohibiting health plans from using these health factors: wellness programs offered by group health plans, which may give participants premium discounts and rebates. Overall, this broad prohibition against using the aforementioned health factors has been particularly important to women, preventing insurers from denying them coverage or charging them more for coverage than they charge men. Before health reform, insurers often based such policies or actions on the premise that women of reproductive age had the ability to become pregnant and bear children, which was, per se, a preexisting condition. The ACA also prohibits health plans from charging higher costs for, denying coverage to, or cancelling the coverage of rape victims.

Prohibiting Discrimination against Health Care Providers

In addition to protecting consumers from certain insurance practices, the ACA protects health professionals by prohibiting insurers from discriminating against them with respect to participation under a plan or coverage, so long as they are acting within the scope of their license or certification under applicable state law. This was included to ensure that insurers cannot exclude certain groups of practitioners, including allied health professionals, from practicing under the capacity of their training and licensure. According to regulators, this provision does not require plans or issuers to accept all types of providers into a network, although insurers are expected to implement the requirements of this section using a "good faith, reasonable interpretation of the law." This provision also does not govern provider reimbursement rates, which may be subject to quality, performance, or market standards and considerations. In other words, it does not prevent a group health plan, a health insurance issuer, or the secretary of health and human services from establishing varying reimbursement rates based on quality or performance measures.

Mandating Essential Health Benefits

The ACA not only increases access to health insurance coverage, but it increases access to coverage that provides a minimum set of benefits. All health plans sold in the new health insurance exchanges or marketplaces, qualified health plans, must provide a broad set of coverage known as "essential health benefits." Each qualified health plan must provide at least a defined minimum benefit in every one of the following ten categories of services:

1. Ambulatory patient services
2. Emergency services
3. Hospitalization
4. Maternity and newborn care
5. Mental health and substance use disorder services
6. Prescription drugs
7. Rehabilitative and habilitative services and devices
8. Laboratory services
9. Preventive and wellness services and chronic disease management
10. Pediatric services, including oral and vision care

To accomplish that, each state begins by selecting what is called a benchmark plan: an existing, popular health insurance plan that will serve as a starting point to define what services will be covered in the essential health benefits package. Those benchmark plans have now been selected by every state and approved by the federal government. The scope (that is, what is covered) and amount (that is, how much is covered) of benefits in each state's benchmark plan largely define the scope and amount of benefits covered in each of the ten categories of essential services. For example, the maternity and newborn care services that a state's benchmark plan covers basically will define the maternity and newborn care services that that state's essential health benefits must cover.

However, in most cases, a state's essential health benefits package also will incorporate the limits on services included in its benchmark plan (i.e., limits on the amount of services and prior authorization requirements). The ACA, though, does prescribe some restrictions on such limits through, for example, "nondiscrimination requirements" that all qualified health plans must meet. Benchmark plan requirements that violate nondiscrimination requirements for essential health benefits cannot be incorporated into that state's essential health benefits package, but state-defined essential health benefits certainly may opt to provide more benefits than those minimum level of benefits required by the ACA. States that exercise this option are financially responsible for the additional costs of additional benefits.

Prevention Is Cheaper Than Cure

One of the major priorities of the health law is prevention of chronic disease and improving public health. In fact, an entire portion of the statute solely focuses on prevention and public health. Before ACA provisions took effect, some health plans already covered preventive services, but millions of Americans were enrolled in plans that did not. One of the most important expansions in the scope of health care coverage under the ACA is the requirement that plans cover preventive services at no additional cost to the beneficiary.

The ACA requires most health plans to offer a nationally consistent set of services that can prevent avoidable long-term health problems that lead to expensive treatment when they go undetected until they worsen. Covered preventive health care services include well-child visits, childhood immunizations, and indicated iron and fluoride supplements; flu shots; Pap smears and mammograms for women; evidence-based screenings and counseling, including colonoscopy screening for colon cancer in adults; behavioral and developmental assessments; and screening for autism, vision impairment, lipid disorders, tuberculosis, and certain genetic diseases in children.[4]

According to the Kaiser Family Foundation's Employer Health Benefits Survey in 2012, more than two workers of every five with employer-sponsored group health plans gained access to expanded preventive services at no cost to themselves. Recent Census Bureau data show that 173 million Americans from birth to age sixty-four are enrolled in private health coverage, suggesting that in 2011 and 2012, more than seventy million Americans received expanded coverage for preventive services with no out-of-pocket costs. Similar changes were authorized for Medicare and Medicaid beneficiaries as well so that older adults enrolled in Medicare no longer had to pay for preventive services as of January 1, 2011. Additionally, the law provided new funding to state Medicaid programs that chose to cover preventive services for patients at little or no cost starting January 1, 2013.

In the beginning of 2010, older adults were also automatically eligible to receive a tax free, one-time $250 rebate check after they reach the Medicare drug coverage gap or the "donut hole." The donut hole refers to a temporary limit on what the plan will cover for drugs. The Centers for Medicare and Medicaid Services has provided the following example to explain this issue:

In 2010, basic Medicare Part D coverage worked like this:

- You pay out-of-pocket for monthly Part D premiums all year.
- You pay 100% of your drug costs until you reach the $310 deductible amount.
- After reaching the deductible, you pay 25% of the cost of your drugs, while the Part D plan pays the rest, until the total you and your plan spend on your drugs reaches $2,800.
- Once you reach this limit, you have hit the coverage gap referred to as the "donut hole," and you are now responsible for the full cost of your drugs until the total you have spent for your drugs reaches the yearly out-of-pocket spending limit of $4,550.
- After this yearly spending limit, you are only responsible for a small amount of the cost, usually 5% of the cost of your drugs.[5]

In 2011 ObamaCare provided even more coverage for individuals with high prescription drug costs by giving them a 50 percent discount on covered brand-name drugs and reduced costs for generic drugs while they are in the donut hole. Between 2012 and 2020, individuals get increasing, continuous Medicare coverage for their prescription drugs and begin paying less for their brand-name Part D prescription drugs in the donut hole. By 2020, the coverage gap or donut hole will be eliminated once and for all and Medicare Part D enrollees will pay only 25 percent out-of-pocket for the total costs of their drugs until they reach the yearly out-of-pocket spending limit.

The law authorized the establishment of the National Prevention, Health Promotion, and Public Health Council to develop the first-ever National Prevention Strategy and made permanent the Community Preventive Services Task Force, which had been established by the CDC in 1996. It also authorized a national outreach and educational campaign on the benefits of preventive services. To strengthen and improve maternal, infant, and early childhood home visiting programs, promote coordination of services, and provide comprehensive services to improve outcomes for families who reside in at-risk communities, the Affordable Care Act authorized $1.5 billion in mandatory funding directly for this issue.

In addition to authorizing various mandatory- and discretionary-funded programs intended to address a variety of critical prevention and public health issues, the ACA established the Prevention and Public Health Fund, which is the nation's first mandatory funding stream dedicated to improving the public health system. The law stipulates that the Prevention Fund must be used "to provide for expanded and sustained national investment in prevention and public health programs to improve health and help restrain the rate of growth in private and public health care costs." Despite mischaracterizations of being a slush fund for the Obama administration, the Prevention Fund actually funded a variety of evidence-based activities, including community and clinical prevention initiatives; research, surveillance, and tracking; public health infrastructure; immunizations and screenings; tobacco prevention; health disparities reduction initiatives; and health workforce and training.

The ACA had authorized and appropriated funding for the $15 billion Prevention Fund, gradually increasing the amount from $500 million in fiscal year 2010 to $2 billion for fiscal year 2015 and every year thereafter. However, in February 2012, when Congress passed the Middle Class Tax Relief and Job Creation Act of 2012, it reduced the amounts that were allocated for the Prevention Fund by a total of $6.25 billion over nine years (FY 2013 through FY 2021), which delayed the Prevention Fund from reaching $2 billion until fiscal year 2022. In the spring of 2013, the amount of funding that was allocated for the Prevention Fund was further decreased by 5.1 percent, or $51 million, as a result of sequestration, or arbitrary cuts to discretionary and mandatory funded federal programs, which went into effect as a result of the Budget Control Act of 2011.

Original Authorization and Appropriation for the Prevention Fund

FY 2010, $500,000,000
FY 2011, $750,000,000
FY 2012, $1,000,000,000
FY 2013, $1,250,000,000
FY 2014, $1,500,000,000
FY 2015 and each fiscal year thereafter, $2,000,000,000

Amended Authorization and Appropriation for the Prevention Fund

FY 2012-2017, $1,000,000,000/FY

FY 2018 and 2019, $1,250,000,000/FY

FY 2020 and 2021, $1,500,000,000/FY

FY 2022 and each fiscal year thereafter, $2,000,000,000

When Congress passed the Consolidated Appropriations Act in 2014, it discontinued the Obama administration's flexible use of the Prevention and Public Health Fund, instead reallocating funds for specific programs. It also required the establishment of a publicly accessible website to track and report the use of funding under the Prevention and Public Health Fund.[6]

Mental Health and Addiction Equity

Historically, health insurance plans (especially employer-sponsored and other private insurance policies) tended to provide a far lower level of coverage for mental health treatment than for other ("physical" or "primary") health care needs. Significant restrictions on behavioral health services, including therapy sessions and prescriptions, were commonplace. During the 1990s and since, a series of national laws and regulatory changes have prodded coverage for mental health and substance use problems to more closely resemble coverage for other health concerns— an equivalency referred to as "parity."

The 2008 Mental Health Parity and Addiction Equity Act ensures that children, youth, and adults with mental and behavioral health disorders, such as anxiety, depression, and substance use disorders, have better access to the treatment they need. It requires private health insurance plans to provide coverage for mental health care that is equivalent to the coverage they provide for physical health care. Adding one more missing piece to the "parity puzzle," the ACA extended application of the act to qualified health plans sold after December 31, 2013, within the health insurance exchanges.

More on Care, Less on Costs

Beginning in calendar year 2011, health plans are required to spend at least 80 percent of their members' health insurance premiums on health services for the individual and small group plans (85 percent for insurers in the large-group market), as opposed to administrative costs such as overhead and profit. However, self-funded health plans, which are plans offered by businesses where the employer assumes the risk for, and pays for, medical care are exempt from this requirement. Medicare health plans were also exempt until 2014.

In any year that an insurance company fails to meet the 80-20 medical loss ratio, it must provide a commensurate rebate to its customers starting in 2012. In 2012, approximately $1.1 billion in rebates were made to 12.8 million individuals using 2011 data. In 2013, more than $500 million in rebates were made to 8.5 million individuals, which averaged $100 per person using 2012 data. Interestingly the declining trend in rebates continued the following year in 2014 when insurers owed $332 million in medical loss ratio rebates to 6.8 million individuals, which averaged $80 per person using 2013 data.[7] This decline shows that more insurers continue to meet the medical loss ratio requirement each year.

Ensuring a Fair and Effective Internal and External Appeals Process

The law requires health plans to establish fair and effective appeals processes with states for coverage determination and claim denial disagreements. This rule provides a way for consumers to appeal through a process outside of their insurance companies. The law also requires health plans available through health insurance exchanges or marketplace in every state to present information to their members using plain language and in a culturally and linguistically appropriate manner, including summary of benefits and coverage and notices about internal and external appeals processes.

Increasing Access to Affordable Health Insurance Coverage

Health plans were generally cost prohibitive for those in the individual or small group markets and created great hardship for millions, often to the point of individuals having to delay or forego necessary health care. To address this problem, the ACA established a series of temporary and permanent programs, mandates, and initiatives to increase access to affordable health insurance coverage for those lacking coverage or having limited coverage.

The two temporary programs, which included the Pre-Existing Conditions Insurance Plan and Early Retiree Reinsurance Program were authorized to provide some level of coverage for people who were most vulnerable and susceptible to losing their coverage especially during the Great

Recession. Both temporary health insurance programs were established in 2010 and no longer accept new enrollees. Instead, individuals who were enrolled in those programs were transferred to permanent programs, including the health insurance exchanges or Medicaid, if they qualified, beginning in 2014.

During the same time the ACA established the two temporary programs, it also made effective one of the first permanent requirements, dependent coverage up to the age of twenty-six. Not only was this designed to increase health insurance coverage, but also limit or prevent a decrease in the number of insured individuals since many young adults had difficulty finding employment that provided health insurance benefits during the Great Recession. Plans that covered dependent children now have to offer that coverage to all eligible dependents up to age twenty-six, including those who are (1) not enrolled in school, (2) not dependents on their parents' tax returns, (3) married, or even (4) eligible for other insurance coverage.[8] Starting in 2014, states are also required to extend Medicaid coverage to young adults up to age twenty-six who have aged out of the foster care system, including those aging out of the Unaccompanied Refugee Minors program. This requirement is quite broad.

The health reform law authorized an increase of federal funding to the US Virgin Islands, Puerto Rico, Guam, American Samoa, and Northern Mariana Islands to establish health insurance exchanges and to help residents pay for their insurance coverage. The law also raised the caps on federal Medicaid funding for each of the territories and ensured their eligibility in programs established under the law.

Health Insurance Exchanges/Marketplaces

After enactment of the ACA, the Obama administration worked diligently on the creation of new health insurance exchanges or marketplaces, which were to be established by October 1, 2013. They would be state based, federally facilitated, or a joint partnership between the state and federal government, depending on whether a state wanted to establish and operate its own exchange or defer to the federal government to operate one for its residents. The law required that these exchanges had to provide individuals and small businesses with a competitive "marketplace" to compare prices and benefits of qualified health plans and purchase health insurance.

The new health insurance exchanges were intended to operate much like popular online travel portals, such as Travelocity and Expedia, and to guarantee that individuals with incomes above the federal poverty level could get insurance, regardless of preexisting conditions, with subsidies available to offset much or most of the cost. This new marketplace was created specifically to help individuals who were unable to obtain coverage through their employers and who did not qualify for certain government-sponsored programs like Medicare or Medicaid obtain affordable and comprehensive coverage. For those who have incomes between 100 percent and 400 percent of the federal poverty level, the law authorized subsidies in the form of tax credits to these individuals and their families so they could purchase insurance through the exchanges and lessen the financial hardship.[9]

To help consumers in every marketplace navigate these new health insurance exchanges and apply for and choose new insurance options, the law authorized several different programs to conduct outreach, education, and enrollment of underserved communities, including navigators, in-person assistance personnel, and certified application counselors. In addition, insurance agents and brokers were also authorized to help consumers enroll in new insurance options. ACA regulations require certain training for navigators to ensure they have expertise in the needs of underserved and vulnerable populations. Federal rules require navigators and other consumer assistance personnel to provide information in a manner that is culturally and linguistically appropriate.[10]

Medicaid Expansion

The ACA also intended to increase health insurance coverage by allowing all individuals under the age of sixty-five with incomes below 138 percent of the federal poverty level to qualify for Medicaid beginning in 2014.[11] So, for the first time, adults without children and who are not pregnant women will be able to secure health insurance coverage through the Medicaid program if they meet the single, uniform income level and age eligibility criteria and their state agrees to expand Medicaid. In June 2012 the US Supreme Court's ruling on the ACA effactually gave each state the option of choosing whether to participate in this Medicaid expansion. As of this writing, thirty states and the District of Columbia have decided to do so, fifteen have decided not to, and six more states are still weighing their options. Some states sought and received permission to begin their Medicaid expansion without waiting until January 2014. There is no actual deadline by which states have to make their decisions, and it is even possible for states to change their decisions over time.

How the ACA Will Change or Is Changing the Paradigm of Medicaid

Since it was first established by Congress in the 1960s, the Medicaid program has become the nation's largest public health insurance program—financing health care services for more than sixty million low-income individuals—70 percent of whom are women. More than two-thirds of Medicaid beneficiaries are low-income families with dependent children, pregnant women, and children under age six with family incomes below 138 percent of the federal poverty line, and the rest are older adults and people with disabilities.

Prior to the enactment of the ACA, the ranks of the uninsured were persistently unacceptably high: there were nearly fifty million uninsured individuals in the United States—almost twenty million of them were women. Yet many of the states that fought to repeal the health reform law and refuse to expand Medicaid are states with the highest uninsurance rates. In fact, 75 percent of the uninsured reside in these states, which are mostly in the South—the majority of these uninsured individuals are racial and ethnic minorities.

Opponents of health reform knew that if they were successful in repealing the ACA or preventing or undermining the expansion of Medicaid, they would have decimated a critical piece of President Obama's efforts to expand coverage. Under the ACA, thirty-two million uninsured or underinsured Americans were expected to gain health insurance coverage—half of these individuals through Medicaid expansion and the other half through the health insurance exchanges or marketplaces. However, because of the Supreme Court ruling in June of 2012, that number is now estimated to be lower than initially thought. For women, people with disabilities, and racial and ethnic minorities, who are the most likely to be uninsured, experience higher unemployment rates, and have lower incomes—which makes it harder to obtain employer-sponsored health insurance coverage—Medicaid expansion would provide these communities access to health services.

Only half of women who are working are able to obtain health coverage through their jobs. The Affordable Care Act is changing and will continue to change the paradigm of Medicaid so that it will provide more comprehensive and meaningful health protections for women and other vulnerable populations. In 2010, 55 percent of women had incomes less than 138 percent of the federal poverty level. This means that seven million women would have been newly eligible for Medicaid coverage in 2014 if all states had expanded their Medicaid programs. In addition, the Mental Health Parity and Addiction Equity Act of 2008, and the Genetic Information Nondiscrimination Act of 2008 would apply to Medicaid expansion, giving new enrollees greater protections. Moreover, primary care providers also benefit from Medicaid expansion, receiving a 73 percent raise because of increases in Medicaid reimbursement.

To fund Medicaid expansion, the federal government would cover 100 percent of the states' costs through 2017, gradually decreasing to 90 percent by 2020 and thereafter. Some opponents of health reform worry, however, that the federal government may significantly reduce its share of the costs once a state decides to expand its Medicaid program. This concern is further exacerbated because of the focus on reducing the federal deficit and debt, which would make the increased federal match for Medicaid expansion a likely target for cuts. Although some have questioned the legitimacy of these concerns, one could reasonably argue that in light of the fact that the Obama administration has previously shown a willingness to reduce Medicaid spending in the past despite statements that those recommendations are no longer on the table, it is a real problem.

Of course, there is nothing to legally stop the federal government from decreasing its share or even clawing back funding for Medicaid expansion. Congress certainly could pass a law changing the federal government's share of the costs of Medicaid expansion, thus increasing a state's burden. Furthermore, although Medicaid is exempt from sequestration under the Budget Control Act of 2011, it should be noted that attempts to reduce spending under Medicaid are still on the table for deficit reduction negotiations moving forward. However, only once has the federal government adjusted its funding levels not to decrease but to increase its share of Medicaid spending during the Great Recession of the late 2000s. Simply stated, there is no precedent for clawing back funding for the Medicaid program and leaving the states on the hook. Federal funding has remained quite consistent in the mid-50 percent range, where on average the federal government pays 57 percent of Medicaid costs in general.

Current Status of Medicaid Expansion

If history is any indication of what to expect in the future, then one might expect a trend similar to what occurred with Medicaid implementation in the 1960s. At that time, we saw mostly northern states implementing Medicaid during the first year they were allowed to, and south-

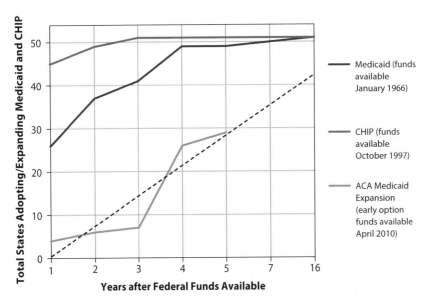

Figure 6.3. State adoption/establishment trends for Medicaid and Children's Health Insurance Programs compared to state trends for Medicaid expansion. Centers for Medicare and Medicaid Services, CHIP State Plan Information; Kaiser Commission on Medicaid and the Uninsured, *Historical Review of How States Have Responded to the Availability of Federal Funds for Health Coverage*; Sommers et al., "Lessons from Early Medicaid Expansions under Health Reform"; and Congressional Research Service, *The ACA Medicaid Expansion.*

ern states implementing Medicaid almost two to four years afterward. Interestingly, there is not a similar pattern with Medicaid expansion. True, many of the same states that delayed Medicaid implementation in the 1960s are now doing the same thing with Medicaid expansion—from North Carolina to Texas, with the exception of Arizona. By the seventh year when both the Children's Health Insurance Program and the original Medicaid program were authorized, virtually all states had established their respective programs. However, this does not seem to be the case with Medicaid expansion. By the fifth year, twenty more states had already established their CHIP and Medicaid programs than is the case with Medicaid expansion.

This is concerning because four of the top five states where uninsured women reside and would benefit tremendously from Medicaid expansion are southern states: Texas, Florida, Georgia, and North Carolina. Also concerning is the fact that nearly 60 percent of African Americans live in the states that have not expanded their Medicaid programs, and they will fall in the health insurance coverage gap. African Americans, Latinos, and people with disabilities tend to have lower employment and higher uninsurance status and would benefit from Medicaid expansion. Currently, there are thirty states that have decided to participate, and almost a third of them have Republican governors, including Arizona, Iowa, Michigan, New Mexico, Nevada, New Jersey, North Dakota, Ohio, and Pennsylvania.

Next Steps for Medicaid Expansion

We are beginning to move into a space that realizes the impact of health disparities that various groups experience and how vital it is for individuals to have access to competent health care that comprehensively addresses their needs. Former secretary of health, education, and welfare Wilbur Cohen, who worked closely with Representative Wilbur Mills and other congressional champions in crafting the Medicaid legislation, wrote, "Many people, since 1965, have called Medicaid the 'sleeper' in the legislation. Most people did not pay attention to that part of the bill."[12] However, Medicaid now represents 40 percent of all federal funding to the states and 51 percent of all total expenditures for long-term services and supports. It has become a state-federal program that has touched many lives and operates to improve the social standing of vulnerable populations, especially those in communities of lower socioeconomic status.

But opponents of health reform continually cite confusion and lack of information or regulations from the administration as a reason for not expanding Medicaid early on. The administration, responding to criticism from opponents, issued a plethora of regulations and subregulations that were intended to ease such concerns and provide better direction to states. However, opponents then argued that the regulations and subregulations were overly burdensome and confusing and still refused to expand their Medicaid programs. Indeed, numerous ACA regulations have been promulgated, but these regulations have punted the health equity provisions to the states and allowed states to determine how to implement these programs. In other instances, federal regulators have reduced the impact that certain health equity provisions could have had by watering them down, or they have chosen to delay or decided not to release regulations touching on the health equity provisions.

Delivery and Payment System Reforms: Integrated Care and Quality Improvements

Senator Bill Frist once stated, "Disparities in care actually are subsets or symptoms of our overall health care quality chasms and challenges. In fact, they are essentially warnings from the most vulnerable of our more widespread challenges."[13] So while health insurance coverage is critically important, just having health insurance does not necessarily equate to access to quality health services and treatments and better outcomes. That is why the ACA included comprehensive reforms to address the fragmentation of health services and to eliminate health disparities among vulnerable populations. Concretized in these reforms is a push-pull mechanism of penalties and incentives intended to help providers cross the quality chasm. And with the law's recognition of the importance of increasing innovation, policy makers established the Center for Medicare and Medicaid Innovation at the Centers for Medicare and Medicaid Services, which is responsible for testing innovative models for the payment and delivery of health services while maintaining and enhancing quality of care.

One of the fastest-growing innovations in health care, the patient-centered medical home, received a huge endorsement from the ACA with strong incentives for its wider adoption. A patient-centered medical home is a team-based approach to health care that includes the person, his or her health care providers, and family members when appropriate. It aims to organize care management, treat each person in a holistic way, and support individuals and families as they work toward self-management goals.[14] Organized care management is especially important for some particular groups of people, including those living with chronic health conditions. Person-centered medical homes can improve health outcomes and reduce expenses associated with a lack of care coordination, frequent visits to the emergency room, and unnecessary hospitalizations. This program was intended to lay the foundation for other delivery and payment system reforms such as accountable care organizations (ACOs), bundled payments, and value based purchasing.

The ACA authorized the establishment of medical homes, also referred to as "health homes," and provided enhanced federal funding for two years for health homes serving Medicaid beneficiaries with chronic conditions, including a mental health condition or a substance use disorder. This optional initiative under the law allows a state to adopt a state plan amendment and has as its core goal

- expanding the traditional medical home models,
- building linkages to other community and social supports, and
- enhancing coordination of medical and behavioral health care, in keeping with the needs of persons with multiple chronic illnesses.

According to CMS, the agency responsible for this initiative, states are expected to operate under a "whole-person" philosophy—caring for an individual's physical condition and providing linkages to long-term community care services and supports, social services, and family services.

The law also authorized community-based health teams to support primary care providers and patient-centered medical homes. These teams consist of health care providers from a variety of disciplines and professions and may include medical specialists, nurses, pharmacists, dentists, nutritionists, social workers, behavioral and mental health providers, licensed doctors of chiropractic, licensed complementary and alternative medicine practitioners, and physician assistants. In collaboration with local health providers, these health teams will coordinate disease prevention, chronic disease management, and the transitioning between health care providers and settings.

To improve communication, the ACA authorized programs to facilitate shared decision making. Disparities in patient-provider communication have affected various cultural groups, resulting in their receipt of poorer patient-centered care and worse health outcomes than the rest of the population. Populations with limited literacy or English proficiency often encounter challenges to getting critical health information.

This idea of shared decision making is essentially a robust informed consent model that actively includes the consumer and provider working in tandem to discuss treatment options. The ACA authorized this program to facilitate communication and collaboration among patients, their families, caregivers, and authorized representatives and their clinicians, so that patients are informed about treatment options, and their preferences and values are incorporated into the medical plan through shared decision making. In addition to promoting shared decision making, the law authorized grants or contracts to nongovernmental entities to develop, update, and produce patient decision aids for preference-sensitive care to assist health care providers in educating patients on the relative safety, effectiveness, and cost of treatment, or where appropriate, palliative care options. The patient decision aids must be age appropriate and adaptable across a variety of cultural and educational backgrounds.

Moving beyond the medical or health home, lawmakers realized that to better coordinate patient care and services and enhance the continuum of care for patients, they needed to provide incentive payments to hospitals, physician group practices, or federally qualified health centers to establish an accountable care organization. Under this voluntary Medicare shared savings pilot program, which began in 2012, integrated groups of hospitals, physicians, community health centers, long-term care facilities, home health agencies, and other health care entities operating as ACOs, assume responsibility and are held accountable for the health of their communities. These ACOs were required to initially manage care for a minimum of five thousand Medicare patients and receive bonus payments for demonstrating higher quality and lower costs. In developing and successfully operating these ACOs, hospitals will need experts from the community to design an effective program that addresses core components of overall health, including behavioral health and oral health.

Another payment system reform intended to reduce fragmentation in care, increase quality, and safely reduce costs that was authorized by the ACA and has been successfully tested in various communities and settings involves the Bundled Payments for Care Improvement. Under this initiative, organizations enter into payment arrangements that include financial and performance accountability for episodes of care—rewarding providers for the quality of care delivered rather than the quantity of care delivered. Historically, Medicare has operated under a fee-for-service model and made separate payments to providers for each of the individual services they furnish to beneficiaries for a single illness or course of treatment. According to CMS, "Research has shown that bundled payments can align incentives for providers—hospitals, post-acute care providers, physicians, and other practitioners—allowing them to work closely together across all specialties and settings."[15]

To increase attention to quality or performance improvement in hospitals, especially those providing inpatient services, the health reform law tied a percentage of a hospital's reimbursement to meeting certain quality benchmarks. The Medicare program known as the Hospital Value-Based Purchasing (VBP) program started in October 2012. As a result, hospitals receive reimbursement for inpatient acute care services based on quality of care—not volume of services. The VBP program is budget neutral because incentives will be offset by a reduction in Medicare base payment rate.[16] Regardless of whether a hospital receives an incentive payment, hospitals will experience a reduction in payments over the following time period: fiscal year 2013, 1 percent; fiscal year 2014, 1.25 percent; fiscal year 2015, 1.5 percent; fiscal year 2016, 1.75 percent; and fiscal year 2017, and beyond 2 percent.

Hospitals are given a hospital performance score, which is used to determine the value-based payment percentage that it receives for a fiscal year. Hospitals with the highest scores will receive the largest value-based incentive payments, and information on each hospital's performance will be made available to the public. Those lower-performing hospitals will see a slight decrease in their reimbursement. Similar VBP programs will be developed for skilled nursing facilities, home health agencies, and ambulatory surgical centers. This is another opportunity for health equity champions to collaborate with their local hospitals to design and implement effective programs to help hospitals address any gaps in health care quality.

The law recognizes that there are significant gaps in quality measures and that a one-size-fits-all approach has not always worked well with diverse population groups. With the prioritization of quality improvement under the Affordable Care Act, standard measurements of quality will be identified to more accurately depict the performance and improvement of health insurance plans, clinicians, health care delivery settings, and the nation's health overall. Grants, contracts, and intergovernmental agreements were authorized to develop quality measures across several priority areas including health outcomes, management and coordination of care, communication between patients or their representatives and their provider, use of health information technology, safety, effectiveness, patient centeredness, appropriateness, timeliness of care, efficiency, equity of health services and reduction health disparities, patient satisfaction, and the use of innovative strategies and methodologies. The law also authorizes technical assistance to health care institutions and providers so that they understand, adapt, and implement practices supported by research conducted by the Center for Quality Improvement and Patient Safety of the Agency for Healthcare Research and Quality.

In addition to the incentive payments given to providers for increasing the quality of care delivered to their patients and the reduction in costs to Medicare and Medicaid, the health law authorized a series of penalties or reductions in reimbursement for not meeting certain benchmarks. To reduce preventable hospital readmissions, the ACA established the Hospital Readmissions Reduction Program, which requires CMS to reduce payments to hospitals with excess readmissions relative to certain conditions, including heart attack, heart failure and pneumonia, chronic obstructive pulmonary disease, and other vascular issues effective for discharges beginning on October 1, 2012.[17] During fiscal year 2013, the payment reduction equated to 1 percent, in fiscal year 2014 the payment reduction equated to 2 percent, and in fiscal year 2015 and beyond the payment reduction is capped at 3 percent. Hospital readmissions rates were also required to be publicly available on the Hospital Compare website hosted by CMS.[18]

By March 2012, the HHS secretary was required by law to make available a program to help reduce readmission rates for those hospitals where they were high. As a result HHS established a Community-Based Care Transitions Program. This five-year, $500 million demonstration program provided funding to eligible hospitals and community-based organizations, and it was charged with providing transition services to improve care to Medicare beneficiaries at high risk for hospital readmission. These at-risk individuals often include those who suffer from chronic conditions or are at risk of having a poor transition to posthospitalized care such as nursing homes. Preference was given to organizations that provide services in medically underserved populations, small communities, and rural areas.

The goals of the Community-Based Care Transitions Program are to

- reduce hospital readmissions,
- test sustainable funding streams for care transition services,
- maintain or improve quality of care, and
- document measureable savings to the Medicare program.

Eligible entities include hospitals with high readmission rates that partner with community-based organizations (CBOs) and CBOs that provide care transition services. CBOs provide transition services across the continuum of care through arrangements with hospitals, and their governing bodies represent multiple health care stakeholders, including consumers. The CBOs use services to effectively manage transitions and report process and outcome measures on their results. CBOs are paid on a per-eligible-discharge basis for Medicare beneficiaries at high risk for readmission, including those with multiple chronic conditions, depression, and cognitive impairments. According to CMS, "From 2007 to 2011, the average monthly 30-day all-cause readmission rate was typically 19 percent or above. Towards the end of 2012, the rate had declined to approximately 18 percent and is now below 18 percent nationally in 2013. If you compare the last 12 months to the baseline in 2010 through 2011, the decrease represents nearly 100,000 Medicare beneficiaries staying home instead of returning to the hospital. This decrease is an early sign that our focus on improving quality and care coordination is beginning to have an impact."[19]

In addition to accruing penalties for preventable readmissions, hospitals were also challenged by another stick in the health care law for hospital acquired conditions (HACs).[20] Beginning in fiscal year 2015, or October 1, 2014, the HAC Reduction Program required the HHS secretary to adjust payments to hospitals whose patients acquire illnesses or infections while in their care, adjusting for risk. Penalties for hospitals scoring in the top quartile of HACs have their Medicare payments reduced by 1 percent beginning in fiscal year 2015. This means that by 2017 lower-performing hospitals could have a potential loss of 6 percent of their Medicare payments due to penalties from VBP, readmissions, and HACs. The ACA also charged CMS with determining the feasibility of extending the HACs program to inpatient rehabilitation facilities, long-term care hospitals, hospital outpatient departments, other hospitals excluded from the acute hospital Inpatient Prospective Payment System, skilled nursing facilities, ambulatory surgical centers, psychiatric hospitals, and health clinics.[21] As with readmissions, the HHS secretary is required to make information relative to HACs available to the public through the Hospital Compare website.

Increasing Access to Health Care

Community health centers, also referred to as federally qualified health centers (FQHCs), provide primary and preventive care to more than twenty million individuals who are often of lower socioeconomic status and are often uninsured, according to the National Association of Community Health Centers.[22] The ACA recognized the critical function these entities play in communities that experience barriers to health care because of economic, geographic, linguistic, and cultural reasons. The law provided $11 billion in new funding over five years to build new community health centers across the country so they can expand operational capacity and enhance their medical, oral, and behavioral health services.

HHS periodically announces demonstration project opportunities where a community organization might be able to team up with a community health center to provide services. One such opportunity was the Federally Qualified Health Center Advanced Primary Care Practice demonstration project, an initiative that allocated an estimated $42 million over three years to up to five hundred FQHCs to coordinate care for Medicare patients. This demonstration project, operated by CMS in partnership with the Health Resources and Services Administration, tested the effectiveness of doctors and other health professionals working in teams to improve care for up to 195,000 Medicare patients. FQHCs that have provided medical services to at least two hundred Medicare beneficiaries in the previous twelve-month period were invited by letter to apply to participate in the demonstration. The demonstrations were conducted September 1, 2011, through August 31, 2014, and the results from this initiative are expected to be published by CMS once it has completed its analysis.

Whereas FQHCs are rewarded under the ACA for the work they are currently doing in terms of providing medical homes for patients with significant funding increases, nonprofit hospitals are asked to do more to increase access and improve the delivery of care. Hospitals that wish to qualify as nonprofit and tax exempt are now required to conduct a community health needs assessment once every three years to determine how well they are meeting the health needs of their community. This expands opportunities for health equity champions to partner with local hospitals to ensure that the health needs of their children and youth are addressed in the course of those assessments.

In addition, nonprofit, tax-exempt hospitals are prohibited from using extraordinary and aggressive collection practices to pursue bad debt and must offer patients financial assistance as well as limit the charges to people who qualify for assistance. Their financial-assistance policies must be posted in places easily accessible to patients and community members. Failure to meet those requirements incurs a $50,000 tax penalty for the hospital.

As health care networks continue to expand and shift to value-based care, population health management and precision medicine have emerged as solutions that can improve quality, lower costs, and improve provider productivity. A major component of these priorities is advancing health equity. By improving health outcomes for a group of people, prioritizing health equity for all groups, and advancing precision medicine (which according to the NIH is an emerging approach for disease treatment and prevention that takes into account individual variability in genes, environment, and lifestyle for each person), we will see a major transformation in the way health care is delivered and received.

Elevating Health Equity in the Federal Agencies

Both eliminating disparities in health status and health care and increasing the cultural competence of service providers are essential to improving health services to underserved children, youth, and adults. This is especially true for children and youth among racial and ethnic minority groups, because evidence shows that behavioral health services currently meet only 13 percent of their needs. Compounding the fact that this group is less likely to receive mental health services, the services they do access tend to be ineffective and of low quality.[23] By contrast, when services are delivered in a culturally and linguistically responsive manner, service utilization increases and the rate of early termination of treatment declines. The lack of attention to the health needs of children, youth, and families who are from racial and ethnic populations, as well as lesbian, gay, bisexual, and transgender, and other vulnerable populations, and the inadequate provision of appropriate health care in these communities, demonstrates a clear need for encouraging collaboration and finding ways to close the gap in care.

The Affordable Care Act addresses the unique health challenges confronting populations, and it carves out critical roles for the government in addressing the issue of disparities in health. The law establishes a priority for health equity among numerous executive agencies within the federal government. One critical office at the HHS that has long been developing appropriate mechanisms to address health disparities and other issues impacting minority health is the Office of Minority Health. The ACA transferred the OMH to the Office of the Secretary of Health and Human Services from the Office of the Assistant Secretary, to be headed by the deputy assistant secretary for minority health. The law retains and strengthens the prior authorities that the OMH had to improve health and the quality of health care that people of color and other vulnerable populations receive, as well as to eliminate racial and ethnic disparities. The OMH now has the authority to engage in quality measure development and determine where there are gaps in health care services for other populations.

Additional Offices of Minority Health

HHS's Office of Minority Health will actually coordinate efforts with an extensive network of agency-specific offices of minority health that were authorized by the Affordable Care Act. Agencies authorized to establish internal offices of minority health include the Centers for Disease Control and Prevention, the Health Resources and Services Administration, the Substance Abuse and Mental Health Services Administration, the Agency for Healthcare Research and Quality, the Food and Drug Administration, and the Centers for Medicare and Medicaid Services.

Office of Women's Health
In addition to elevating the OMH to the Office of the Secretary of HHS, the ACA established an Office of Women's Health in the Office of the Secretary of HHS and charged it with the following:

- Developing short- and long-range goals and objectives that relate to disease prevention, health promotion, service delivery, research, and public and health care professional education
- Providing expert advice and consultation regarding scientific, legal, ethical and policy issues relating to women's health
- Monitoring activities concerning women's health
- Establishing the HHS Coordinating Committee on Women's Health
- Establishing the National Women's Health Information Center

The ACA also strengthened existing authority for offices of women's health at the Centers for Disease Control and Prevention, Food and Drug Administration, and Health Resources and Services Administration, as well as the Office of Women's Health and Gender-Based Research at the Agency for Healthcare Research and Quality.

National Institute of Minority Health and Health Disparities
In what was once only a vision, the National Center on Minority Health and Health Disparities at the National Institutes of Health was also elevated to institute status. This effort took twenty years from the time the Office of Research on Minority Health was established to when it was elevated to a center to finally reaching the pinnacle of an institute. The resultant National Institute of Minority Health and Health Disparities manages expanded research endowments and will lead, coordinate, review, and evaluate NIH's research and activities on minority health and health disparities.

Improving Data Collection and Reporting
Although there were attempts by White House officials to scrap the data collection provision during intense health reform negotiations, one year after the bill passed, Assistant Secretary of Health Dr. Howard

Koh wrote a blog celebrating the fulfillment of the ACA's data collection requirement, by stating that they were now collecting demographic data in federal surveys.[24]

While health equity champions in Congress and outside of Congress were working hard to increase attention to this matter and win support for its inclusion in the health care law, the Institute of Medicine released a major report in 2009. It highlighted the absence of a comprehensive national system to accurately track disparities in health status and health care and gauge the level of health care and preventive services that vulnerable populations are receiving.[25] The report argued for more and better data collection and reporting. Without accurate, detailed demographic data, advocates argued that it is difficult to properly track health disparities and develop culturally and linguistically effective strategies to counter existing disparities.

Acknowledging an expanding body of evidence demonstrating the pervasiveness of health disparities in the United States, the ACA included a robust data collection and reporting requirement. In particular, the statute required the secretary of Health and Human Services to ensure that by 2012 any federally conducted or supported public health or health care program (including Medicaid and CHIP), activity, or survey collects data on five self-reported variables:

1. Race
2. Ethnicity
3. Gender
4. Primary language
5. Disability status

The ACA authorizes the collection of data on subgroups, if practicable, and any other demographic data deemed appropriate by the secretary, including immigrant and underserved rural and frontier populations. HHS has chosen to approach this work in phases and started with federal public health and health care surveys in 2012. Standards related to gender identity and sexual orientation will be developed and field tested for inclusion in later surveys. Many vulnerable populations experience inequitable care, but inadequate and inaccurate data collection and reporting has hidden the facts. The ACA's data collection provisions will help to reduce these disparities because health providers will no longer be allowed to make judgments about an individual's race or ethnicity, primary language, and disability status based on their perceptions, or take the collection of data for granted. Instead, health providers will have to take steps to ensure that patients report demographic data themselves and that it is documented accurately.

Enhancing Health Disparities Research

Significant gaps and gray areas in data have limited our understanding of the nature and extent of health care disparities. The ACA provided an important impetus to develop new research opportunities that can underpin improvements in the health care and health status of diverse groups in the future. HHS reported in 2001 that rates of mental disorders are not adequately studied in many racial and ethnic groups, both indigenous (American Indians, Alaska Natives) and immigrant (Asian Americans, some Pacific Islanders), yielding a scarcity of quality research. Studies have recognized that epidemiological studies often fail to include data on vulnerable, high-risk subgroups such as persons who are exposed to violence or who are homeless, incarcerated, institutionalized, or in foster care. The Institute of Medicine noted in 2011 that studies examining issues impacting LGBT individuals have failed to adequately include adolescents as well as bisexual and transgender individuals. Those research gaps can have significant implications on health care. Diagnostic criteria developed with one racial group may not be directly and simply applicable to other racial groups, such that instruments of assessment and diagnosis may be less appropriately applied in different groups.[26]

The Affordable Care Act provides unique opportunities to expand the scope of research related to health disparities, as well as opportunities to identify, develop, and disseminate appropriate pathways to reduce those disparities. President Obama and Congress recognized that a "one-size-fits-all" approach is ineffective in both understanding the impact of certain chronic diseases on vulnerable populations and in developing proper treatments for diverse individuals.

The ACA established the Patient-Centered Outcomes Research Institute (PCORI), a private, nonprofit institute that is now responsible for identifying and carrying out national research priorities in comparative effectiveness research, in which two or more health care treatments, services, or items are compared for their effectiveness, risks, and benefits.[27] Research might be generated, for example, to test the effectiveness of two drugs created to treat schizophrenia and their impact on various populations or the effectiveness of two drugs created to treat an infectious disease on various populations.

PCORI research findings will be used to inform patients, clinicians, purchasers, and policy makers of the best health care practices available to treat health problems across the full spectrum of America's diversity. The systematic reviews of existing research, randomized clinical trials, observational studies, and other research will, as appropriate, take into account differences in the effectiveness of treatment, services, and items across populations, including racial and ethnic groups, women, people of varying ages, and groups with different medical conditions, genetic sub-types, or quality of life preferences.

PCORI has adopted a rigorous stakeholder-driven process that empha-sizes patient engagement and uses forums and formal public comment opportunities to increase awareness of its work and obtain public input and feedback prior to adoption of priorities, agendas, methodological stan-dards, peer review processes, or dissemination strategies.[28] This will help to increase evidence-based policy making, but, like the Agency for Health-care Research and Quality, PCORI has continuously been targeted by op-ponents of the ACA who are opposed to its purpose.

Enhancing Nondiscrimination Protections

One prominent health equity champion in Congress once stated, "Lawsuits will not eliminate health disparities."[29] While this may be true, it still does not hurt to provide individuals with a private right of action to enforce their rights and protect them from disparate and dis-criminatory services and treatment. Several existing laws address a vari-ety of discriminatory practices in the health care system, but the Afford-able Care Act obligates health care providers to take more active roles in eliminating health disparities among vulnerable groups in the United States, by now prohibiting discrimination based on gender identity and sex stereotyping, race and ethnicity, or disability. Coupled with the new data collection actions, the ACA's Section 1557 nondiscrimination provision now provides consumers and providers with a legal enforcement mecha-nism to ensure that their rights under the law, including protection from certain discriminatory practices, are upheld.

The ACA strengthens and expands protections under section 1557, which is enforced by the HHS Office of Civil Rights, for population groups that have long endured discrimination in access to health care. It does so by prohibiting their exclusion from participating in, being denied the benefits of, or being subjected to discrimination under, any health program or activity, any part of which is receiving federal financial assistance, including credits, subsidies, or contracts of insurance. This prohibition extends to any program or activity administered by any executive agency or by any entity established under the Affordable Care Act. The ACA also allows states to choose to provide additional protections.

National Strategies to Reduce Health Disparities

In addition to all of the aforementioned policies, several national strategies were commissioned by the health reform law or by executive order, and these are the first-ever comprehensive strategies to address health disparities focused on quality, prevention and public health, workforce, HIV/AIDS, health literacy, and health information technology. These strategies provide communities with model plans and information that may be used to coordinate action to reduce disparities in health status and health care. These strategies also provide insight into the federal government's efforts to reduce disparities and help communities tailor their grant applications based on these focus areas.

National Strategy of Quality Improvement in Health Care

The health reform law required the development of a national strategy to improve health outcomes, efficiency, and patient-centered care for all Americans. The plan, which will be updated annually, must address ways to reduce health disparities and the gaps in quality across populations and geographic areas, improve research on best practices to improve patient safety, and reduce medical errors, preventable admissions and readmissions, and hospital infections. Five years after enactment of the Affordable Care Act, it was the only strategy that had failed to meaningfully address the statutorily mandated prioritization of health equity and the reduction of health disparities, until CMS released a separate equity plan for quality improvement in the fall of 2015.

National Prevention and Health Promotion Strategy

The health reform law required the development of a national prevention, health promotion, public health, and integrative health care strategy. The development of this strategy was led by the eighteenth US surgeon general, Dr. Regina Benjamin, who effectively ensured that it meaningfully prioritized health equity and incorporated the most effective and achievable means of improving the health status of all Americans. It also prioritized reducing the incidence of preventable illness and disability in the United States. This strategy is required to be reviewed and revised periodically and prioritize the reduction of health disparities as the nation moves toward better health outcomes for all population groups.

HHS Action Plan to Reduce Racial and Ethnic Health Disparities and National Stakeholder Strategy for Achieving Health Equity

For the first time in this country's history, the health reform law recognized the severity of health disparities, and HHS released two significant strategies for addressing racial and ethnic health disparities and for the achievement of health equity. Together, they provide a common set of goals and objectives for public and private sector initiatives and partnerships to help racial and ethnic minorities—and other underserved groups—reach their full health potential. Communities may use these strategies to identify which goals are most important for them and adopt the most effective strategies and action steps to help reach them.

National HIV/AIDS Strategy

This strategic plan is the first-ever comprehensive, coordinated HIV/AIDS roadmap, created to achieve clear and measureable targets by 2015. This strategy incorporated provisions around behavioral health and has three overarching goals: (1) reducing HIV incidence, (2) increasing access to care and optimizing health outcomes, and (3) reducing HIV-related health disparities. On July 30, 2015, a strategy updated to 2020 was released by the White House. It retained the three overarching goals and added a fourth delineated goal, achieving a more coordinated national response. The updated strategy details eleven new steps and thirty-seven new action steps that focus on the "right people, right places, right practices" as well as clear outcomes that are expected by 2020.[30]

National Action Plan to Improve Health Literacy

This action plan was developed to engage interested stakeholders in a comprehensive effort to improve health literacy. The plan is based on the principles that everyone has the right to health information that helps them make informed decisions and health services should be delivered in ways that are understandable and beneficial to health, longevity, and quality of life.

Federal Health IT Strategic Plan

The Office of the National Coordinator for Health Information Technology published a final version of the Federal Health IT Strategic Plan 2011-2015, which underscored the importance of addressing the digital divide in underresourced communities. This plan reflects a coordinated strategy between the public and private sector to improve the quality, efficiency, safety, and patient centeredness of health care through use of information and technology. A key area of this plan aims to leverage health information technology to address pressing health disparities in communities across the country. The plan was updated to 2020 and again made clear its expectation that "successful implementation of the Plan will also mean that health IT is culturally and linguistically sensitive, safe, accessible for everyone (including those with limited English proficiency or with disabilities), intuitive, functional, and provides a rewarding user experience."[31]

CMS Equity Plan for Improving Quality in Medicare

On September 8, 2015, CMS released its first-ever plan to address health equity in Medicare, the CMS Equity Plan for Improving Quality in Medicare.[32] It focuses on six priority areas and aims to reduce health disparities in four years by focusing on Medicare populations that experience disproportionately high burdens of disease, lower quality of care, and barriers accessing care. These include racial and ethnic minorities, sexual and gender minorities, people with disabilities, and those living in rural areas. The six priority areas include the following:

1. Expand the collection, reporting, and analysis of standardized data
2. Evaluate disparities impacts and integrate equity solutions across CMS programs
3. Develop and disseminate promising approaches to reduce health disparities
4. Increase the ability of the health care workforce to meet the needs of vulnerable populations
5. Improve communication and language access for individuals with limited English proficiency and persons with disabilities
6. Increase physical accessibility of health care facilities

Key Department and Agency Roles in Implementing Health Equity–Related Provisions in Health Reform

Department/Agency	Responsibilities	Key Roles in Health Reform	Contact
Department of Health and Human Services (HHS)	Protect and promote the nation's health and provide essential human services Oversee Medicare and Medicaid programs and the US Public Health Service	Oversees most of the implementation for Health Reform provisions (See specific divisions) Provides online interactive education tools on health reform Data collection and reporting Section 1557 nondiscrimination enforced by the Office of Civil Rights Grant program to support school-based health centers Patient-Centered Outcomes Research Institute (PCORI) in conjunction with the comptroller Grant program to promote small business wellness programs Office of Minority Health transferred to the Office of the Secretary of Health and Human Services Indian Health Care Improvement Act implementation through the Indian Health Service Establish health teams to support the patient-centered medical home Programs to facilitate shared decision making Establish the National Prevention, Health Promotion, and Public Health Council Establish the Prevention and Public Health Investment Fund to provide for expanded and sustained national investment in prevention and public health programs Establish an independent Preventive Services Task Force Advancing Research and Treatment for Pain Care Management	877-696-6775 www.hhs.gov

Agency	Mission	Programs/Offices	Contact
HHS Administration on Aging (AoA)	Develop a comprehensive, coordinated and cost-effective system of home and community-based services for the senior population	Community-Based Care Transition Program Advisory Board on Elder Abuse, Neglect and Exploitation	202-401-4634 www.aoa.gov
HHS Administration of Children and Families (ACF)	Promote the economic and social well-being of families, children, individuals, and communities	Grant program for home visitation program Grant program for personal responsibility education Demonstration projects to address health professions workforce needs	877-696-6775 www.acf.hhs.gov
HHS Agency for Healthcare Research and Quality (AHRQ)	Improve the quality, safety, efficiency, and effectiveness of health care	Primary Care Extension Program to educate providers National Strategy for Quality Improvement in Healthcare in conjunction with CMS Quality improvement technical assistance and implementation Development of quality measures AHRQ Office of Minority Health AHRQ Office of Women's Health and Gender-Based Research	301-427-1104 www.ahrq.gov
HHS Centers for Disease Control and Prevention (CDC)	Provide information and tools people and communities need to protect their health and prevent disease Monitor health, detect and investigate health problems, conduct prevention research, promote healthy behaviors, foster safe and healthful environments	CDC Office of Minority Health CDC Office of Women's Health Community Preventive Services Task Force Community Transformation Grants Grant program to increase epidemiology and laboratory capacity Oral Healthcare Prevention Education Campaign Grant program for community-based diabetes prevention Funding for Childhood Obesity Demonstration Project Breast Cancer Education Campaign Education and Outreach Campaign Regarding Preventive Benefits	800-232-4636 www.cdc.gov

(continued)

Key Department and Agency Roles in Implementing Health Equity-Related Provisions in Health Reform

Department/Agency	Responsibilities	Key Roles in Health Reform	Contact
HHS **Centers for Medicare and Medicaid Services (CMS)** (Includes the Center for Consumer Information & Insurance Oversight [CCIIO], which was created by the ACA)	Provide effective health care coverage and promote quality care for Medicare and Medicaid beneficiaries	Medicare and Medicaid related provisions on health insurance reforms and prescription drugs Health insurance exchanges/marketplaces Value-based purchasing programs Community-Based Care Transitions Program Medicaid Quality Measurement Program Fraud protection program CMS Office of Minority Health Enrollment outreach targeting low income populations, including navigators, certified application counselors, and champions for coverage Funding Outreach and Assistance for Low-Income Programs Increase federal funding for US territories by $2 billion and raises the caps on federal Medicaid funding for each of the territories; allows each territory to elect to operate a health benefits exchange	877-267-2323 Or your State Medicaid Office www.cms.gov
HHS **Center for Medicare & Medicaid Innovation (CMMI)—created by the ACA**	Develop and fund demonstration projects to improve patients' quality of care	Bundled Payments for Care Improvement Health Care Innovation Challenge Grants Pioneer accountable care organization (Pioneer ACO)	www.innovation.cms.gov/
HHS Food and Drug Administration (FDA)	Assure the safety, efficacy, and security of drugs, biological products, medical devices, the nation's food supply, cosmetics, and products that emit radiation	FDA Office of Minority Health FDA Office of Women's Health	888-463-6332 www.fda.gov

HHS **Health Resources and Services Administration (HRSA)**	Regulate manufacturing, marketing and distribution of tobacco products		
	Improve access to health care services for people who are uninsured, isolated or medically vulnerable	Title VII and Title VIII health professional pipeline programs, including Health Careers Opportunity Program, Area Health Education Centers, and Centers of Excellence Loan repayment programs to recruit primary care, public health, nursing, psychology, social work, counseling and other behavioral health professions students to practice in underserved communities State Healthcare Workforce Development Grants Workforce education and training programs established or enhanced, including • Family medicine, general internal medicine, general pediatrics, and physician assistantship • Rural physicians training • Direct care workers providing long-term care services and supports • General, pediatric, and public health dentistry • Alternative dental health care provider • Geriatric education and training for faculty in health professions schools and family caregivers • Mental and behavioral health education and training grants to schools for the development, expansion, or enhancement of training programs in social work, graduate psychology, professional training in child and adolescent mental health, and preservice or in-service training to paraprofessionals in child and adolescent mental health • Cultural competency, prevention, public health, and individuals with disabilities training • Advanced nursing education grants for accredited nurse midwifery programs • Nurse education, practice, and retention grants to nursing schools to strengthen nurse education and training programs and to improve nurse retention • Nurse practitioner training program in community health centers and nurse-managed health centers • Nurse faculty loan program for nurses who pursue careers in nurse education • Grants to promote the community health workforce to promote positive health behaviors and outcomes in medically underserved areas through use of community health workers	888-464-4772 www.hrsa.gov

(continued)

Key Department and Agency Roles in Implementing Health Equity-Related Provisions in Health Reform

Department/Agency	Responsibilities	Key Roles in Health Reform	Contact
(HRSA, continued)		Student loan forgiveness for nursing and medical school faculty	
		Promoting diversity in the workforce	
		HRSA Office of Minority Health	
		HRSA Office of Women's Health	
		National Health Service Corp	
		Nurse-managed health clinics	
		Federally qualified health clinics	
		School-based health centers	
		Maternal, Infant and Early Childhood Home Visiting Programs	
		Grants to promote community health workforce	
HHS **Indian Health Service** **(IHS)**	Promote the health of American Indians and Alaska Natives	Office of Indian Men's Health, Indian Health Service Program for treatment of child sexual abuse Indian Health Service Mental Health Technician Training Program	301-443-3593 www.ihs.gov
HHS **National Institutes** **of Health (NIH)**	Set national medical research agenda Largest source of funding for medical research in the world	Grants for Cures Acceleration Network Grant Program to promote Centers of Excellence for Depression National Center on Minority Health and Health Disparities elevated to an institute	301-496-4000 www.nih.gov
HHS **Substance Abuse and** **Mental Health Services** **Administration (SAMHSA)**	Reduce the impact of substance use and mental illness on communities	SAMHSA Office of Behavioral Health Equity Grants to develop and implement health disparity reduction initiatives Community mental health centers	877-726-4727 www.samhsa.gov
Department of Education **(ED)**	Promote student achievement and preparation for global competitiveness	Investment in HBCUs and Minority Serving Institutions	800-872-5327 www.ed.gov

Agency	Mission	Responsibilities	Contact
Department of Labor (DOL)	Foster and promote the welfare of employees and advance job opportunities for those who are in the job market	Health insurance exchanges/marketplaces Cultural and linguistic competence trainings grants Guidelines for health insurance issuers to utilize value-based insurance designs	866-487-2365 www.dol.gov
Department of the Treasury (DOT)	Maintain a strong economy and financial security	Oversee funds including the Patient Outcomes and Research Trust Fund and the Class Independence Funds Program for Advance Determination of Tax Credit Eligibility	202-622-2000 www.treasury.gov
Federal Trade Commission (FTC)	Enforce consumer protection and competition jurisdiction in broad sectors of the economy	Oversee some aspects of accountable care organizations Fraud and abuse prevention efforts aimed at keeping consumers protected while health reform is implemented	877-382-4357 www.ftc.gov
Government Accountability Office (GAO)	Independent, nonpartisan agency that works for Congress to investigate how federal tax dollars are spent	National Health Care Workforce Commission Advisory Board State Cooperatives Consumer Advisory Council for Independent Payment Advisory Board Private Purchasing Council for State Cooperatives Patient-Centered Outcomes Research Institute (PCORI) Drug discounts through the 340B program extended to inpatient drugs	202-512-3000 www.gao.gov
Internal Revenue Service (IRS)	Help individuals understand and meet their tax responsibilities and enforce federal tax laws	Community health needs assessment for nonprofit hospitals Nonprofit hospital financial aid policies Excise tax on indoor tanning services Small employer health care tax credit Individual and employer mandate—collection and enforcement of tax or penalty	800-876-1715 www.irs.gov
Office of Personnel Management (OPM)	Recruit and train federal workforce	Advisory board for multistate health plans	202-606-1800 www.opm.gov

(continued)

Key Department and Agency Roles in Implementing Health Equity-Related Provisions in Health Reform

Department/Agency	Responsibilities	Key Roles in Health Reform	Contact
State Agencies		Office of health insurance consumer assistance or an ombudsman program	Please contact state agencies. Most programs and initiatives will be implemented by state health departments.
		State authority to purchase recommended vaccines for adult programs	
		Medicaid State Offices:	
		Medicaid preventive and obesity-related services awareness campaigns	
		Medicaid coverage of tobacco cessation services for pregnant women	
		Elimination of exclusion of coverage of certain drugs in Medicaid	
		CHIP (Child Health Insurance Program) obesity demonstration program	
		Various Funding opportunities:	
		Grant program to plan health care workforce development	
		Grant program for providers who treat a high percentage of medically underserved populations	
		Grant program for maternal, infant, and early childhood home visitation program	
		Community Transformation Grants	
		Grants for school-based health centers	
		Oral Healthcare Prevention Demonstration Program	
		Immunization Coverage Improvement Program	
		Epidemiology and laboratory capacity grants	
		Healthy Aging, Living Well Public Health Grant Program	
		Grants to promote community health workforce	

NOTES

1. Sen. Kirk cosponsored an amendment to include physician rural training grants, Sen. Bennett offered changes to the SBHC program, Sen. Coburn offered one to make sure comparative effectiveness research could not be used for cost and coverage decisions.

2. The individual mandate is also referred to as the individual responsibility requirement.

3. The Children's Health Insurance Program (CHIP) was created in 1997 to assist states in providing health insurance for low-income children who lack the financial ability to pay for private insurance and who are not eligible for Medicaid. Under the ACA, federal funding for CHIP was extended from 2015 to 2019.

To meet the requirement of "minimum essential coverage," coverage must be affordable and comprehensive. Employers must allow employees an opportunity to enroll in a plan that will pay at least 60 percent of medical expenses on average and ensure that an employee's premium contribution for the lowest-cost health plan does not exceed 9.5 percent of the employee's household income. If any of these requirements are not met, then the employer has failed to provide minimum essential coverage.

4. For a complete list of covered services, visit the United States Preventive Services Task Force (see "A and B" recommendations) at http://www .uspreventiveservicestaskforce.org/.

5. Blum, "What Is the Donut Hole?"

6. US Department of Health and Human Services, "Prevention and Public Health Fund," http://www.hhs.gov/open/recordsandreports/prevention/ or http://www.hhs.gov/open/recordsandreports/prevention/announcements.html.

7. US Department of Health and Human Services, *The 80/20 Rule: Providing Value and Rebates to Millions of Consumers*; Centers for Medicare and Medicaid Services, *80/20 Rule Delivers More Value to Consumers in 2012*; Centers for Medicare and Medicaid Services, *2013 MLR Refunds by State*.

8. There have been some exceptions to this requirement for some "grandfathered" plans, but those exceptions will cease by the first plan renewal date after January 1, 2014.

9. Using 2014 figures, individuals with incomes between $11,670 and $46,680—and families of four with incomes between $23,850 and $95,400—were eligible for subsidies to help them afford health insurance coverage in the marketplace exchanges.

10. Consumer Assistance Tools and Programs of an Exchange; Affordable Care Act §1311(i)(3) and 45 CFR §155.210(e).

11. Using 2014 figures, this would mean an individual making less than $15,521 per year.

12. Cohen, "Reflections on the Enactment of Medicare and Medicaid."

13. Frist, "Overcoming Disparities in US Health Care."

14. "Patient centered" is sometimes referred to as "person centered." The Agency for Healthcare Research and Quality defines a health home as "model for transforming the organization and delivery of primary care that is patient-centered, comprehensive, coordinated, accessible, and continuously improved." *Patient Centered Medical Home Resource Center.*

15. Centers for Medicare and Medicaid Services, "Bundled Payments for Care Improvement (BPCI) Initiative."

16. Measures cannot be selected for VBP until they have been adopted for the hospital Inpatient Quality Reporting Program and posted on the Hospital Compare for one year prior to the start of the VBP performance period. Calculations of budget neutrality exclude indirect medical education (IME), disproportionate share hospital (DSH), and other payments.

17. This does not apply to IME, DSH, or other payments.

18. https://www.medicare.gov/hospitalcompare/search.html.

19. *U.S. Efforts To Reduce Healthcare-Associated Infections Before United States Senate Committee on Health, Education, Labor & Pensions* (statement by Patrick Conway).

20. HACs may include foreign object retained after surgery, air embolism, blood incompatibility, Stage III and IV pressure ulcers, falls and trauma, manifestations of poor glycemic control, catheter-associated urinary tract infection (UTI), vascular catheter-associated infection, surgical site infection, deep vein thrombosis (DVT)/pulmonary embolism (PE) following certain orthopedic procedures, iatrogenic pneumothorax with venous catheterization. CMS has defined HACs as those conditions that (1) are high cost and/or high volume, (2) result in the diagnosis of a case to DRG that has a higher payment when present as a secondary diagnosis, and (3) could reasonably have been prevented through the application of evidence-based guidelines.

21. According to CMS, a prospective payment system is a method of reimbursement in which Medicare payment is made based on a predetermined, fixed amount. The payment amount for a particular service is based on the classification system of that service (for example, diagnosis-related groups for inpatient hospital services). CMS uses separate prospective payment systems for reimbursement to acute inpatient hospitals, home health agencies, hospice, hospital outpatient, inpatient psychiatric facilities, inpatient rehabilitation facilities, long-term care hospitals, and skilled nursing facilities.

22. America's Health Centers, National Association of Community Health Centers Fact Sheet.

23. Stagman and Cooper, *Children's Mental Health*; Cooper et al., *Unclaimed Children Revisited.*

24. Koh, "Improving Health Disparities Data for a Healthier Nation."

25. Institute of Medicine, *Race, Ethnicity, and Language Data.*

26. US Department of Health and Human Services, *Mental Health*; American Psychological Association, "Psychological and Behavioral Perspectives on Health Disparities"; Institute of Medicine, *The Health of Lesbian, Gay, Bisexual and Transgender People*; Low and Hardy, "Psychiatric Disorder Criteria and Their Application to Research in Different Racial Groups."

27. According to the Agency for Healthcare Research and Quality, comparative effectiveness research "is designed to inform health-care decisions by providing evidence on the effectiveness, benefits, and harms of different treatment options. The evidence is generated from research studies that compare drugs, medical devices, tests, surgeries, or ways to deliver health care." For more information about comparative effectiveness research, see "What Is Comparative Effectiveness Research?"

28. For more information on comparative effectiveness research, grant opportunities, or to learn more about PCORI's comparative effectiveness research initiatives and provide input and feedback, please visit www.pcori.org.

29. Frist, "Overcoming Disparities in US Health Care."

30. US Department of Health and Human Services, *National HIV/AIDS Strategy*; White House, National HIV/AIDS Strategy for the United States.

31. US Department of Health and Human Services, *Federal Health IT Strategic Plan*.

32. Centers for Medicare and Medicaid Services, The CMS Equity Plan for Improving Quality in Medicare.

BIBLIOGRAPHY

Affordable Care Act §1311(i)(3) and 45 CFR §155.210(e).

Agency for Healthcare Research and Quality. *Patient Centered Medical Home Resource Center*. https://pcmh.ahrq.gov/.

———. "What Is Comparative Effectiveness Research?" http://www .effectivehealthcare.ahrq.gov/index.cfm/what-is-comparative-effectiveness -research1/.

American Psychological Association. "Psychological and Behavioral Perspectives on Health Disparities." Communique, 2009. Washington, DC.

America's Health Centers. National Association of Community Health Centers Fact Sheet. National Association of Community Health Centers, Bethesda, MD, July 2012.

Blum, Jonathan. "What Is the Donut Hole?" *Medicare Blog*, August 2010. http:// blog.medicare.gov/2010/08/09/what-is-the-donut%C2%A0hole/.

Centers for Disease Control and Prevention. *National Health Interview Survey*. Washington, DC, 2014.

Centers for Medicare and Medicaid Services. "Bundled Payments for Care Improvement (BPCI) Initiative: General Information." http://innovation.cms .gov/initiatives/bundled-payments/.

——. CHIP State Plan Information. http://www.medicaid.gov/chip/state
-program-information/chip-state-program-information.html.

——. The CMS Equity Plan for Improving Quality in Medicare. Baltimore,
September 2015. https://www.cms.gov/About-CMS/Agency-Information
/OMH/OMH_Dwnld-CMS_EquityPlanforMedicare_090615.pdf.

——. *80/20 Rule Delivers More Value to Consumers in 2012*. Baltimore, MD, July
2013. https://www.cms.gov/CCIIO/Resources/Forms-Reports-and-Other
-Resources/Downloads/2012-medical-loss-ratio-report.pdf.

——. *2013 MLR Refunds by State*. Baltimore, MD, July 2014. https://www.cms
.gov/CCIIO/Resources/Data-Resources/Downloads/2013_MLR_Refunds_by
_State.pdf.

Cohen, Wilbur. "Reflections on the Enactment of Medicare and Medicaid."
Supplement, *Health Care Financing Review* (December 1985): 3-11. http://
www.ncbi.nlm.nih.gov/pmc/articles/PMC4195078/.

Congressional Research Service. *The ACA Medicaid Expansion*. Washington, DC,
December 30, 2014.

Consumer Assistance Tools and Programs of an Exchange. 45 CFR § 155.205(d)
and (e).

Cooper, J., Y. Aratani, J. Knitzer, A. Douglas-Hall, R. Masi, P. Banghart, and
S. Dababnah. *Unclaimed Children Revisited: The Status of Children's Mental
Health Policy in the United States*. New York: National Center for Children in
Poverty, 2008.

Dawes, D., and N. Jarrett. *Understanding Health Reform: A Community Guide for African
Americans*. Washington, DC: Congressional Black Caucus Foundation, 2010.

Dawes, D., F. Rider, and L. Lambert. *Health Reform and Immigrant Children, Youth,
and Families: Opportunities and Challenges for Advancing Behavioral Health*.
Washington, DC: Technical Assistance Partnership for Child and Family
Mental Health, 2013.

Frist, William H. "Overcoming Disparities in US Health Care." *Health Affairs* 24,
no. 2 (March 2005): 445-451.

Institute of Medicine. *The Health of Lesbian, Gay, Bisexual and Transgender People:
Building a Foundation to Better Health*. Washington, DC: National Academies
Press, 2011.

——. *Race, Ethnicity, and Language Data: Standardization for Health Care Quality
Improvement*. Washington, DC: National Academies Press, 2009.

Kaiser Commission on Medicaid and the Uninsured. *A Historical Review of How
States Have Responded to the Availability of Federal Funds for Health Coverage*.
Washington, DC, August 2012. https://kaiserfamilyfoundation.files
.wordpress.com/2013/01/8349.pdf.

Koh, Howard. "Improving Health Disparities Data for a Healthier Nation." The
White House. November 2, 2011. http://www.whitehouse.gov/blog/2011/11
/02/improving-health-disparities-data-healthier-nation.

Low, N., and J. Hardy. "Psychiatric Disorder Criteria and Their Application to Research in Different Racial Groups." *BMC Psychiatry* 7, no. 1 (2007). doi: 10.1186/1471-244X-7-1.

Sommers, Benjamin D., Emily Arntson, Genevieve M. Kenney, Arnold M. Epstein, Harvard School of Public Health–Department of Health Policy & Management, Urban Institute. "Lessons from Early Medicaid Expansions under Health Reform: Interviews with Medicaid Officials." *Medicare & Medicaid Research Review* 3, no. 4 (2013): E1–E19.

Stagman, S., and J. Cooper. *Children's Mental Health: What Every Policymaker Should Know.* New York: National Center for Children in Poverty, 2010.

US Department of Health and Human Services. *The 80/20 Rule: Providing Value and Rebates to Millions of Consumers.* Washington, DC, June 21, 2012. http:// www.hhs.gov/healthcare/facts/factsheets/2012/06/mlr-rebates06212012a .html.

———. *Federal Health IT Strategic Plan: 2015–2020.* Washington, DC, 2015. http://www.healthit.gov/sites/default/files/federal-healthIT-strategic-plan -2014.pdf.

———. *National HIV/AIDS Strategy: Updated to 2020 What You Need to Know.* Washington, DC, July 2015.

———. "Prevention and Public Health Fund." http://www.hhs.gov/open /prevention/index.html.

US Department of Health and Human Services, Public Health Service, Office of the Surgeon General. *Mental Health: Culture, Race and Ethnicity—a Supplement to Mental Health: A Report of the Surgeon General.* Rockville, MD, 2001.

U.S. Efforts To Reduce Healthcare-Associated Infections Before United States Senate Committee on Health, Education, Labor & Pensions. September 24, 2013. Statement by Patrick Conway. http://www.hhs.gov/asl/testify/2013/09 /t20130924.html.

White House. National HIV/AIDS Strategy for the United States: Updated to 2020. Washington, DC, July 2015.

Moving Health Equity Forward
Current Issues and the Struggle Ahead

What we need are leaders who care enough, know enough, do enough, and persist enough.—*Dr. David Satcher, 16th US Surgeon General*

My best friend, Philip Baker, whom I have known since we were children, often questioned the need for comprehensive health reform. Late one evening in 2009, in the midst of the frenzy of health reform negotiations, I got a call from Philip while on the Metro on my way home from work. When I answered, he asked, "How is everything going? Do you think you guys are going to be successful with the health reform bill?" I answered yes and asked him what was up, as it was unusual for him to call so late. He asked if I was sitting down, then told me to take a seat. I immediately felt ill and told him to just spit out whatever news he was about to give me. He then said, "I don't know how to say this Daniel . . . I was recently diagnosed with stage four colon cancer. They are telling me that I may have six months to live."

I was shocked and devastated and hoped it was just a terrible joke. Philip told me it was not and explained that for some time he had been experiencing severe abdominal pain. He had been to the emergency room several times, each time being told by doctors that they could not find anything wrong and it was all in his head. Finally, after having lost fifteen pounds, he went to the hospital again during another episode of severe abdominal pain. This time he refused to leave until they did a comprehensive exam. Once they did, the doctors discovered that he had colon cancer, which by this point had metastasized to his liver and lungs. They had caught it too late, but Philip was determined to fight his cancer for as long as he could.

One year later, Philip called me to catch up as we had every week. We chatted about new news, old news, and his status. We joked as usual, but this time his tone got more serious. Philip had been terrified of losing his insurance throughout his ordeal and having to go on COBRA.[1] But even with that fear he was grateful because he had suitable health insurance coverage, and he told me he could not fathom how much worse this situation would be for a person who was uninsured. He said, "Daniel, I never quite understood what it is you do or why you cared so much about health care access until now. I want you to promise me that you will continue advocating, that you guys will implement this health care bill. It's important for people like me not to have to work our butts off at the same time we are trying to get care and treatment. I now get it." Philip passed away three weeks later at the age of twenty-nine, one year after the Patient Protection and Affordable Care Act was enacted into law.

The Affordable Care Act, while not a cure-all, has already demonstrated great success. By March 2014, at the end of the first enrollment period, the Obama administration touted figures showing that more than 8 million Americans had purchased coverage through both state-based and federally facilitated health insurance marketplaces.[2] Although later figures showed fewer enrollees—the Centers for Medicare and Medicaid Services administrator Marilyn Tavenner in September 2014 shared data showing that there were actually 7.3 million enrollees, and two months later the Secretary of Health and Human Services Sylvia Mathews Burwell announced that the enrollment figure was standing at 7.1 million enrollees—most still deemed the law's efforts a huge success. Moreover, despite later revelations that CMS had included approximately 380,000 stand-alone dental plans in the count, the figures were still impressive, and the attrition rate was lower than many expected. By March 2015, the US Department of Health and Human Services released another report showing that approximately 11.7 million people had purchased health insurance through both state-based and federally facilitated marketplaces in the second enrollment period, which again showed positive gains.

Overall, the Affordable Care Act's efforts to increase health insurance coverage have benefitted all racial and ethnic groups and are helping to decrease disparities in access to care in the United States. Five years after its passage, more than sixteen million uninsured people gained health insurance coverage, with African Americans and Latinos having seen the greatest decline among all racial groups. According to the White House, "Since the Marketplaces opened and Medicaid expansion began, the uninsured rate among African Americans has dropped 41% and Latinos declined 29%, with an estimated 2.3 million African

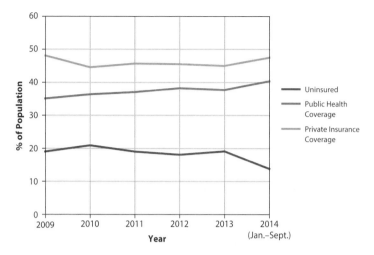

Figure 7.1. African American health coverage rates. Centers for Disease Control and Prevention, National Health Interview Survey, 2014.

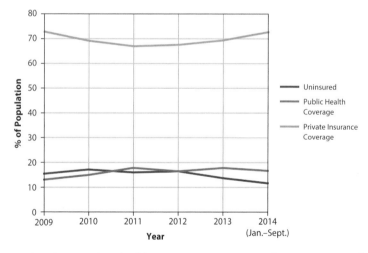

Figure 7.2. Asian American health coverage rates. Centers for Disease Control and Prevention, National Health Interview Survey, 2014.

American adults gaining coverage, and about 4.2 million Latino adults gaining coverage."[3]

In addition to providing coverage to millions of Americans who were previously uninsured, the Affordable Care Act has eased the financial bur-

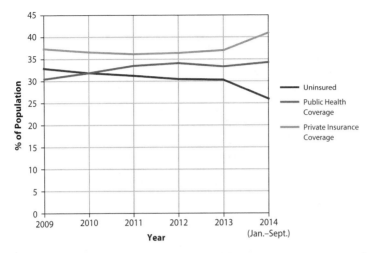

Figure 7.3. Hispanic or Latino health coverage rates. Centers for Disease Control and Prevention, National Health Interview Survey, 2014.

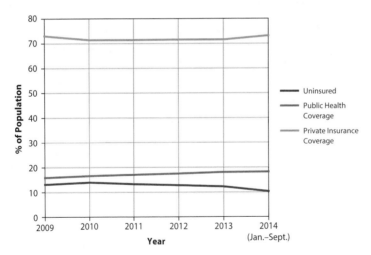

Figure 7.4. Caucasian health coverage rates. Centers for Disease Control and Prevention, National Health Interview Survey, 2014.

den on many individuals who had to pay hundreds of dollars in insurance premiums every month. Today, we can see the tremendous impact the ACA is having on people across the country with numerous stories of uninsured individuals benefitting from premium and cost-sharing subsidies allowing

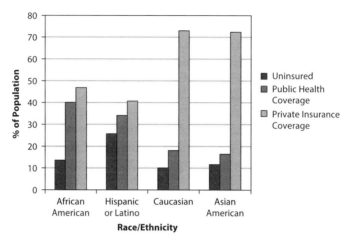

Figure 7.5. 2014 (Jan.-Sept.) coverage rates for populations under age 65. Centers for Disease Control and Prevention, National Health Interview Survey, 2014.

them to access health insurance coverage they can afford. One single mother and cancer survivor in Pennsylvania saw her premium payments fall from $880 a month before the Affordable Care Act to $22 after enactment of the health care law.[4]

Even physicians have remarked how ObamaCare has positively impacted the lives of their patients—not only helping to improve their health outcomes but saving their lives. Dr. Donovan D. Taylor, a physician in Miami, Florida, recounted an episode where one patient decided to comply with the mandate to purchase health insurance. He was able to purchase affordable health insurance coverage through the exchange. Sometime later, this gentleman started experiencing night sweats and feeling lethargic, so he came in to Dr. Taylor's office for a checkup. Once the examination was over and the test results came back, it was clear that they had to immediately get him into treatment. He had cancer, but they were able to catch it right in time before it metastasized further.[5]

Before the health insurance marketplace opened for business and states decided to expand their Medicaid programs, the law was already benefiting Americans by providing them with consumer rebates from insurance companies, ensuring that children with preexisting conditions were no longer denied coverage, providing free comprehensive women's preventive services, closing the Medicare prescription drug donut hole for older adults, ending lifetime limits on coverage, and providing small businesses with a health care tax credit, along with other benefits. The Affordable Care Act also incorporated numerous provisions that have and will serve as a bridge to effectively and efficiently address health disparities and achieve health equity. Although there were previous laws that addressed discrimination in health care access, disparate treatment between protected classes in health services, and parity between mental and substance use benefits and medical and surgical benefits, no other law has prioritized health equity and the reduction of health disparities to this extent.

Another bright spot for the Affordable Care Act has been the general slowing of the growth of medical costs. While health care costs are still increasing, the rate of increase has slowed since 2010. Certainly, one could argue that other factors have also contributed to the lowering of health care spending, such as patients deferring elective procedures as well as the proliferation of cheaper, generic drugs. But one would be hard pressed to ignore the fact that the average rate of health care cost increases since the law's enactment has been less than half the average in the prior forty years, which is due in part to the Affordable Care Act lowering the annual increases that Medicare pays to hospitals, home health agencies, and private insurance plans.[6] The health care law also disincentivizes lower-quality care and places an emphasis on value-based care, so payments are made based on value, not volume. In such a system, providers are rewarded for keeping their patients healthy rather than for the frequency of their patients' hospital visits.

• • •

Despite all of these successes, opponents have continued to fight against ObamaCare in the public arena, employing creative scare tactics to put the law in a negative light. In July 2014, a nonprofit called Generation Opportunity installed a "Creepy Carenival" on the National Mall in Washington, DC, featuring clowns, jugglers, and amusements, intended to "educate and mobilize young Americans to kick the ObamaCare disaster out of their towns."[7] The same group previously posted ads on the Internet showing "Creepy Uncle Sam" intruding on patients as they await medical examinations, closing with the message "Don't let the government play doctor." Interestingly, this is the argument that was used to successfully bring down the Clinton plan, so why not recycle it and promulgate it again to intensify the opposition's fears?

While opponents continue politicking against the Affordable Care Act, the vitriolic rhetoric that has been amplified by certain individuals could have deadly consequences. The anti-ObamaCare wave, although festering in some parts of the country, continues to spread across communities. Sound bites have become gospel for some, from "death panels" to "government takeover of health care" to arguing that it is akin to "slavery" instead of turning to the very source—the law—to learn what it really contains. Indeed, the Affordable Care Act is not a perfect law and could be strengthened in some respects, but attacking the law for the sake of partisan political gain helps no one.

Opponents have taken advantage of the complexity of health law and policy in general as well as the backpedaling by some politicians who voted in favor of the bill to create confusion and bolster their arguments. Opponents have used the mass confusion to their advantage, realizing that few have the time or wherewithal to dig deeper to come to the truth. This wave could continue to cause harm unless we see increased bipartisan collaboration at the helm of government.

On the state level, opponents of the Affordable Care Act have taken advantage of the Supreme Court's ruling that participating in the Medicaid expansion should be optional. As of 2015, approximately twenty states still refused to expand Medicaid coverage. State governors who have refused the expansion have cited economic concerns, stating that the Medicaid expansion would burden state budgets. The governors of Louisiana and Florida asserted that the expansion would cost their states $1 billion and $5 billion respectively, and the former Alaska governor Sean Parnell expressed concerns about the federal budget: "at this point, the federal government cannot even say with certainty that it can meet its obligations to cut welfare checks on April 1, let alone finance Medicaid expansion."[8]

By contrast, a small number of Republican governors, such as Brian Sandoval of Nevada and Jack Dalrymple of North Dakota, agreed to expand Medicaid in their states for the benefit of their citizens. Even the once-staunch opponent of ObamaCare, Arizona's former governor Jan Brewer agreed to expand Medicaid in her state after a fierce battle that divided the state's Republican Party, saying at the time of signing, "This legislation will protect Arizona's hospitals, it will create thousands of jobs and it will save lives."[9] She believed that since the federal law allowed permanent legal residents under the federal poverty level to get subsidies to purchase health insurance on the exchanges, and US citizens were not authorized to receive such subsidies if they were under the federal poverty level, then it made sense to expand Medicaid so citizens below 100 percent of the federal poverty level could gain access to health services.

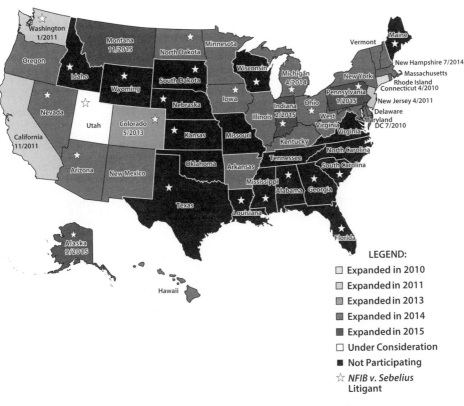

Figure 7.6. States expanding Medicaid coverage as of 2015

In addition to refusing to participate in the Medicaid expansion, certain state governors and legislatures have been taking additional steps to obstruct the implementation of the Affordable Care Act. From the law's enactment in 2010 to 2015, lawmakers in forty-seven state legislatures *proposed* bills to limit, alter, or oppose policies stemming from the Affordable Care Act, and at least twenty-two state legislatures *enacted* laws challenging or opting out of various health reform provisions.[10] The national trend has shown a remarkable decline in enacting bills opposing ObamaCare. Instead, there has been an increase in legislation signed into law to help take advantage of some of the funding opportunities resulting from the ACA. Of the enacted laws against the ACA, however, eighteen different states challenged the ACA's individual and employer coverage mandates, with laws providing that the state government will not enforce them. These contradictory state laws have no effect on the Affordable Care Act provisions, however, because of the Supreme Court's June 2012 decision upholding the mandates.

Six states have passed laws requiring the state legislature's approval before any steps are taken to comply with the ACA. And at least seventeen states have passed laws restricting the use of navigators, the federal program intended to assist Americans in understanding the new health insurance marketplace and purchasing coverage. Republican lawmakers have cited privacy concerns in enacting these restrictions, arguing that the navigators could steal applicants' private information. Despite some legitimate concerns with privacy, however, many states have passed obstructionist laws requiring that navigators, who are often members of community groups or staff at health clinics, obtain separate certifications and licenses, in addition to the requirements already imposed under federal law. In one of these cases, it was revealed that the state department that was responsible for developing this exam admitted to erasing the name of the insurance agent test and writing "navigator test" on it.[11]

These exacting requirements have impeded the ability of many navigators to perform their role and in some cases led to groups returning their grants and dropping out of the navigator program. Dr. Louis Sullivan, former Health and Human Services secretary under George H. W. Bush, has urged Republicans to stop fighting the Affordable Care Act because it includes priorities that they previously advocated. Dr. Sullivan pointed out that the individual mandate—arguably the most opposed provision of the law—was initially proposed by Republicans in 1991, and asked, "If they were supportive of it then, why are they so opposed to it now?"[12]

On the federal level, the implementation of the Affordable Care Act has also been met with many challenges, which is perhaps unsurprising with a law so sweeping and complex. Many Americans have a limited understanding of or mistaken assumptions about health insurance in general, a problem compounded by the raucous rhetoric of ObamaCare opponents. This problem is even further exacerbated for a large portion of the population with limited English proficiency. And perhaps the most infamous obstacle the ACA has faced to date was the launch of healthcare.gov, the new national website for the purchase of health insurance in the marketplace.

The website launched on October 1, 2013, and it was immediately plagued with errors and site downtime. The site's software and systems were not built to withstand the large number of visitors, and only a small number of applicants were able to purchase insurance in the first month.

Opponents sharply criticized the Obama administration and called for the resignation of HHS secretary Kathleen Sebelius. The administration appointed a contractor to fix the website's problems, and by December more than 365,000 Americans had successfully purchased coverage through healthcare.gov. The Obama administration acknowledged the mistakes made with the site's rollout, with Secretary Sebelius describing the initial launch as "flawed, frustrating and unacceptable."[13] She would eventually be vindicated by the successful enrollment figures after the enrollment period ended in March 2014.

Despite its bumpy beginnings, the Affordable Care Act is indeed the law of the land, and, four years after its enactment, opponents appeared to be losing steam. Republican campaign ads for the 2014 midterm elections in North Carolina, Arkansas, and Louisiana showed much less emphasis on attacks of the Affordable Care Act.[14] With uninsured rates going down significantly, some Republicans seemed to be shying away from vilifying the law. However, there has been notable criticism regarding the unexpected Medicaid enrollments seen in many states in 2015 where enrollment was hundreds of thousands beyond initial projections. Opponents of the Affordable Care Act have cited this as evidence that their concerns about states being unable to afford implementing ObamaCare were warranted to begin with.

As discussed in an earlier chapter, there are distinct parallels between public attitude toward Social Security and Medicare in the past and the Affordable Care Act now. Those programs endured a great deal of opposition that eventually faded, so it is probable the opposition to the ACA will do the same. One particularly encouraging point came from a poll conducted by the Commonwealth Fund in 2014, which showed that even Republicans who signed up for health insurance through the marketplace were satisfied with their coverage.[15] So, as time passes and Americans continue to benefit from the law, we may see opposition to the Affordable Care Act die out completely.

. . .

Human progress never rolls in on wheels of inevitability; it comes through the tireless efforts of men willing to be coworkers with God, and without this hard work, time itself becomes an ally of the forces of social stagnation.—*Dr. Martin Luther King Jr.*

Chris Koyanagi, writing for the Kaiser Family Foundation, observed, "Administrations come and go at all levels of government and priorities can change within administrations as well. This makes it hard to ensure sustained commitment. Changing gears, reducing funding or simple neglect could undermine policy . . . in the future. Public support is perhaps the best hedge against these swings in policy, but to inform the public and policy makers, continued evaluations, research and policy advocacy will be essential."[16] Overall, the efforts of the National Working Group on Health Disparities and Health Reform were hugely successful. Our achievements, in helping to include health equity-focused provisions in the Affordable Care Act, are a testament to the power of collaboration and our determination to address pervasive health disparities among vulnerable populations. But, lest we forget Ms. Koyanagi's declaration to always remain vigilant, health equity advocates could easily lose many of the gains we have achieved over the years or lose opportunities to advance health equity even further than we ever imagine possible in public policy.

In November 2012, the US Senate Democratic Steering Committee, for the first time, invited health equity leaders from various organizations to present our ideas for advancing health equity. Dr. Elena Rios of the National Hispanic Medical Association, Kathy Ko Chin of the Asian & Pacific Islander American Health Forum, and I, representing the National Working Group, were asked to open the roundtable by highlighting issues that the committee should consider moving forward to advance health equity. Senators reassured us that health equity was still being prioritized in federal policy. However, despite these reassurances and the fact that health equity advocates achieved a great deal with the enactment of the health reform law, without continued diligence, we could lose all the progress that has been made. This becomes clear when looking at the frequency of bills involving disparities that have been introduced in Congress. The number of bills was steadily increasing up until 2010, when the Affordable Care Act passed, then started declining and has continued to do so. This is particularly troubling, because while the Affordable Care Act does comprehensively address the issue of health disparities, it will not completely fix the problem.

As health equity advocates know too well, the improvements and changes to health care and public health systems will not occur overnight but will take several years to materialize. The health equity provisions in the Affordable Care Act, found in the quality improvement, prevention and wellness, data collection, comparative effectiveness research, workforce

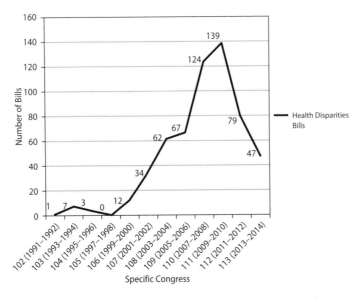

Figure 7.7. Trend for introduction of bills addressing health disparities by Congress

development, and health insurance sections are intended to address inequities in a comprehensive manner. However, these provisions are only a fraction of the public policies needed to achieve health equity and improve the health of all communities in the United States.

Health reform in some form is here to stay, but there will be years of fixes and adjustments, especially as these provisions are implemented. As a result, there is still much work to do to develop, strengthen, and implement public policies that aim to achieve health equity for vulnerable populations. Federal budget constraints will continue to apply pressure to reduce health care costs, opponents of health equity will try to continue chipping away at the Affordable Care Act, and there will be additional hurdles to overcome politically, legally, and administratively.

After one has participated in the policy-making process, one cannot help but gain new reverence for the law—for the policies that have been meticulously developed, negotiated, tested, vetted, and revised internally and externally hundreds of times, in many cases, before the final product is introduced or reintroduced and ultimately passed. Consequently, because of the investment in time and energy it took to pass this law, health equity advocates—whether students, faculty, consumers, community leaders, faith leaders, business leaders, or health professionals—will need to invest similar time and energy to see it successfully implemented.

This should involve advocating for adequate funding from Congress and the White House for the many health equity provisions that fall under discretionary funding and to protect programs that receive mandatory appropriations under the law. Advocates should frame the health equity issue so it will resonate in these austere times, including figuring out the economic impact of disparities at the most granular level—by states, by districts, by counties, by cities—and determine how disparities are contributing to the high costs of health care, in terms of lives lost and funds expended. Equally important is the need for advocates to elevate health equity in local and state policies because advances in state health policies lead to advances in health policy around that given issue at the federal level too. Oftentimes, states are the incubators of new policies that are then adopted by federal policy makers.

In addition, advocates should continue providing sound information and feedback to regulators who are and will be drafting the regulations to implement the law so that health equity and the reduction of disparities remain a priority. One of the major areas that has been neglected in health reform involves the nexus between quality improvement and health equity. For the first time since it began releasing separate annual reports on health care quality and health care disparities in 2003, the federal Agency for Healthcare Research and Quality in 2015 combined both reports into one, giving readers a better snapshot of how these two issues intersect across the country.[17]

In general, the report showed an interesting trend—states with higher health care quality scores tended to show higher disparities in care among racial and ethnic groups. States with lower health care quality scores tended to show lower disparities in care among racial and ethnic groups, meaning that in these states all racial and ethnic groups receive lower-quality care.[18] As policy makers push for increasing health information technology and the adoption of electronic health records as well as improving the quality of health care, there is a real possibility that this may exacerbate disparities. With the American Recovery and Reinvestment Act, the Affordable Care Act, and the Medicare Access and CHIP Reauthorization Act of 2015 steering us away from a fee-for-service system to a system focused on quality, value, and accountability, there is concern that this could lead to a separate and unequal health care system, a system resulting in striking

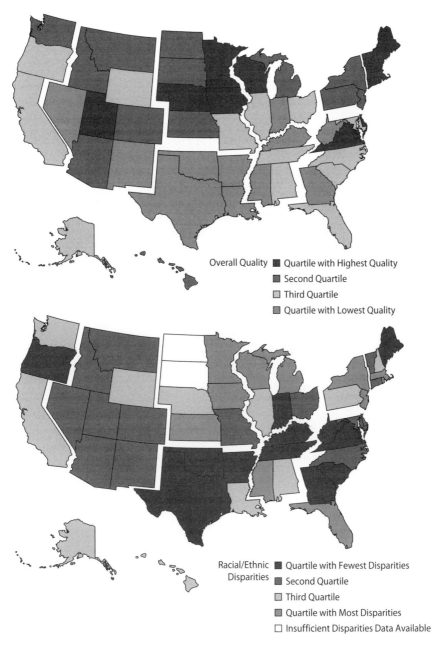

Figure 7.8. Quality disparities: overall quality and racial/ethnic disparities varied widely across states and often not in the same direction. States sorted by overall quality (top) and average differences among blacks, Hispanics, and Asians compared with whites (bottom). Source: Agency for Healthcare Research and Quality, 2013 State Snapshots.

differences in the provision of health care services based on one's racial and ethnic background or geographic location.[19] Therefore, more attention is needed in this area to ensure that consumers, as well as the providers and payers that serve these communities, are not unfairly penalized. This must entail bringing all communities to the table and working collaboratively to design models that are focused on achieving equity in health care.

Health equity advocates should also make sure they are aware of key advisory groups, commissions, and task forces that were established by the law to ensure proper representation of the issues impacting vulnerable populations. They should make sure that they are participating in the development of national strategies relative to health disparities reduction, so that their voices are heard. Lastly, advocates should keep a watchful eye on political and legal efforts to amend health reform to make sure that these efforts do not weaken the protections secured under the law for the most vulnerable individuals.

Former majority leader and distinguished US senator Bill Frist recognized the significant advancement of policies and laws prioritizing health equity over the last four decades when he declared, "I am confident that our generation can meet the challenge posed by the 'unfinished work' of health disparities. I am also confident that one day all Americans regardless of skin color or social status, will have equal opportunity to prevent and overcome disease and live longer, happier, and healthier lives."[20] With the passage of the Affordable Care Act, the realization of this goal seems closer than it ever has before.

Unlike earlier proposed or repealed health policies, the Affordable Care Act has been given a chance to prove its worth. Public policies such as Dorothea Dix's mental health proposal, or President Carter's Mental Health Systems Act could have had an enormous positive effect on the health and well-being of Americans, but they were never given the chance to do so. The Affordable Care Act has been buffeted by a constant tide of opposition while hanging in the balance, but it will take deliberate and diligent action to ensure that its policies increasing access to care and treatments, improving quality, prioritizing prevention and early interventions, and advancing health equity will be fully realized and enjoyed by generations of Americans for the next 150 years.

Lest one think ObamaCare has reached the point where no policy maker would dare dismantle this law, it is worth remembering the fate that befell the Freedmen's Bureau, which reached its seventh birthday before it was terminated indefinitely. It was not the US Supreme Court that had repealed it or substantially undermined it, nor was it the US Supreme Court that repealed the Carter mental health reform law. In both instances, their demise was achieved through the political process. For the rest of the major health policies that passed the US Congress and were allowed to be implemented, the US Supreme Court did not rule against them when challenges to these statutes were brought before it. The Court continued to follow this trend with the Affordable Care Act, making it very clear to opponents that they would have to use the political process to repeal or undermine ObamaCare.

As our nation moves to make health care more accessible, of higher quality, and more patient centered over the next 150 years, it is worth noting that while laws and public policies can have a positive impact and help us attain improved population health outcomes, developing and executing private policies to address the health care challenges vulnerable populations often face is also critical. Consequently, it is worth remembering, while championing health equity, Justice Thurgood Marshall's admonition that laws and policies do have limitations: "the legal system can force open doors and sometimes even knock down walls, but it cannot build bridges. That job belongs to you and me."[21] It will certainly take the power of collaboration from the grassroots to the grasstops, at every level, to ensure continued success of the health equity movement.

NOTES

1. Under the Consolidated Omnibus Budget Reconciliation Act of 1985 (COBRA), employees may continue their health insurance coverage under certain situations after leaving employment.

2. US Department of Health and Human Services, "Enrollment in the Health Insurance Marketplace Totals over 8 Million People."

3. White House, "Building Ladders of Opportunity in Underserved Communities."

4. Calandra, "Clients Save, Insurers Get Boost from Affordable Care Act."

5. Personal interview at his medical practice, May 22, 2015, Miami, Florida.

6. Cutler, "Health-Care Law's Success Story."

7. Johnson, "New Anti-Obamacare Stunt."

8. After the November 2014 elections, Bill Walker, an independent who supported Medicaid expansion, won the governor's race in Alaska, and on July 16, 2015, he announced he would expand Medicaid using his executive power to approximately forty thousand residents on September 1, 2015. Jindal, "To Fix Medicaid, Listen to Governors"; "White House Says Medicaid Expansion

Would Boost Florida's Health and Finances"; Bohrer, "Parnell Opposed to Medicaid Expansion Now."

9. Reinhart, "Brewer Signs into Law Arizona's Medicaid Program."

10. National Conference of State Legislatures, *Health Reform Database.*

11. Kennedy, "Study"; Bookman, "Ga. Insurance Chief Brags about Sabotage of ObamaCare."

12. Potter, "Bush Health Secretary Louis Sullivan Is One Republican Who Supports Obamacare."

13. Somashekhar, "Enrollment up, HealthCare.gov Back on Track, Sebelius Testifies."

14. Przybyla, "Obamacare Losing Power as Campaign Weapon in Ad Battles."

15. Collins, Rasmussen, and Doty, "Gaining Ground."

16. Koyanagi, *Learning from History.*

17. Unfortunately, since the passage of the Affordable Care Act, the AHRQ has been the target of repeated attempts to dismantle it or significantly decrease its appropriations. Advocates should be concerned with this because AHRQ's research has tremendously helped to advance evidence-based policy making, especially as related to health disparities. Without this critical agency, it would be difficult to track the disparities in health care on an annual basis and determine where policy makers should focus their efforts.

18. While southern states in general show lower quality care and fewer disparities in care, interestingly the South has higher and costlier disparities in health status, which is overwhelmingly borne by African Americans.

19. Also referred to as the "Doc Fix," the legislation addressed the sustainable growth rate, which threatened physician Medicare reimbursement for nearly eighteen years. In essence, it reauthorized many of the programs that had expired in the Affordable Care Act and demonstrated support for many of the delivery and payment system reforms espoused in the ACA. One could argue that the American Recovery and Reinvestment Act laid the foundation for the Affordable Care Act, and the Medicare Access and CHIP Reauthorization Act of 2015 paved the way for these reforms to more easily get implemented.

20. Frist, "Overcoming Disparities in U.S. Health Care," 450.

21. Marshall, "Acceptance Speech for the Liberty Medal."

BIBLIOGRAPHY

Agency for Healthcare Research and Quality. 2013 State Snapshots. Rockville, MD, 2013.

Bohrer, Becky. "Parnell Opposed to Medicaid Expansion Now." *Alaska Journal of Commerce*, March 1, 2013. http://www.alaskajournal.com/Alaska-Journal-of -Commerce/March-Issue-1-2013/Parnell-opposed-to-Medicaid-expansion -now/.

Bookman, Jay. "Ga. Insurance Chief Brags about Sabotage of ObamaCare." *Atlanta Journal-Constitution*, August 29, 2013. http://www.ajc.com/weblogs /jay-bookman/2013/aug/29/ga-insurance-chief-brags-about-sabotage -obamacare/.

Calandra, Robert. "Clients Save, Insurers Get Boost from Affordable Care Act." *Philly.com*, April 6, 2014. http://articles.philly.com/2014-04-06/news/48912148 _1_independence-blue-cross-premium-payment-ibc.

Collins, Sara, Petra W. Rasmussen, and Michelle M. Doty. "Gaining Ground: Americans' Health Insurance Coverage and Access to Care after the Affordable Care Act's First Open Enrollment Period." *Commonwealth Fund*, July 2014. http://www.commonwealthfund.org/~/media/files/publications /issue-brief/2014/jul/1760_collins_gaining_ground_tracking_survey.pdf.

Cutler, David. "The Health-Care Law's Success Story: Slowing down Medical Costs." *Washington Post*, November 8, 2013. http://www.washingtonpost .com/opinions/the-health-care-laws-success-story-slowing-down-medical -costs/2013/11/08/e08cc52a-47c1-11e3-b6f8-3782ff6cb769_story.html.

Frist, William H. "Overcoming Disparities in US Health Care." *Health Affairs* 24, no. 2 (March 2005): 445–451.

Galloway, Jim. "Ralph Hudgens: No Longer an Obamacare 'Obstructionist.'" *Atlanta Journal-Constitution*, August 21, 2014. http://politics.blog.ajc.com/2014 /08/21/ralph-hudgens-i-cant-be-an-obamacare-obstructionist/.

Jindal, Bobby. "To Fix Medicaid, Listen to Governors." Op-Ed. *Washington Post*, January 28, 2013. https://www.washingtonpost.com/opinions/bobby-jindal -to-fix-medicaid-listen-to-governors/2013/01/28/ff5c8e5e-6711-11e2-85f5 -a8a9228e55e7_story.html.

Johnson, Benny. "New Anti-Obamacare Stunt: A Creepy Carnival on the National Mall." *Buzzfeed*, July 7, 2014. http://www.buzzfeed.com /bennyjohnson/new-anti-obamacare-stunt-a-creepy-carnival-on-the-national -m#12vn4ur.

Kennedy, Kelly. "Study: Navigator Laws Limit Health Exchange Outreach." *USA Today*, January 14, 2014. http://www.usatoday.com/story/news/nation/2014 /01/14/navigator-laws-limit-health-outreach-efforts/4462759/.

Koyanagi, Chris. *Learning from History: Deinstitutionalization of People with Mental Illness as Precursor to Long-Term Care Reform*. Kaiser Family Foundation, August 2007.

Marshall, Thurgood. "Acceptance Speech for the Liberty Medal." Given at Independence Hall on July 4, 1992, in Philadelphia, PA. http:// constitutioncenter.org/libertymedal/recipient_1992_speech.html.

National Conference of State Legislatures. *Health Reform Database*. http://www .ncsl.org/research/health/new-health-reform-database.aspx.

Potter, Wendell. "Bush Health Secretary Louis Sullivan Is One Republican Who Supports Obamacare." *Huffington Post*, March 31, 2014. http://www

.huffingtonpost.com/wendell-potter/bush-health-secretary-lou_b_5063071
.html.

Przybyla, Heidi. "Obamacare Losing Power as Campaign Weapon in Ad Battles."
Bloomberg, August 19, 2014. http://www.bloomberg.com/news/2014-08-19
/obamacare-losing-punch-as-campaign-weapon-in-ad-battles.html.

Reinhart, Mary K. "Brewer Signs into Law Arizona's Medicaid Program." *Arizona
Republic,* June 18, 2013. http://www.azcentral.com/news/politics/articles
/20130617brewer-signs-law-arizona-medicaid-program.html.

Somashekhar, Sandhya. "Enrollment up, HealthCare.gov Back on Track,
Sebelius Testifies." *Washington Post,* December 11, 2013. http://www
.washingtonpost.com/national/health-science/sebelius-launches-review-of
-botched-launch-of-obamacares-healthcaregov/2013/12/10/ec75df52-61e3
-11e3-8beb-3f9a9942850f_story.html.

US Department of Health and Human Services. "Enrollment in the Health
Insurance Marketplace Totals Over 8 Million People." Press release, May 1,
2014. http://www.hhs.gov/news/press/2014pres/05/20140501a.html.

White House. "Building Ladders of Opportunity in Underserved Communities."
May 11, 2015. https://www.whitehouse.gov/sites/default/files/docs/051115
_ladders_of_opportunity_guidance_final_0.pdf.

"White House Says Medicaid Expansion Would Boost Florida's Health and
Finances." *Sun Sentinel,* June 4, 2015. http://www.sun-sentinel.com/news
/local/florida/fl-fed-report-medicaid-impact-florida-20150604-story.html.

Acknowledgments

The completion of this book is the culmination of years of research, analysis, and writing and I could not have succeeded without the cooperation, support, and diligence of some incredible friends, colleagues, and leaders. I will always be grateful to these individuals in my life who continue to believe in me and support me on this journey to improve the health of all communities, eliminate health disparities, and advance health equity both nationally and globally in all public laws and policies. I particularly want to thank all of the associations, coalitions, and organizations around the country representing diverse stakeholders for the incredible work you did to help advance a health equity agenda in the Affordable Care Act. The stories of so many individuals who struggle to attain quality health care and preventive services are what motivate me every day to advocate on their behalf.

Successful advocacy entails enormous teamwork and the collective efforts of a committed community. I want to express my heartfelt thanks to everyone who has helped to mold and shape me into the person I am today and those who have shown me unwavering support. To God, my family, and community, who early on taught me that all lives matter and instilled in me a deep respect for all human beings, I thank you. I credit you all for lighting this unyielding passion within me for gaining knowledge and finding the truth and for sharing that knowledge and truth with those who desire it. Thanks to all of my family for their patience, understanding, and generous support during the writing of this book. I especially want to recognize and thank my wife, Dr. Nedeeka Dawes; my sons, Raymond Edward Dawes and Marc Daniel Dawes; my grandmother, Maudelyn Dawes; my father, Edward Dawes; my mother, Mernel Dawes; my brothers, Patrick and David; my father-in-law, Dr. Raymond Ramsay; my mother-in-law, Merna Ramsay; my brother-in-law, Jermaine Ramsay; my uncle Leslie Dawes, my aunt Delrene Dawes, and my uncle Bertram Dawes; my uncle

Peter Gordon, my aunt Sonia Gordon, my uncle Ian Wint, my aunt Correl Wint, and Jeannette Hind; Nicole Green; Fritz and Angela Hind; Elrado Ramsay; Dr. Creaton and Valerie Francis; Dr. Anthon and Nalda Francis; Dr. Kahilah Whyte; Kellon Jones; Kevin Cambridge; Dr. Maxine and Maurice Theriot; Joyce Williams; Daniel and Karen Negron; Dawn Williams-Bobo; Katrine Williams; Paul and Clover Williams; Shanelle and Mikalei Gordon; Shelly Ann Grant; Kian Wint; Dr. Terry Ann and Jason James; Jhanelle Dawes; Leslie Dawes Jr.; Ionie Goldson; and Tyrone and Lisa Backers, who never failed to help me when I needed them the most.

To my dear aunt Dr. Marvel Jones, whose generous spirit is a constant reminder to me why we are on this earth—to "defend the cause of the weak and fatherless; maintain the rights of the poor and oppressed." Thank you for your consistent words of encouragement and for showing us how to fight for what we believe in.

To my wonderful friends who provided a constant stream of encouragement during this process and who through the years have never given up on me, I thank you and cherish you: Edward Flood, Esq.; Dr. Anneline Flood; Dr. Lyndon and Monique Riviere; Kay-Kay Tong; Ki-Cha Flash-Zapata; Dr. Jerry Chia; Justin and Maria Gularek; Byron and Dr. Kari Barnes; Natilia Chambers; Jennifer Gray, Esq.; Cathy Jose; Danielle Revilien; June Reid; Marcus and Justin Newton; and Jason and Maureen Wheeler.

Thank you to Krista Morrison, Esq., who provided me with invaluable feedback and assistance and worked with me day and night to bring these chapters to life on the page. Many thanks for helping me to think through ideas and ways to organize the book and making sure this project came together nicely. I could not have completed this book on time without your kind assistance. To Kenneth Pass, I will forever be grateful for your tremendous assistance with researching and organizing the information. Thank you for being dependable and for always paying attention to the details. I also want to acknowledge the incredible support and assistance I received from Erika and Anthony Pringle, who helped review and edit the final draft manuscript. I appreciate the time you took to help me enhance the book. Your help toward the end proved invaluable. Thank you for putting up with my constant need for perfection!

To the incredible teachers at Nova Southeastern University who taught me to never shy away from the truth, to pursue excellence in scholarship, and to promulgate the evidence in a manner that is appropriate and accessible, even though it may be controversial. Dr. Suzanne Ferriss, you are one of a kind, and I thank you for your words of wisdom and encouragement as well as your acts of kindness past, present, and future. My thanks to you and Dr. Steven Alford for providing exceptional feedback and guidance to me during this challenging process.

To the incredible scholars at the University of Nebraska College of Law, I thank you for exposing me to the law, opening my eyes to the impact of laws and policies on vulnerable populations, and arming me with the knowledge and skills to help effectuate the changes that underserved, vulnerable, and marginalized groups desperately need. I especially want to recognize and thank Professor Stefanie Pearlman for taking the time to review my manuscript and for providing substantive feedback and critical edits. I appreciate you very much.

I owe a debt of gratitude to Dr. William McDade at the University of Chicago, who early on told me that I owed it to the next generation to write this book and share insights into a process that is often misunderstood and perceived as cloaked in secrecy. The book would not be a reality if it were not for Dr. McDade's encouragement, constant support, and unwavering commitment to creating and advancing health equity. Your mentorship and leadership is truly valued.

Thank you to Congressman Louis Stokes, Congresswoman Donna Christensen, Congressman John Lewis, Congresswoman Robin Kelly, Congressman Bobby Scott, Ambassador Andrew Young, Dr. Louis Sullivan, Dr. Garth Graham, Dr. David Satcher, the Honorable Kathleen Sebelius, Jeffrey Crowley, James Albino, Liliana Ranon, David Mineta, Sherice Perry, Dr. Millicent Gorham, Dr. Britt Weinstock, the Honorable Calvin Smyre, Senator Edward M. Kennedy, Congressman Hank Johnson, Congressman Patrick Kennedy, and others for your tremendous support before, during, and after the health reform negotiations. I also want to thank you for generously sharing your time with me and for trusting me to tell your stories accurately and fairly. You all are remarkable leaders, trailblazers, mentors, and courageous individuals whose roles in the health equity movement are an inspiration to all who care deeply about advancing health equity in our country.

Thanks to another one of my heroes, Dr. Regina Benjamin, who steadfastly labored to ensure that the National Public Health and Prevention Plan prioritized health equity when she served as the eighteenth US surgeon general. I have never forgotten your words of wisdom nor your counsel. Thanks to Dr. Renard Murray at CMS, who always works to ensure that health equity is front and center in the debate and who sacrificed his time, leaving Atlanta to go to Baltimore to help establish the CMS Office of Minority Health. You have been a true friend to me and one of our nation's health equity leaders whom I most admire. Dr. Nadine Gracia and Dr. Pamela Roshell, you are both role models to all of us, and we are certainly more blessed because of your leadership at HHS. Thank you for your unwavering support and mentorship.

Thanks also to Dr. Larke Huang and Dr. Teresa Chapa, who from the very beginning convened a group at HHS to ensure that they were informed about how the Affordable Care Act advanced a health equity agenda. Dr. Huang and Dr. Chapa are those quiet champions who deserve our thanks and praise for moving our nation one step closer to behavioral health equity.

I wish to also pay special tribute to the Honorable Kendrick Meek, A. Shuanise Washington, Dr. Elsie Scott, Tasha Cole, and the entire team at the Congressional Black Caucus Foundation for their unyielding support. I am indebted to the foundation for giving me the opportunity of a lifetime to serve as a Louis Stokes Health Policy Fellow and learn firsthand how the legislative process really works. I am blessed to have incredible friends and mentors through this program, including Dr. Marjorie Innocent; Dr. Lynn Jennings; Aranthan Jones; Dr. William Garner; Lisa Bediako; Virgil Miller; David Johns; Alex Johnson; Camille Sealy; Julia Elam; Jerrica Mathis; Waverly Gordon, Esq; Brandon Garrett; Brandon Webb; and Timothy Robinson, Esq.

To my colleagues, mentors, and friends at the Morehouse School of Medicine who are a constant source of encouragement and strength, I thank you from the bottom of my heart for pushing me to excel and granting me the opportunity to help our nation realize the vision of health equity for all. I especially want to thank the following colleagues and mentors for their support and feedback during the writing of this book: President and Dean Valerie Montgomery Rice, MD; former president John E. Maupin Jr., DDS, MBA; Art Collins; Susan Grant; Tony Welters, JD; Dr. Rhonda Medows; Desiree Ramirez; Dr. Sandra Harris-Hooker; Dr. Martha Elks; Dr. Ngozi Anachebe; Dr. Derrick Beech; Santhia Curtis, JD; Dr. Kisha Holden; Dr. Rachel Harris; Drs. Peter and Marlene MacLeish; Dr. Gary Gibbons; Dr. Camera P. Jones; Dr. Reinetta Waldrop; Dr. Robert Mayberry; Dr. Roland Matthews; Dr. Cheryl Franklin; Dr. Yolanda Wimberly; Dr. Harry Heiman; Dr. Daniel Blumenthal; Dr. Elizabeth Ofili; Dr. Dominic Mack; Ronna Charles Nu'Man; Dr. John Patrickson; Dr. George Rust; Dr. Beverly Taylor; Dr. Stephanie Miles-Richardson; Dr. Tabia Akintobi; Yvonne Kirkland; Megan D. Douglas, Esq.; Dr. Jammie Hopkins; Dr. Brian McGregor; Dr. Glenda Wrenn; Daniel Walls; Gayle E. Rutledge; Dr. Virginia Floyd; Dr. Willie Clemons; and Dr. Shanell McGoy.

I will always be grateful to the great author David Chanoff for his incredible mentorship and support during the writing and publishing of this book. Your guidance, advice, and support motivated me to keep pressing forward and produce an important resource for health equity champions. Thank you and Lisa for your friendship.

I especially want to recognize and thank my friends Dr. Ken Martinez, Dr. Octavio Martinez, Dr. Mario Hernandez, Scott Bryant-Comstock, and Rick Ybarra, MA, who have been a constant source of mentorship and motivation before, during, and after writing this book. I will never forget your kindness.

I also wish to acknowledge and thank the following individuals for their incredible support, mentorship, and assistance during the writing of this book: Day Al-Mohamed, Esq.; Dr. Renaisa Anthony; Dr. Adam Aponte; Christopher R. Banks; Tammy Barnes; Nicky Bassford; Luis Belen; Dr. Georges Benjamin; Dr. Gary Blau; Linda Blount; N. Renee Brown; Nathaniel Brown; Natalie Burke; Rashad Burgess; Dr. Jonca Bull; Jeff Caballero; Robin H. Carle; Roberta Carlin, MS, JD; Jovita Carranza; Ja'net Carter; Tracy Carter; Blair Childs; Kathy Ko Chin; Oral and Ornell Christie; Patrick and Rebecca Cokley; Corinne Colgan; Andrea Collier; Dr. Nakela Cook; Dr. Joia Crear-Perry; Jeffrey Crowley; Dr. Dennis Cryer; Donna Cryer, Esq.; Michelline Davis, Esq.; Dr. Esther R. Dyer; William Emmet; Ron Frieson; Lark Galloway-Gilliam; Rep. Pat Gardner; Dr. Connie Garner; Elizabeth Goodman, Esq.; Dr. Margaret Grey; Dr. Mary Gullatte; Anton Gunn; Dr. Barbara Guthrie; Chanelle Hardy, Esq.; Dan Hawkins; Sinsi Hernández-Cancio, JD; Priscilla Huang, Esq.; Dr. Dora Hughes; Dr. Christopher Hulin; Andy Imparato; Carlos Jackson; Iyanrick John; Ronald Johnson; Dr. Holly Powell Kennedy; Barbara L. Kornblau, JD, OTR; Joyce Larkin; Dr. Thomas LaVeist; Dr. L. Toni Lewis; Jennifer Lubin; Brigette Mack; Dr. Beverly Malone; Dr. Pierluigi Mancini; Professor Dayna Matthew; Dr. LaShawn McIver; Dr. Flavia Mercado; Dr. Faith Mitchell; Dr. Eduardo Montana; Christine Montgomery; Cathy Morales; Marc Morial, Esq.; Dr. Sandra B. Nichols; Dr. Marc Nivet; Dr. Elena Ong; Dr. Kavita Patel; Kermit Payne; Duanne Pearson; Gilda (Gigi) Pedraza; Ruth Perot; Marcos Pesquera; Dr. Gary Puckrein; Margaret Reagan; Deborah Reid, Esq.; Dr. Elena Rios; Dr. Maya Rockeymoore; Dr. Clarke Ross; Dr. Fred Rottnek; Charmaine Ruddock; Dr. John Ruffin; Pastor Frederick Russell; Dr. Dirk Schroeder; Dr. Bernard Shore; Dr. Brian Smedley; Caren Street; Dr. Donovan Taylor; Dr. Erica Taylor; Dr. Kalahn Taylor-Clark; Mathew and Sheila Thornton; Annie Toro, Esq.; Dr. Jaime Torres; Tonya

French Turner; Gretchen Wartman; Professor Sidney Watson; Gina Eleane Wood; Dr. Ronald Wyatt.

I wish to pay special tribute to my Nebraska mentors, family, and friends who have long supported and encouraged me to pursue excellence in scholarship: Professor Anna Shavers; Professor Catherine Wilson; Professor Craig Lawson; Professor Steve Willborn; Patrick Campbell, Esq.; Thomas and Brenda Christie; Yohance Christie, Esq.; Kelli King; Toyin, Olamide, and Bode Alabi; Jai Kim, Esq.; Jerry Brooks, Esq.; Rebekah Caruthers, Esq.; Keillen Curtis, Esq.; Odies Williams IV, Esq.; Oscar and Deah Harriott; Dave, Judith, and Aaron Fintel; Richard and Judy Weill; Professor Sandra Placzek; Professor John Snowden; Professor John Gradwohl; Hon. Jan Gradwohl; Hon. Vernon Daniels; Eugene Crump, Esq.; Linda Crump, Esq.; Glenda Pierce, Esq.; Jeff Kirkpatrick, Esq.; and Dean Susan Poser.

Finally, I want to thank my editor, Robin W. Coleman, and the entire team at Johns Hopkins University Press, who early on recognized the importance, novelty, and authority of the work and provided tremendous guidance and support during this process. I will forever be grateful to you as well as Gregory M. Britton, Juliana McCarthy, Kerry Cahill, Isla Hamilton-Short, Hilary S. Jacqmin, Carrie Watterson, Andre Barnett, Becky Clark, Gene Taft, Tom Broughton-Willett, and others who labored assiduously to produce this book at JHUP.

There are certainly others who have been very supportive and helpful to me during the development of this book who are not listed, and I hope that they know how truly grateful I am to them. Please forgive this omission and know that it was an inadvertent mistake.

Appendix

Key Federal Health Equity Policy Timelines

Universal Health Policy Timeline
Mental Health Policy Timeline
Minority Health Policy Timeline
American Recovery and Reinvestment Act, Affordable Care Act, Medicare Access and CHIP Reauthorization Act

1798 - President John Adams signed into law the Act for Relief of Sick and Disabled Seamen
1854 - Congress passed the Bill for the Benefit of the Indigent Insane, but it was vetoed by President Pierce
1865 - The Freedmen's Bureau Act was signed into law
1869 - Congress failed to reauthorize Freedmen's Bureau
1872 - Freedmen's Bureau officially closed
1875 - Civil Rights Act of 1875 was signed into law
1883 - Civil Rights Act of 1875 ruled unconstitutional by the US Supreme Court
1896 - *Plessy v. Ferguson* decided by the US Supreme Court promoting "separate but equal" doctrine
1912 - President Theodore Roosevelt endorsed social insurance as part of his platform, including health insurance, but lost election
1912 - President William Taft established the Children's Bureau, which began a nation-wide investigation of maternal and infant mortality rates
1915 - National Negro Health Week established
1921 - President Warren G. Harding signed the Sheppard-Towner Maternity and Infancy Protection Act, which provided funding to states to establish and run prenatal and child health centers based on the work done by the Children's Bureau; it expired eight years later in 1929 and was not reauthorized due to the stock market crash
1927 - President Calvin Coolidge established the Committee on the Cost of Medical Care to investigate the health care system, but recommendations from this committee were put on hold due to the stock market crash in 1929
1932 - USPHS opened the Office of Negro Health Work

1935 – President Franklin Delano Roosevelt signed the Social Security Act but abandoned the inclusion of national health insurance coverage because of the strong opposition

1936 – President Franklin Delano Roosevelt established by executive order the Interdepartmental Committee to Coordinate Health and Welfare Activities to assess the health care needs of the people

1940 – President Franklin Delano Roosevelt enacted the Lanham Act, which provided federal funding to communities impacted by the defense industry so that they could improve their infrastructure, including health care facilities

1942 – President Franklin Delano Roosevelt signed Executive Order 9079, Making Certain Public Health Service Hospitals Available for the Care and Treatment of Insane Persons

1945 – President Harry Truman argued that the federal government should play a role in health care during a special address to Congress; after his speech the Murray-Wagner-Dingell bill authors redrafted their legislation to include President Truman's health care proposal

1946 – President Harry Truman signed the Hospital Survey and Construction Act, also referred to as the Hill-Burton Act

1946 – President Harry S. Truman signed the National Mental Health Act into law

1949 – National Institute of Mental Health established

1955 – President Dwight D. Eisenhower signed the Mental Health Study Act, leading to the establishment of the Joint Commission on Mental Illness and Mental Health

1956 – President Dwight D. Eisenhower argued for federal reinsurance under which the federal government would subsidize partial payment of premiums for low-income individuals

1956 – Eaton v. Board of Managers of the James Walker Memorial Hospital initiated by NAACP to challenge the separate-but-equal doctrine supported by the Hill-Burton Act

1960 – President-elect John F. Kennedy appointed a presidential Task Force on Health and Social Security for the American People, which recommended private health insurance for older adults

1961 – Eisenhower's Joint Commission on Mental Illness and Mental Health released comprehensive report

1962 – *Simkins v. Moses H. Cone Memorial Hospital* initiated by the NAACP to challenge the separate-but-equal doctrine in health care privileges

1963 – President John F. Kennedy signed the Mental Retardation Facilities and Community Mental Health Centers Construction Act

1964 – Civil Rights Act of 1964 signed into law

1965 – President Lyndon B. Johnson signed the Medicare and Medicaid legislation into law

1971 – Senator Edward Kennedy introduced a health insurance reform statute, which was countered by a proposal from President Richard Nixon a few months after, titled National Health Insurance Partnership Act

1971 - Congressional Black Caucus established
1973 - President Nixon signed into law the Health Maintenance Organization Act
1974 - Gerald Ford became president after Nixon's forced resignation; he prioritized universal health insurance and set a goal of passing the Kennedy-Mills plan that year
1976 - Congressional Hispanic Caucus established
1977 - President Carter issued an executive order establishing the President's Commission on Mental Health
1978 - President's Commission on Mental Health produced a seminal report
1978 - Congressional Black Caucus Health Braintrust established
1979 - President Jimmy Carter developed national health insurance plan and delivered it to Congress
1979 - First Hearing on Minority Health held in the United States Senate by Senator Edward Kennedy
1979 - Patricia Roberts Harris appointed first African American US secretary of health, education, and welfare
1980 - President Carter signed the Mental Health Systems Act
1981 - President Reagan signed the Omnibus Reconciliation Act, which rendered most of the Mental Health Systems Act moot
1983 - External groups presented reports on minority health and health disparities to Secretary of HHS Margaret Heckler
1983 - Secretary Heckler realized significant gaps in minority health
1984 - Secretary Heckler established the Task Force on Black and Minority Health
1985 - The Emergency Medical Treatment and Active Labor Act was signed into law
1985 - Landmark *Report of the Secretary's Task Force on Black and Minority Health* released
1986 - Office of Minority Health created at HHS
1989 - President George H. W. Bush developed a comprehensive health insurance proposal, but it was set aside because of pressing international issues
1989 - Minority Health Bill introduced by Representative Louis Stokes and Senator Edward Kennedy
1990 - President George H. W. Bush signed into law the Americans with Disabilities Act
1990 - *Healthy People 2000* released, prioritizing "reduction of health disparities"
1990 - Congress passed the Disadvantaged Minority Health Improvement Act of 1990 and appropriated $1 million to support health disparities research the following year
1990 - The Office of Research on Minority Health was established
1991 - Congress appropriated $1 million to support health disparities research
1992 - The Minority Health Initiative was launched and allocated $45 million for programs geared to addressing health disparities
1993 - President Clinton convened the White House Task Force on Health Reform, a group of more than five hundred policy experts, physicians, and other health professionals, and appointed First Lady Hillary Clinton as chair

1993 – Democratic senator George Mitchell introduced a 1,370-page bipartisan bill with twenty-nine cosponsors, titled the Health Security Act, which was the embodiment of the Clinton plan. That same day, Republican senator John Chafee introduced the bipartisan Health Equity and Access Reform Today Act of 1993—with twenty cosponsors. The Clinton plan was defeated in 1994.

1994 – Congressional Asian Pacific American Caucus established

1996 – President Bill Clinton signed into law the Mental Health Parity Act

1998 – Minority HIV/AIDS Initiative began with $156 million in funding from Congress

1999 – The REACH program was created at the Centers for Disease Control and Prevention

2000 – *Healthy People 2010* released, prioritizing "elimination of health disparities"

2000 – Congress passed the Minority Health and Health Disparities Research and Education Act, which directs AHRQ to conduct assessment of health care disparities, the IOM to produce a report, establish Centers of Excellence (COEs) on health disparities research

2001 – Institute of Medicine released report *Crossing the Quality Chasm: A New Health System for the 21st Century*

2001 – Surgeon General released major report, titled *Mental Health: Culture, Race and Ethnicity*

2002 – President George W. Bush announced the establishment of the New Freedom Commission on Mental Health

2002 – IOM released landmark report, titled *Unequal Treatment: Confronting Racial and Ethnic Disparities in Health Care*

2003 – The New Freedom Commission on Mental Health released landmark report, titled *Achieving the Promise: Transforming Mental Health Care in America*

2003 – AHRQ released the first *National Healthcare Disparities Report*

2003 – The NIH *Strategic Research Plan and Budget to Reduce and Ultimately Eliminate Health Disparities* was issued

2007 – President George W. Bush proposed a plan to address health insurance coverage, but it was never acted upon by Congress

2008 – President George W. Bush signed into law the Paul Wellstone and Pete Domenici Mental Health Parity and Addiction Equity Act

2008 – President George W. Bush signed into law the Americans with Disabilities Act Amendments Act

2009 – President Obama signed the American Recovery and Reinvestment Act, also referred to as the stimulus law, laying the foundation for health reform

2009 – National Working Group on Health Disparities and Health Reform created to advocate for a health equity agenda in health reform legislation

2009 – President Obama and Tri-Caucus congressional members declared support for addressing health disparities in a comprehensive health reform package

2009 - The Joint Center released landmark report, titled *The Economic Burden of Health Disparities in the United States*

2010 - President Obama signed the Patient Protection and Affordable Care Act (ACA) into law, the first time that comprehensive health reform has been enacted into law

2010 - *Healthy People 2020* released, prioritizing achievement of health equity, elimination of disparities, and improvement in the health of all groups

2015 - President Obama signed into law the Medicare Access and CHIP Reauthorization Act, which extends many of the health reform programs from the ACA and expands delivery and payment reforms

National Working Group on Health Disparities and Health Reform Membership

AARP
Adventist HealthCare
Advocates for Youth
Aetna
AIDS Action Council
AIDS Institute
Allergy and Asthma Network
American Academy of Child and
  Adolescent Psychiatry
American Academy of Pediatrics
American Academy of Physician
  Assistants
American Association for Health
  Education
American Association for Marriage
  and Family Therapy
American Association of Orthopedic
  Surgeons
American Association of Pastoral
  Counselors
American Association of People with
  Disabilities (AAPD)
American Association on Health and
  Disability
American Cancer Society Cancer
  Action Network
American Counseling Association
American Dental Association
American Dental Education
  Association
American Diabetes Association

American Dietetics Association
American Group Psychotherapy
  Association
American Heart Association
American Hospital Association
American Kidney Foundation
American Kidney Fund
American Medical Student Association
American Music Therapy Association
American Nurses Association
American Occupational Therapy
  Association
American Physical Therapy
  Association
American Psychiatric Association
American Psychological Association
American Psychotherapy Association
American Public Health Association
American Social Health Association
American Stroke Association
America's Health Insurance Plans
  (AHIP)
Amputee Coalition of America
Anxiety Disorders Association of
  America
Asian American Justice Center
Asian & Pacific Islander American
  Health Forum
Asian & Pacific Islander Wellness Center
Asian Pacific Islander Caucus in
  official relations with APHA

Association for Ambulatory
  Behavioral Healthcare
Association of American Medical
  Colleges
Association of Asian Pacific
  Community Health Organizations
  (AAPCHO)
Association of Clinicians for the
  Underserved (ACU)
Association of Minority Health
  Professions Schools (AMHPS)
Association of Nurses in AIDS Care
Association of Professional Chaplains
Association of Public Health
  Laboratories
Association of University Centers on
  Disabilities (AUCD)
Autism Society of America
Bazelon Center for Mental Health Law
Beckett Family Consulting
Brain Injury Association of America
Brooklyn Task Force on Infant and
  Maternal Mortality and Family
  Health
California Black Health Network
California Center for Public Health
  Advocacy (CCPHA)
California Immigrant Policy Center
California Pan-Ethnic Health Network
California Partnership
California Primary Care Association
Campaign for Mental Health Reform
Carter Center
Catholic Healthcare West
C-Change-Collaborating to Conquer
  Cancer
Center for Advancing Health
Center for Clinical Social Work/ABE
Center for Integrated Behavioral
  Health Policy
CHADD—Children and Adults with
  Attention-Deficit/Hyperactivity
  Disorder
Children's Health Group
Child Welfare League of America
Clinical Social Work Association

Coalition of National Health
  Education Organizations
Coalition on Human Needs
Colorado Progressive Coalition
CommonHealth Action
Communities Advocating Emergency
  AIDS Relief (CAEAR) Coalition
Communities Advocating Emergency
  AIDS Relief (CAEAR) Foundation
Community Catalyst
Community Health Councils
Community HIV/AIDS Mobilization
  Project (CHAMP)
Community Voices
Consumers Union
Council of Schools and Programs of
  Professional Psychology (NCSPP)
Council on Social Work Education
Defeat Diabetes Foundation
Depression and Bipolar Support
  Alliance (DBSA)
Disparities Solutions Center at
  Massachusetts General Hospital
Epilepsy Foundation
External Partners Group of the
  National Center on Birth Defects
  and Developmental Disabilities
Faithful Reform in Health Care
Families USA
Family Equality Council
Foundation for Mental Health
Having Our Say
Health and Medicine Council of
  Washington
Healthcare Equality Project
Health Care for America Now (HCAN)
Health Professions and Nursing
  Education Coalition
Hepatitis B Foundation
Hepatitis Foundation International
Hispanic Federation
HIVictorious, Inc.
HIV Medicine Association
Howard University
Human Rights Campaign
Idaho Community Action Network

Institute for the Advancement of
Social Work Research
Institute of Medicine
ISAIAH: Faith in Democracy (MN)
Japanese American Citizens League
(JACL)
Joint Center for Political and
Economic Studies
Kaiser Family Foundation
Ke Ali'i Maka'ainana Hawaiian Civic
Club
Kellogg Health Scholars Program
Khmer Health Advocates
Korean Resource Center
La Fe Policy Research and Education
Center
Language Access Coalition
Latino Agenda for Healthcare Reform
Latino Caucus in official relations
with the APHA
Latinos for National Health Insurance
League of United Latin American
Citizens (LULAC)
Maine People's Alliance
Make the Road New York
Massachusetts Immigrant & Refugee
Advocacy Coalition
Medicare Rights Center
Meharry Medical College
Mental Health America
Mental Health Liaison Group
Michigan Positive Action Coalition
(MI-POZ)
Montanans for Health Care
Morehouse School of Medicine
National Academy of Public
Administration
National Alliance for Hispanic Health
National Alliance for Thrombosis and
Thrombophilia
National Alliance of State and
Territorial AIDS Directors
National Alliance on Mental Illness
(NAMI)
National Alliance to End
Homelessness

National Asian American Pacific
Islander Mental Health Association
National Asian Pacific American
Families Against Substance Abuse
National Asian Pacific American
Women's Forum
National Association for the
Advancement of Colored People
(NAACP)
National Association of Anorexia
Nervosa and Associated Eating
Disorders
National Association of Chronic
Disease Directors Health Equity
Council
National Association of Community
Health Centers (NACHC)
National Association of County
Behavioral Health and
Developmental Disability
Directors
National Association of People With
AIDS (NAPWA)
National Association of Public
Hospitals and Health Systems (now
America's Essential Hospitals)
National Association of School
Psychologists
National Association of Social
Workers
National Black Gay Men's Advocacy
Coalition
National Black Nurses Association
National Cambodian American Health
Initiative
National Center for Children in
Poverty
National Coalition for LGBT Health
National Coalition of STD Directors
(NCSD)
National Committee to Preserve
Social Security and Medicare
National Council of Jewish Women
National Council of La Raza (NCLR)
National Council of Urban Indian
Health

National Dental Association
National Federation of Families for Children's Mental Health
National Foundation for Mental Health
National Health Equity Coalition
National Health Law Program
National Hispanic Medical Association
National HIT Collaborative for the Underserved
National Immigration Law Center
National Indian Project Center
National Kidney Foundation
National Korean American Service and Education Consortium (NAKASEC)
National Latina Institute for Reproductive Health (NLIRH)
National Latino Behavioral Health Association (NLBHA)
National Latino Tobacco Control Network
National League for Nursing
National LGBT Health Coalition
National Medical Association
National Minority AIDS Council
National Minority AIDS Education and Training Center
National Network to Eliminate Behavioral Health Disparities
National Partnership for Women and Families
National Puerto Rican Coalition, Inc.
National REACH Coalition
National Urban League
National WIC Association
National Women's Health Network
National Women's Law Center
Native Research Network, Inc.
New Age Services Corporation
New Hampshire Health Care for America Now Coalition
New York Immigration Coalition
New York Lawyers for the Public Interest
Northeast Action

Northwest Federation of Community Organizations
Novo Nordisk
Ocean State Action
Oregon Action
Out of Many, One Coalition
Papa Ola Lokahi
Parents, Families and Friends of Lesbians and Gays (PFLAG) National
Physician Assistant Education Association
Premier Health Alliance
Prevention Institute
Project Inform
Psychologists in Indian Country
Raising Women's Voices for the Health Care We Need Coalition
Researchers against Inactivity-related Disorders (RID)
San Francisco AIDS Foundation
Service Employees International Union (SEIU)
Society for Public Health Education (SOPHE)
South Dakotans for Health Care Solutions
Southeast Asia Resource Action Center (SEARAC)
Special Olympics
Strategic Health Resources
Summit Health Institute for Research and Education
Take Action Minnesota
Tenants and Workers United
Thresholds
Trust for America's Health
Visiting Nurse Association of America
Washington Community Action Network
WE ACT for Environmental Justice
Wexler and Walker
Women Heart-National Coalition for Women with Heart Disease
Zero to Three

Where to Find Additional Information on Health Reform

- For more information and regular updates on health reform from the federal government, including the available insurance options under the new health care law and the opportunity to compare the quality of care of facilities across the country, visit www.healthcare.gov.

- For a timeline of when key provisions in the law go into effect, visit http://www.hhs.gov/healthcare/facts/timeline/timeline-text.html.

- For more information on proposed and final regulations on the health reform law, visit www.regulations.gov or www.federalregister.gov.

- For more information on health reform grants that are forthcoming, visit http://www.acf.hhs.gov/hhsgrantsforecast/.

- For more information on health reform grants that have been released, visit www.grants.gov.

- To get a better understanding of the health reform law, track the implementation of the health equity provisions, access analysis and news regarding the impact of the ACA in each state, and join a network of health equity champions committed to advancing evidence-based health equity-focused policies in each state, visit www.healthequitynetwork.org.

- For more information specifically focused on the health reform law's impact on disparities in mental and behavioral health, visit www.nned.net and search for "health reform."

- For more information on the Substance Abuse and Mental Health Services Administration's initiatives relating to behavioral health equity, visit http://www.samhsa.gov/health-disparities.

- To get a better understanding of health reform's impact on racial and ethnic minorities and other vulnerable populations, visit http://minorityhealth.hhs.gov/.

- For more information about how health reform will affect Medicaid and Medicare populations and for other general information regarding health reform, visit http://healthreform.kff.org.

- For information about innovative health equity–focused programs, studies, analyses and information from organizations across the United States, visit http://www.rwjf.org/en/our-topics/topics/health-disparities.html or https://www.aetna-foundation.org/grants-partnerships/health-care-equity.html.

- To access studies on the ACA and research on various population groups relative to health care disparities and quality initiatives, visit http://www.ahrq.gov/health-care-information/topics/topic-affordable-care-act.html.

- To track more than 3,500 state legislative actions related to health reform, the National Conference of State Legislators (NCSL) has developed an online database at http://www.ncsl.org/research/health/health-reform.aspx.

- For thoughtful analyses and reports on policy issues impacting the health care system in general and specific to the ACA, including information from important research studies, demonstrations, and innovative community efforts, visit https://www.nhpf.org/.

- For more information on the impact of the ACA on consumers in general and analysis of contemporary issues impacting the implementation of the health care law, visit www.familiesusa.org/health-reform-central/.

- For more information on the tax provisions of the Affordable Care Act, visit http://www.irs.gov/Affordable-Care-Act.

- For more information on the implementation of Affordable Care Act provisions that are related to private health insurance, including regulations and subregulations, visit the Center for Consumer Information and Insurance Oversight (CCIIO) at www.cciio.cms.gov.

- To access resources focused on health reform and children's mental health, visit www.cmhnetwork.org. Click on Resources and select "Health Care Reform" under Resource Topics.

Index

Page numbers in bold indicate text in figures.